Research Coproduction in Healthcare

Research Coproduction in Healthcare

EDITED BY

Ian D. Graham
University of Ottawa, Ontario, Canada

Jo Rycroft-Malone
Lancaster University, Lancaster, UK

Anita Kothari
Western University, Ontario, Canada

Chris McCutcheon
Ottawa Hospital Research Institute, Ontario, Canada

WILEY

Registered Offices
John Wiley & Sons, Inc., 111 River Street, Hoboken, NJ 07030, USA
John Wiley & Sons Ltd, The Atrium, Southern Gate, Chichester, West Sussex, PO19 8SQ, UK

Editorial Office
9600 Garsington Road, Oxford, OX4 2DQ, UK

For details of our global editorial offices, customer services, and more information about Wiley products visit us at www.wiley.com.

Wiley also publishes its books in a variety of electronic formats and by print-on-demand. Some content that appears in standard print versions of this book may not be available in other formats.

Library of Congress Cataloging-in-Publication Data
Print ISBN: 9781119757238
ePdf: 9781119757245
ePub: 9781119757252
oBook: 9781119757269

Cover image: Courtesy of Peter Rhee
Cover design by Wiley

Set in 10.5/13pt and STIXTwoText by Integra Software Services Pvt. Ltd, Pondicherry, India
Printed and bound by CPI Group (UK) Ltd, Croydon, CR0 4YY

C9781119757238_290422

Contents

Foreword

What a joy to read a book devoted entirely to research coproduction.

It's timely for such a guide to have emerged. As coproduction has become increasingly widespread in research and implementation, it has become ever more obvious that it is a difficult beast to grasp. Its complexity is often obscured by the misguided notion that, because coproduction is a natural, human process it can be easily achieved. Nothing could be further from the truth. As with all human interactions, the coproduction of research needs careful crafting, cajoling, and coaxing if it is to be successful. This book, with its accessible content, both theoretical and practical, can be read at many levels – from brief readings of abstracts and learning points, to selective explorations of just the chapters relevant to one's role, to detailed study of material that authoritatively covers every conceivable angle. All in all, the book helps us not only to understand how to coproduce research but also to appreciate that effective coproduction requires imagination and courage as well as clear techniques. The authors offer a wide range of well-evidenced pointers that will help anyone involved to capitalize on its obvious benefits, and to avoid the pitfalls. There is plenty of good advice – and plenty to debate – for all concerned, be they researchers, practitioners, service users, managers, evaluators, educators, or funders. After all, representatives from many of these groups have collaborated to write such comprehensive chapters.

When writing this foreword, we ourselves embraced the book's central tenets. We were not, of course, strictly engaged in coproduction, which requires bringing together researchers and research users. Rather, we collaborated: we discussed ideas, advocated contrasting approaches, tussled over how best to craft our words, and finally agreed what we would and wouldn't say. Doing so was much more difficult than writing as individuals but worth striving for, since the point of coproduction is to bring together different, and sometimes differing, perspectives to co-create a better result – just like the research that should result when readers have absorbed this well-constructed and highly accessible book.

The key to any collaboration is to develop and maintain open and trusting social, intellectual, and practical relationships. But as the authors repeatedly – and rightly – emphasize, this becomes even harder to do in coproduction, where one is striving to inclusively involve people who have divergent knowledge, experiences and skills, or even conflicting goals, values and cultures. So, at its heart, coproduction inevitably becomes a *relational* exercise that requires a wide range of interpersonal and organizational skills. Perhaps that explains why terms like mutual respect, mutual learning, trust, transparency, flexibility, open communication, shared knowledge, common commitment, inter-personal skills, and open dialogue are a leitmotif through so many of the chapters. Such principles are necessary to help meet the challenge of sharing control, of democratizing the research process. As the authors underline, they require not just skill and good will, but time, resources, and training. Genuine coproduction is hard won, and often requires systemic organizational change to support the necessary shifts in relationships.

One of the driving forces for coproduction has been the conviction that engaging a range of active participants will help when it comes to implementing the study's findings. If coproducers develop a sense of empowerment and ownership, they will help ensure that the research is relevant and responsive to the full context of policy and practice. They should also be best placed to have the networks and influence to enable the findings, if appropriate, to become widely accepted and used. Not surprisingly, therefore, implementation and impact form another leitmotif of the book. It is easy to assume, though, that coproduction will lead naturally to implementation and impact. It may not. The energy of the early and middle phases of coproduction often wanes before the final implementation and maintenance stages when we most need it to make a real sustainable difference. Woven throughout this volume are many well-founded clues as to how to make those final stages a success too.

Coproduction is not a rapid sprint to findings; it's a steady stroll from early design through to eventual implementation, impact, and sustainability. Coproduction will always be a craft – a complex art – that is vital to doing good research and implementing the findings. That craft will be all the stronger thanks to this group of authors. We can all learn much from their book. Enjoy it.

Andrée le May
Professor Emerita of Nursing at the University of Southampton.
Editor-in-Chief for several of the National Institute of Health Research's
Library Journals and Co-editor of the Journal of Research in Nursing

John Gabbay
Professor Emeritus at the University of Southampton.
With Andrée le May, Implementation Co-lead for the East of England
Applied Research Collaboration, and Honorary Senior Visiting Fellow at
Cambridge Public Health

About the Chapter Authors

Davina Banner, RN, PhD
Associate Professor, School of Nursing, University of Northern British Columbia, Prince George
British Columbia, Canada

Shauna Best, RN
IWK Health, Halifax, Nova Scotia, Canada

Ingrid Botting, PhD
Corporate Secretary, Winnipeg Regional Health Authority
Winnipeg, Canada

Sarah Bowen, PhD
Applied Research and Evaluation Consultant
Nova Scotia, Canada

Christopher R. Burton DPhil, PGCertHE, BN, RGN
Professor, School of Allied and Public Health Professions, Canterbury Christ Church University, Canterbury, UK

Fred Carden, PhD
Principal, Using Evidence Inc
Board Chair, Partnership for Economic Policy
Ottawa, Canada

Christine E. Cassidy, BScN, PhD
Assistant Professor, Dalhousie University
Affiliate Scientist, IWK Health
Halifax, Nova Scotia, Canada

Cheyne Chalmers, BHlthSc(Nsg), MHlthServMt
Chief Operations Officer, Ryman Healthcare
Christchurch, New Zealand
Adjunct Professor, School of Nursing and Midwifery
Deakin University, Melbourne, Australia

Jo Cooke, B. Nurs, MA
University of Sheffield, Health Sciences School, Barber Annex House
Sheffield, UK

Ian D Graham, PhD, FCAHS, FNYAM, FRSC
Distinguished University Professor, School of Epidemiology and Public Health
School of Nursing, University of Ottawa
Senior Scientist, Ottawa Hospital Research Institute
Ottawa, Canada
Honorary Professor, School of Nursing and Midwifery, Deakin University
Melbourne, Victoria, Australia

Susan Hampshaw, PhD, MSc, BA (Hons)
Head of Public Health (Delivery), Doncaster Council
Doncaster, UK
Honorary Research Fellow, School for Related Research
The University of Sheffield
Sheffield, UK
Honorary Research Fellow Rotherham, Doncaster and
South Humber NHS Foundation Trust, UK

Femke Hoekstra, PhD
Post doctoral Fellow, School of Health and Exercise Sciences, Faculty of Health
and Social Development, University of British Columbia
Kelona, B.C., Canada

Bev J Holmes, PhD
Adjunct Professor, SFU Faculty of Health Sciences; UBC School of Population
and Public Health
CEO, Michael Smith Foundation for Health Research
Vancouver, Canada

Alison M Hutchinson, BAppSc(Adv Nsg), MBioeth, PhD
Chair in Nursing, Monash Health
Alfred Deakin Professor of Nursing, School of Nursing and Midwifery, Centre
for Quality and Patient Safety Research, Institute for Health Transformation
Deakin University
Melbourne, Australia

Chonnettia Jones, PhD
Vice President, Research
Michael Smith Foundation for Health Research
Vancouver, Canada

Sarah Knowles, PhD, MSc
Knowledge Mobilisation Research Fellow
Centre for Reviews and Dissemination
York University
York, UK

Anita Kothari, PhD
Full Professor, School of Health Studies, University of Western Ontario
London, Canada

Joe Langley, PhD, MEng
Lab4Living, Sheffield Hallam University
Sheffield, UK

Claire Ludwig, RN, MA, PhD (Candidate)
School of Nursing, University of Ottawa
Ottawa, Ontario, Canada

Anne MacFarlane, BA, MA, PhD
Professor, Primary Healthcare, Public and Patient Involvement Research Unit
School of Medicine, University of Limerick
Limerick, Ireland

Susan J Mawson, Bsc Hon, PhD
Professor of Health Services Research, The University of Sheffield
School of Health and Related Research (ScHARR)
Innovation Centre, Sheffield, UK

Chris McCutcheon, MA, PhD (Candidate)
University of Ottawa
Research Programme Manager, Ottawa Hospital Research Institute
Ottawa, Ontario, Canada

Robert K.D. McLean, MSc, PhD
Senior Evaluation Specialist, International Development Research Centre
Ottawa, Canada

Tone Elin Mekki, RN, PhD
Associate Professor, Center for Care Research, Western Norway
Western Norway University of Applied Sciences
Bergen, Norway

Kelly Mrklas, BSc (Zool), BSc (Psych), MSc (Hospital Epi), PhD Health Services Research (Candidate)
Knowledge Translation Implementation Scientist, Strategic Clinical Networks, Provincial Clinical Excellence Alberta Health Services
Calgary, Canada

Katrina Nankervis, BA, DipAppSci(Nsg), MNSc
Executive Director of Residential and Support Services and Chief Nursing and Midwifery Officer, Monash Health
Adjunct Professor, School of Nursing and Midwifery, Deakin University
Melbourne, Australia

Sume Ndumbe-Eyoh, HonsBSc, MHSc
Director, Black Health Education Collaborative
Assistant Professor, Clinical Public Health Division
(Formerly National Collaborating Centre for Determinants of Health)
Dalla Lana School of Public Health, University of Toronto
Toronto, Ontario, Canada

Nicole (Nikki) M. Phillips, PhD, MNS, GDipAdvNurs(Ed), BN
Professor of Nursing and Head, School of Nursing and Midwifery
Centre for Quality and Patient Safety Research
Institute for Health Transformation
Deakin University
Melbourne, Australia

Katrina Plamondon, PhD, MSc, RN
Assistant Professor & Michael Smith Health Research BC Scholar
Faculty of Health & Social Development, School of Nursing, The University of British Columbia
Kelowna, BC, Canada
Co-Chair, University Advisory Council, Canadian Association for Global Health

Emily R Ramage, BaPhysio(Hons), PhD (Candidate)
University of Newcastle
Callaghan, NSW, Australia
Supported by an Australian Government Research Training Program Scholarship

Jo Rycroft-Malone, RN, BSc(Hons), MSc, PhD
Distinguished Professor and Dean, Faculty of Health and Medicine
Lancaster University, Lancaster, UK

Jonathan Salsberg, PhD
Senior Lecturer, Primary Healthcare, Public and Patient Involvement Research Unit, School of Medicine, University of Limerick
Limerick, Ireland

Sana Shahram, PhD, MPH
Assistant Professor & Michael Smith Health Research BC Scholar
Faculty of Health & Social Development, School of Nursing, The University of British Columbia
Kelowna, BC, Canada
Collaborating Scientist, Canadian Institute for Substance Use Research
University of Victoria
Victoria, BC, Canada

Kathryn M Sibley, PhD
Associate Professor, Department of Community Health Sciences
University of Manitoba
Director, Knowledge Translation, George & Fay Yee Centre for Healthcare Innovation
Winnipeg, Canada

Sandy M. Steinwender, OT Reg (Ont.), MSc, PhD (Candidate)
Western University, London Health Sciences
London, Ontario

Vicky Ward, PhD, MA
Reader in Management and Director of the Research Utilisation
School of Management, University of St. Andrews
St. Andrews, Scotland

Editors

Ian D Graham
Distinguished University Professor, School of Epidemiology and Public Health
University of Ottawa
Senior Scientist, Ottawa Hospital Research Institute
Honorary Professor, Deakin University, Melbourne
Centre for Practice Changing Research
Ottawa, ON, Canada

Jo Rycroft-Malone
Professor, Department of Health Research
Dean, Faculty of Health & Medicine
Lancaster University
Lancaster, UK

Anita Kothari
Professor School of Health Studies
Faculty of Health Sciences
Epidemiology and Biostatistics, Schulich School of Medicine & Dentistry
Western University
London, ON, Canada

Chris McCutcheon
Research Programme Manager, Integrated Knowledge Translation Research Network
Centre for Practice-Changing Research, Ottawa Hospital Research Institute
Ottawa, ON, Canada

Acknowledgements

The creation of this work was supported in part by a Canadian Institutes of Health Research Foundation grant entitled, Moving Knowledge into Action for More Effective Practice, Programs and Policy: A Research Program Focusing on Integrated Knowledge Translation (FDN# 143237). We express our appreciation to all the chapter authors who, despite the challenges imposed by the COVID-19 pandemic, prepared their chapters in a timely manner and responded to our editorial suggestions with alacrity. Emma Richard did an amazing job desiging the book cover for us. We are grateful to Meg Carley for expertly undertaking the final editing and formatting of the chapters.

About the Companion Website

This book is accompanied by a companion website which includes a number of resources created by the authors for students and instructors that you will find helpful.

https://iktrn.ohri.ca/

CHAPTER 1

Introduction

Anita Kothari, Jo Rycroft-Malone, Chris McCutcheon, and Ian D. Graham

BACKGROUND: WHAT IS THIS BOOK ABOUT?

Research coproduction is a collaborative way to plan and implement healthcare research. Instead of the researcher working alone, driven by academic curiosity, those who will use the research – called knowledge users – are part of the research team. A researcher *or* a knowledge user can initiate the research project. The idea is that multiple perspectives about a research problem will result in research that is more relevant to programs, policies, practice, patients, and communities. The findings will be more feasible to implement, eventually resulting in better health services and improved health and wellness. In this book we define **research coproduction** as a model of collaborative research that explicitly responds to knowledge user needs in order to produce research findings that are useful, useable, and used. Collaboration in coproduction research is characterized by shared decision-making between knowledge users and researchers, mutual learning, and respect.

This emerging approach is receiving strong attention in healthcare for a number of reasons. One motivation is the indicators that research findings are not finding their way into practice, programs, or policy, suggesting a lag time between research findings and their application (Health Economics Research

Research Coproduction in Healthcare, First Edition. Edited by
Ian D. Graham, Jo Rycroft-Malone, Anita Kothari, and Chris McCutcheon.
© 2022 John Wiley & Sons Ltd. Published 2022 by John Wiley & Sons Ltd.

Group et al. 2008). This gap in implementation of research results has been noticed by governments and research funders, who need to demonstrate a return on investment. Historically and theoretically, the problem has been called the two-community problem, characterized by differences in timelines, jargon, and performance rewards between the researcher and knowledge user communities (Dunn 1980). Two solutions have been presented for this lag time in research application. First, knowledge transfer strategies have focused on improved tailoring and dissemination efforts of research findings for knowledge users, starting from the assumption that knowing and practice are two separate epistemologies; in this worldview, using research findings to make healthcare decisions is seen as rational behavior. The second solution is about a different way to generate knowledge, a collaborative way that assumes knowledge and practice are linked, and hence coproduction approaches will result in research findings that are more feasible and relevant for practice (Greenhalgh and Wieringa 2011). In this book, we spotlight the latter approach to knowledge generation. The assumption is that research coproduction will result in research that is relevant and usable in particular (practice/policy/patients/community) contexts, thus accelerating the application of research findings to solve real-world problems.

Another motivation for research coproduction is the conceptual shift, from patient to *consumer* of healthcare, which has led to the recognition from healthcare organizations for patient, caregiver, and public involvement in research. Endeavors such as the INVOLVE initiative (INVOLVE 2012), Patient-Centred Outcomes Research Initiative (PCORI) (Selby 2013), and Strategy for Patient Oriented Research (SPOR) (Canadian Institutes of Health Research 2014) were created, and they aligned with the patient and consumer activism movement in research, often termed patient and public engagement or involvement. Major funders, like the UK's National Institute of Health Research and PCORI in the USA, signaled their support for this partnered approach by requiring patient or public participation in research projects from the outset. In shifting from patients to consumers, this movement acknowledges patient/public agency and power in health and social care processes.

The broader societal shift around re-defining "the expert" and democratizing science also motivates the turn to research coproduction. This agenda has a broad focus, whether that be related to institutions (through which knowledge production is supported) (Hutchinson et al. Chapter 3.5), decision-making (for which research findings are considered along with lay persons' knowledge) (Ludwig and Banner Chapter 3.2), or determining scientific impact (where societal outcomes are counted along with contributions to science) (McLean et al. Chapter 4.3). The important lesson is that this agenda, which is complementary to the consumerism movement, strives to rebalance the privileging of science. Research coproduction is a way to give power to citizens and their values by creating an inclusive and deliberative knowledge-generation process with equal contributions from multiple types of knowledge (Ritter et al. 2018).

Often there is ambiguity in the broader literature about exactly who the *stakeholders* are in contrast to *knowledge users* (McGrath and Whitty 2017). We define stakeholders as all individuals and groups who might be interested in, or affected by, the research findings, such as funders or managers in the wider healthcare community. Knowledge users are a special set of stakeholders who use research findings to make healthcare or system decisions over which they have control; these knowledge users are sometimes called "decision makers." They include, but are not limited to, policy makers, clinicians, health system managers, the public, patients, and researchers from different fields or industries. A second group of stakeholders is not in a position to make decisions but is affected by the decisions that knowledge users make, and by the research. The third group of stakeholders does not make decisions and is not directly impacted, but is generally interested in research findings.

In terms of their role within a research team, knowledge users are considered research partners (essentially, co-investigators or research team members on research projects or research programs); they are *necessary* for research coproduction. Stakeholders from groups two (affected by the research findings) or three (interested in the findings) could be included as research partners, but often they are not. Stakeholders from any of the three groups could also be included as advisors (advisory committee members to projects or individuals consulted by the research team to elicit their unique perspectives) to the research process or the dissemination of project findings (McCutcheon et al. Chapter 4.2). As advisors, they might provide guidance to the research team at key decision points about methodology, dissemination, or implementation, but they are not as closely integrated with the research process as the knowledge user partners, nor are they considered equal partners with researchers on the team. Figure 1.1 depicts these possible different groups, where stakeholders operating as knowledge user partners is a necessary condition for research coproduction.

Understanding these distinctions among knowledge user partners, knowledge user advisors, and stakeholders can be extremely useful in understanding the different perspectives each brings to the coproduction process. Armed with this understanding, coproduction research teams can consider the possible need for different levels of involvement depending on the stage of the research process. For example, some stakeholders might be engaged broadly through surveys or workshops, but the team might decide that stakeholders also need to be aware of ongoing project findings throughout the research, using tailored dissemination strategies. We encourage the coproduction team to attend to each category of involvement and engagement by thinking about what to measure, engagement processes and related barriers, information and dissemination needs, and sustainability issues.

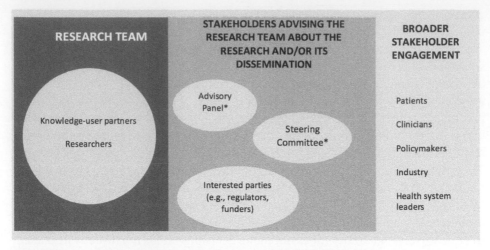

FIGURE 1.1   The coproduction research team and stakeholders.
* could include knowledge users and other stakeholders who are impacted and/or interested in the research findings. Adapted from: Reszel J, Sprague AE, Darling EK, on behalf of the Ontario Birth Centre Demonstration project evaluation team. An integrated knowledge translation approach to evaluate the first year of operations of two new freestanding, midwifery-led birth centers in Ontario. In: McCutcheon C, Reszel J, Kothari A, Graham ID, editors. *How We Work Together: The Integrated Knowledge Translation Research Network Casebook.* Volume 4. Ottawa, ON: Integrated Knowledge Translation Research Network. 2021; 11–15.

FOCUS OF THE CHAPTER: WHAT DO WE MEAN BY RESEARCH COPRODUCTION?

This book focuses on coproduction during the research endeavor (a model of collaborative research that explicitly responds to knowledge user needs in order to produce research findings that are useful, useable, and used). Research coproduction is an approach that can be superimposed on any study design or research methodology and associated method (e.g., see Baumbusch et al. (2018) for an account of research coproduction and ethnography). Therefore, we position it as a lens but not quite yet as a philosophy accompanied by a particular epistemology, as others have defined partnered research (Frank et al. 2020). This lens can be layered on top of other paradigms and ontologies. Research coproduction can be characterized as taking up a problem and using deliberative processes to turn it into a question that is useful for, or derived from, the practice/policy field and from gaps in knowledge. Research coproduction adopts a participatory approach. Team members – researchers and knowledge users – are equal partners with respect to research and dissemination decisions, drawing on everyone's expertise. Research coproduction usually originates in one of three ways: 1) researchers initiate a discussion with knowledge users about a potential research question or problem, 2) researchers and knowledge users collectively come up with a research question or problem, or 3) knowledge users initiate discussion with researchers about a research question or problem of interest to them. Researcher-initiated coproduction is the most common way researcher–knowledge user partnerships are developed. Because knowledge user partners are invested in the research question, and see the research-generating solutions to their problems/issues, they can easily use the findings in practice or policy. Research coproduction is also about mutual learning – through a research project a researcher learns about the knowledge user partner context and the knowledge user learns about research.

One way to understand research coproduction is to contrast the approach with traditional, researcher-driven research (Bowen and Graham 2013) that uses knowledge translation strategies to get research findings in the hands of knowledge users. Bowen and Graham (2013) have framed the problem as the failure to effectively communicate research findings and with the research generation process itself; research coproduction is positioned as a solution. The authors state that researcher-driven research is fueled by curiosity, while research coproduction is usually motivated by knowledge user-identified problems. Unlike researcher-driven research, in research coproduction the team is composed of researchers and knowledge users, all of whom decide on the research question, data collection approaches including analysis, outcome measures, and implementation approaches. Knowledge users are equal partners on the team, and their insights are valued in research discussions. This implies that what counts as evidence in research coproduction can often go beyond research findings (researcher-driven) to also include expert knowledge, local knowledge, cultural knowledge, and patient/caregiver experiential knowledge, especially when data are interpreted in discussions using this knowledge. Finally, another important difference is that researcher-driven research focuses on generalizable findings that can be applied across contexts, while research coproduction is focused on findings that are feasible and most often relevant for application in a particular context, yet theoretically transferable to other contexts.

As shown in Chapters 2.3 (Effects, Facilitators, and Barriers), 5.3 (Role of Funders), and elsewhere (Campbell and Vanderhoven 2016), there are many benefits to research coproduction. In 2012, the Canadian Institutes of Health Research released a report of an evaluation of CIHR's Knowledge Translation Funding Program (McLean and Tucker 2013). This was, and remains, the largest and most comprehensive evaluation of a health funder's research coproduction funding program. CIHR uses the term integrated knowledge translation (IKT) in a way that aligns with research coproduction. The evaluation revealed that the grants funded through the IKT funding program that required knowledge-user co-investigators or co-principal investigators were just as likely to generate the same number of academic outputs (e.g., peer-reviewed publications, books), more likely to engage highly trained personnel (students, postdoctoral fellows), and more likely to produce knowledge translation or dissemination outputs (e.g., websites, decision tools) compared to more traditional researcher-driven project grants funded by CIHR (i.e., with no knowledge users on the research team). It has also been shown that IKT projects tend to be based on what researchers and knowledge users refer to as meaningful partnerships, which they consider to be "a catalyst for increasing both the relevance of research and the use of research," (McLean and Tucker 2013, p. ii). Evaluation findings demonstrated that the involvement of partners in research happened more often with IKT structured grants; these grants were more likely to influence the behavior of knowledge user partners and lead to the creation of real-world relevant applications.

The take-home message from this evaluation is that coproduction grants are complementary to traditional researcher-driven grants. It takes time and effort to develop productive relationships with knowledge user partners to plan and execute coproduction grants. However, these grants have the potential to influence uptake and the impact of the research findings and, from a researcher's perspective, produce similar or more academic outputs, highly qualified personnel, and knowledge translation products than traditional grants.

KNOWN FROM THE LITERATURE: INTELLECTUAL ORIGINS AND HISTORICAL TRADITIONS

Research coproduction can trace its intellectual development and departure from traditional research approaches to a range of disciplines and fields. To describe these threads, Nguyen et al. (2020) examined five specific collaborative research approaches: IKT, engaged scholarship, Mode 2 research, coproduction, and participatory research. Nguyen and colleagues noted more similarities than differences across these five approaches, based on interviews with experts in the field. The identified common elements included: an orientation towards true partnerships and collaborations, the need for extensive time and financial resources, and similar core values and principles. Participants also focused on the "essential components and processes rather than labels" (Nguyen et al. 2020, p. 2). Below we describe each of these five approaches to contribute to our conceptualization of research coproduction.

The concept of research coproduction is very closely aligned with the Canadian term IKT, the first partnership approach examined by Nguyen *et al.*, defined as a "model of collaborative research, where researchers work with knowledge-users who identify a problem and have the authority to implement the research recommendations" (Kothari et al. 2017, p. 299). IKT "...represents a different way of doing research and involves active collaboration between researchers and research users in all parts of the research process, including the shaping of the research questions, decisions about the methods involvement in the data collection and tools development, interpretation of the findings and dissemination and implementation of the research results," (Graham and Tetroe 2007, p. 21). In some cases, the co-development of an intervention (service/treatment/implementation strategy) is considered research coproduction, but it would not be considered research coproduction from an IKT perspective as this would represent coproduction of only one phase of the research process rather than the entire research process.

Nguyen and colleagues included engaged scholarship as another collaborative approach in their study. The driver behind engaged scholarship is the gap between theory and practice, albeit from a management perspective. Boyer (1996) and Van de Ven (Van de Ven 2018; Van de Ven and Johnson 2006) have developed the concept of engaged scholarship: an identity or positionality between researchers and their communities, which forms a learning community through negotiation and mutual respect – a research model where others (i.e., relevant non-researcher perspectives) contribute whose voices are valued. Van de Ven offers at least four different forms of engaged scholarship depending on the type of research (e.g., description, action intervention) and whether the researcher is located externally, like a consultant, or internally within an organization (Cuthill 2008). Engaged scholarship relationships can include research, teaching, and service activities to benefit communities (Bowen 2015).

Mode 2, the third collaborative approach examined by Nguyen and colleagues, is another influential view alongside research coproduction. In the 1990s, Gibbons and Nowotny developed the concept of Mode 2 research to differentiate it from what they called Mode 1 research (Gibbons 1999; Nowotny et al. 2003). The former concept reflects a reinvigorated social contract between universities and society in which research is based on social problems. In addition, Mode 2 research is seen as transdisciplinary, scientifically valid, and socially robust. The research process is conducted with engagement of knowledge users, including industry partners. Thus, research is conducted with an eye to application. Mode 1 research, on the other hand, represents traditional, curiosity-driven university research that takes the position of objectivity as scientifically valid. Subsequently, Mode 3 research (Carayannis et al. 2016) – basic research in the context of application – was proposed to work by supporting diverse knowledge production and innovation or application approaches, such as across Modes 1 and 2.

A historical lens shows how the general term "coproduction," the next approach examined by Nguyen *et al.*, was developed in the field of economics. Ostrom and colleagues used it to stress the need to include consumers in the production and consumption of public services, specifically police services (Ostrom 1973; Ostrom et al. 1978). Scholars then extended the concept to other public services. The general premise was that consumers or clients have local knowledge and resources that are just as important as the expert skills held by practitioners. It was envisioned that, with this knowledge, consumers would be able to design services for better outcomes. The original definition of coproduction was the "...process through which inputs used to produce a good or service are contributed by individuals who are not 'in' the same organization" (Ostrom 1996, p. 1073). This broader view of coproduction for applied health services continues to be popular in several countries.

The tradition of involving the community in the process of health research encompasses a number of sub-genres, such as action research or community-based participatory research. This entire body of literature is vast and well developed. While each sub-genre has developed its own nuanced method, the broad tradition of participatory research rests on the principles of social justice, community expertise and capacity-building. Nguyen et al. (2020) describe the two major branches of participatory research known as the Northern and Southern Traditions. The former, originally developed in the US and the UK based on Lewin's work, can be characterized as cycles of reflection and action with community members who are positioned as co-researchers (Lewin 1946). Through collaborative efforts, problems that concern community members are addressed with community-generated solutions. The Southern tradition, credited to Freire (1970), is rooted in emancipation of disadvantaged groups through their engagement in research and change. Much of this original work can be traced to South America, Africa and Asia. Participatory research has a strong focus on process as well as on power: humility is needed to reflect authentically on privilege and power (Nguyen et al. 2020).

Nguyen and colleagues found that IKT, engaged scholarship, Mode 2 research, coproduction, and participatory research share more similarities than differences. They vary in the extent to which they are concerned with emancipation, building the capacity of knowledge users to become researchers in their own right, or relinquishing complete power to knowledge users. They share a common view on being action-oriented, facilitating authentic partnering and involvement with non-researcher partners, and embracing diverse sources of knowledge (Bowen 2015). Essentially, these collaborative research approaches acknowledge and value the different knowledge, skills, and lived experiences brought to the research partnership by researchers and knowledge user partners.

It is likely that other collaborative approaches will also shape how we think about research coproduction. These models influence how we conceptualize the relationship, the partnering, and the partners; how we think about power within this process; and how collective efficacy is actualized. Research coproduction is a cross-disciplinary and pluralistic approach with its roots embedded in many traditions. The relationship between researchers and knowledge users within a coproduction approach represents shared expertise through a research process, where both are equal partners. Researchers bring their expertise in conducting research; knowledge users bring their expertise, including lived experience of the research issue and implementation know-how. These different perspectives enrich the research project and generate synergistic effects.

SCOPE OF THE BOOK

The collection of chapters in this book presents both the scholarship and application of coproduction for researchers, knowledge users, funders, organizations and coproduction teams. Chapter authors discuss coproduction occurring in projects, programs of research, at an organizational or geographical level. Most chapters focus on high-income countries. The use of examples, key learnings, and the development of a slide presentation for each chapter is intended to ensure the chapters are practical and useful for a range of audiences. The chapters stand on their own, which means readers might notice some overlapping content or different interpretations of concepts. For example, some authors present slightly different "principles" for coproduction (Plamondon et al. Chapter 2.2; Sibley et al. Chapter 2.3; Langley et al. Chapter 3.3; Hutchinson et al. Chapter 3.5). Our response is that readers do not try to locate the perfect set of principles but rather use them to frame their partnership planning and discussions. In addition, research coproduction includes some skills that are not emphasized in traditional research training, like building trust through humility, ongoing communication, and emotional intelligence. These "soft skills," discussed by Sibley and colleagues (Chapter 2.3), Hutchison et al. (Chapter 3.5), and others (Hoekstra et al. 2020) are important for the relational aspects of successful research collaboration between very different groups.

Section 2 of the book lays down the foundations of research coproduction. Salsberg and MacFarlane start Chapter 2.1 by making the case for the importance of developing a theory of coproduction. To support this development, they discuss the concepts underlying coproduction, such as power and tokenism, complemented by a description of the key literature theorizing research coproduction. Plamondon and colleagues, in Chapter 2.2, elaborate on the notions of power and equity as the touchpoints of social systems, structures, and human interactions. They highlight coproduction's transformative potential for social change. The concluding Chapter (2.3), by Sibley and colleagues, presents research coproduction facilitators and barriers, organized as individual, relationship, process, and system factors, as identified in the published literature. The effects of coproduction are also described.

The theme of Section 3 is the structures and processes related to working with a range of knowledge users. Cooke et al. provide some helpful approaches in Chapter 3.1, using case examples to initiate a research coproduction relationship at both project and program levels. What becomes clear is that spending time on relationship infrastructure, like developing a joint vision and doing some relationship building, is important at both levels. Chapter 3.2, by Ludwig and Banner, takes up patients and caregivers as coproduction partners, noting the barriers to partnering meaningfully with this knowledge user category. Strategies that researchers and patients can use to build an effective research partnership are offered. In the chapter that follows, 3.3, Langley and colleagues direct their comments at researchers to advance a principles-based approach to research coproduction. The five principles are accompanied by resources to assist in the application of the principles. Next, in Chapter 3.4, Bowen et al. direct their comments at organizations (i.e., health leaders and managers) who wish to be more savvy in their coproduction involvement. They encourage organizations to clearly specify the role they wish to play in research, and then ensure that policies, structures, and processes are established to avoid any nega-tive consequences to partnering. Research coproduction can also occur when universities and health service organizations partner, as described by Hutchison et al. in Chapter 3.5. Similarly to the previous chapter, this one presents practical strategies in the area of partnership management, sustainability, and evaluation to mitigate any possible challenges to a productive relationship; these strategies are based on the underlying principles of mutual respect, trust, transparency, flexibility, open communication, shared knowledge, and commitment.

The chapters in Section 4 address the planning, doing, and evaluating of research coproduction. In Chapter 4.1, Graham and colleagues write about how to write a successful research coproduction proposal. They draw on guides from funders, their own experience as funders and peer reviewers, the published literature, and tips from Twitter colleagues to put together a comprehensive blueprint with several key learnings for grant writers. Next, in Chapter 4.2, McCutcheon et al. take and adapt current guidance on dissemination to reflect when knowledge users and researchers also collaborate on the dissemination plan, in addition to the knowledge generation. Even researcher-driven research might benefit from a coproduced dissemination plan. In Chapter 4.3, McLean and colleagues focus on measuring coproduction impact using the RQ+ methodology.

Capacity-building and infrastructure are discussed in Section 5. In the first chapter of this section (5.1), Burton and Elin discuss research coproduction and implementation competencies related to mastery of research, personal effective-ness, public involvement, and impact generation. Next, as trainees, Cassidy and colleagues are offering their perspective in Chapter 5.2 to provide a much-needed roadmap to other trainees wanting to move into the research coproduction space. Chapter 5.3 focuses on the role of funders and speaks to how funding agencies can support research coproduction at program design, application review, project facilitation, and reporting stages. Holmes and Jones suggest that funders can promote research coproduction on multiple levels.

We end the book with a reflective chapter to reveal overarching themes of several chapters and identify some essential building blocks of research copro-duction. Readers might be interested in how chapter authors presented research coproduction as a lens (rather than a method), and correspondingly, that involve-ment with knowledge users and stakeholders ought to remain flexible. We describe the strong push for meaningful and authentic partnerships. In parallel, authors situated research coproduction partnerships within contextual layers, each with its own challenges and opportunities. Other considerations include the need to build individual and system-level competencies for coproduction. Finally, we propose that, when properly understood, we have entered the fourth generation of knowledge to action, called "democratization," that builds on and evolves the earlier generations of linear, relational, and systems knowledge to action thinking.

REFERENCES

1. Baumbusch, J., Wu, S., Lauck, S.B., Banner, D., O'Shea, T., and Achtem, L. (2018). Exploring the synergies between focused ethnography and integrated knowledge translation. *Health Research Policy and Systems/BioMed Central* 16: 103. doi: 10.1186/s12961-018-0376-z.

2. Bowen, S. (2015). The relationship between engaged scholarship, knowledge translation and participatory research. In: *Participatory Qualitative Research Methodologies in Health* (ed. G. Higginbottom and P. Liamputtong), 183–199. SAGE Publications Ltd.

3. Bowen, S.J. and Graham, I.D. (2013). From knowledge translation to engaged scholarship: promoting research relevance and utilization. *Archives of Physical Medicine and Rehabilitation* 94: S3–8. doi: 10.1016/j.apmr.2012.04.037.

4. Boyer, E.L. (1996). The scholarship of engagement. *Bulletin of the American Academy of Arts and Sciences* 49: 18–33. doi: 10.2307/3824459.

5. Campbell, H.J. and Vanderhoven, D. (2016). Knowledge That Matters. Realising the Potential of Co-production. Manchester: N8 Research Partnership. https://eprints.whiterose.ac.uk/99657/1/FinalReport-Co-Production-2016-01-20.pdf.

6. Canadian Institutes of Health Research. (2014). *Strategy for Patient-oriented Research – Patient Engagement Framework*. [Online]. https://cihr-irsc.gc.ca/e/45851.html (accessed 31 August 2021).

7. Carayannis, E.G., Campbell, D.F.J., and Rehman, S.S. (2016). Mode 3 knowledge production: systems and systems theory, clusters and networks. *Journal of Innovation and Entrepreneurship* 5. doi: 10.1186/s13731-016-0045-9.

8. Cuthill, M. (2008). Review of engaged scholarship: a guide for organizational and social research by Andrew H. Van de Ven. *Gateways: International Journal of Community Research and Engagement* 1: 200–201. doi: 10.5130/ijcre.v1i0.892.

9. Dunn, W.N. (1980). The two-communities metaphor and models of knowledge use: an exploratory case survey. *Science Communication* 1: 515–536. doi: 10.1177/107554708000100403.

10. Frank, L., Morton, S.C., Guise, J.M., Jull, J., Concannon, T.W., and Tugwell, P., and Multi Stakeholder Engagement Consortium. (2020). Engaging patients and other non-researchers in health research: defining research engagement. *Journal of General Internal Medicine* 35: 307–314. doi: 10.1007/s11606-019-05436-2.

11. Freire, P. (1970). *Pedagogy of the Oppressed*. New York: Herder & Herder.

12. Gibbons, M. (1999). Science's new social contract with society. *Nature* 402: C81–4. doi: 10.1038/35011576.

13. Graham, I.D. and Tetroe, J. (2007). How to translate health research knowledge into effective healthcare action. *Healthcare Quarterly* 10: 20–22. doi: 10.12927/hcq.18919.

14. Greenhalgh, T. and Wieringa, S. (2011). Is it time to drop the "knowledge translation" metaphor? A critical literature review. *Journal of the Royal Society of Medicine* 104: 501–509. doi: 10.1258/jrsm.2011.110285.

15. Health Economics Research Group, Office of Health Economics and RAND Europe. (2008). *Medical Research: What's It Worth? Estimating the Economic Benefits from Medical Research in the UK*. London, UK: Evaluation Forum. https://mrc.ukri.org/publications/browse/medical-research-whats-it-worth.

16. Hoekstra, F., Mrklas, K.J., Khan, M., McKay, R.C., Vis-Dunbar, M., Sibley, K.M., Nguyen, T., Graham, I.D., SCI Guiding Principles Consensus Panel, and Gainforth, H.L. (2020). A review of reviews on principles, strategies, outcomes and impacts of research partnerships approaches: a first step in synthesising the research partnership literature. *Health Research Policy and Systems / BioMed Central* 18: 51. doi: 10.1186/s12961-020-0544-9.

17. INVOLVE. (2012). *Briefing Notes for Researchers: Involving the Public in NHS, Public Health and Social Care Research*. Eastleigh, UK: INVOLVE. https://www.invo.org.uk/wp-content/uploads/2014/11/9938_INVOLVE_Briefing_Notes_WEB.pdf.

18. Kothari, A., McCutcheon, C., and Graham, I.D. (2017). Defining integrated knowledge translation and moving forward: a response to recent commentaries. *International Journal of Health Policy and Management* 6: 299–300. doi: 10.15171/ijhpm.2017.15.

19. Lewin, K. (1946). Action research and minority problems. *Journal of Social Issues* 2: 34–46. doi: 10.1111/j.1540-4560.1946.tb02295.x.

20. McGrath, S.K. and Whitty, S.J. (2017). Stakeholder defined. *International Journal of Managing Projects in Business* 10: 721–748. doi: 10.1108/IJMPB-12-2016 0097.

21. McLean, R.K.D. and Tucker, J. (2013). *Evaluation of CIHR's Knowledge Translation Funding Program*. Canadian Institutes of Health Research. https://cihr-irsc.gc.ca/e/documents/kt_evaluation_report-en.pdf.

22. Nguyen, T., Graham, I.D., Mrklas, K.J., Bowen, S., Cargo, M., Estabrooks, C.A., Kothari, A., Lavis, J., Macaulay, A.C., MacLeod, M., Phipps, D., Ramsden, V.R., Renfrew, M.J., Salsberg, J., and Wallerstein, N. (2020). How does integrated knowledge translation (IKT) compare to other collaborative research approaches to generating and translating knowledge? Learning from experts in the field. *Health Research Policy and Systems/BioMed Central* 18: 35. doi: 10.1186/s12961-020-0539-6.

23. Nowotny, H., Scott, P., and Gibbons, M. (2003). Introduction: "Mode 2" revisited: the new production of knowledge. *Minerva* 41: 179–194. doi: 10.1023/A: 1025505528250.

24. Ostrom, E. (1973). *Community Organization and the Provision of Police Services*. Beverly Hills: Sage Publications.

25. Ostrom, E. (1996). Crossing the great divide: coproduction, synergy, and development. *World Development* 24: 1073–1087. doi: 10.1016/0305-750X(96)00023-X.

26. Ostrom, E., Parks, R.B., Whitaker, G.P., and Percy, S.L. (1978). The public service production process: a framework for analyzing police services. *Policy Studies Journal* 7: 381–381. doi: 10.1111/j.1541-0072.1978.tb01782.x.

27. Ritter, A., Lancaster, K., and Diprose, R. (2018). Improving drug policy: the potential of broader democratic participation. *The International Journal on Drug Policy* 55: 1–7. doi: 10.1016/j.drugpo.2018.01.016.

28. Selby, J.V. (2013). PCORI's strategic plan: setting the framework for success. [Online]. https://www.pcori.org/blog/pcoris-strategic-plan-setting-framework-success [accessed 21 September 2021].

29. Van de Ven, A.H. (2018). Academic-practitioner engaged scholarship. *Information and Organization* 28: 37–43. doi: 10.1016/j.infoandorg.2018.02.002.

30. Van de Ven, A.H. and Johnson, P.E. (2006). Knowledge for theory and practice. *Academy of Management Review* 31: 802–821. doi: 10.5465/amr.2006.22527385.

Foundations of Research Coproduction

2.1 Conceptualizing and Theorizing for Research Coproduction

Anne MacFarlane and Jon Salsberg

Key Learning Points

- The theory of research coproduction is important to improve our conceptual understanding about, and support, the practices and processes of meaningful research partnerships.
- Theorizing about research coproduction is underway and is essential for clarifying conceptual ambiguities about what research coproduction is and for understanding relationships and mechanisms between its core concepts.
- Combining knowledge about the theory and concepts of research coproduction with implementation theories will enrich our understanding of what it takes to co-generate, implement and sustain new knowledge in routine practice, programmes and policy in health care settings.

Research Coproduction in Healthcare, First Edition. Edited by
Ian D. Graham, Jo Rycroft-Malone, Anita Kothari, and Chris McCutcheon.
© 2022 John Wiley & Sons Ltd. Published 2022 by John Wiley & Sons Ltd.

INTRODUCTION

In this chapter, we use the term coproduction broadly to encapsulate research approaches that meaningfully engage and empower a broad range of stakeholders, particularly those who must use or stand to benefit from the research process. Research coproduction is an extrapolation of Ostrom's (1996) original proposition of coproduction as a synergistic collaboration between public providers and service users/consumers in the coproduction of public services (Ostrom 1996). Research coproduction in the field of healthcare integrates stakeholders and knowledge users from community, clinical, policy, and academic settings into the knowledge creation process to maximize the chance of using that knowledge to achieve outcomes such as changes in health policy and/or healthcare practice (Nguyen et al. 2020 and see Chapter 1). The process of research coproduction emphasizes equality among stakeholders and knowledge users by placing a value on the diversity of experiences and knowledge. The emphasis is on *giving voice to all involved* so that their expertise is acknowledged and incorporated into the research process. This adds breadth and depth to more traditional forms of research, which have privileged academic knowledge only (Nguyen et al. 2020; Wallerstein and Duran 2010). Thus, research coproduction leads to more comprehensive and inclusive knowledge that can be used to improve health status and health (Nguyen et al. 2020; Wallerstein and Duran 2010). This is beneficial for all research but has particular significance for research with people who are underserved, harmed by the research process itself, experience marginalization and inequitable health outcomes (e.g., people of color), Indigenous communities, and migrants (Macaulay et al. 1999; Wallerstein and Duran 2010 and see Chapter 2.2).

The key issue arising from this basic premise is that research coproduction needs to be *meaningful* to combat the problem of tokenistic participation. This is important because too often stakeholders and knowledge users are involved in events and activities by researchers in order to "tick a box," to say that there was participation, when in fact there was none: decisions had already been taken, or the process used limited the scope for stakeholders and knowledge users to deliberate and share decision-making (Clarke et al. 2019; Cornwall 2002). There is a history of "helicopter research:" researchers swoop in "from above" and extract data from patient or community groups at a distance without understanding their experiential knowledge and context (Macaulay 2017). This leads to disappointment, distrust, and research fatigue – particularly among people of color, Indigenous communities, and migrants – as it repeats a pattern of institutional injustice whereby there is a lack of respectful attention to the plurality of knowledge and practices within, and across, social and cultural groups (see Chapter 2.2). Further, it means that important knowledge from key stakeholders is missing from the analysis, so the quality, sustainability, and overall impact of research is diminished (Wallerstein and Duran 2010).

The historical origins of research coproduction are diverse, and have been shaped by the influence of concepts and theories about power, ethics, equity, context, and sustainability from a variety of disciplines (Nguyen et al. 2020). These include the organizational action reflection cycle (Lewin 1946), engaged scholarship (Boyer 1996), health equity-related theories of conscientization, emancipation, and power for individual and structural change (Freire 1970), and post-colonial psychology (Duran and Duran 1995). Within some academic traditions (e.g., Duran and Duran 1995; Freire 1970), issues of social justice and inequity are central as they focus on power differentials linked with gender, class, ethnicity, and other intersectional characteristics, as well as indicators of social deprivation or marginalization.

These underlying concepts and theories are important to consider in our work because they are the *foundations of research coproduction* that can guide our thinking and practice in terms of designing partnerships, projects, and their evaluation. Importantly, however, this is a *foundation of ever-evolving knowledge*: while we can certainly seek guidance from underlying concepts and theories, our work can also contribute further to their refinement, relevance, and impact. Indeed, arguably an important goal would be to develop an overarching, contemporary theory (or theories) of research coproduction to provide a robust, conceptual synthesis and explanation of when and how research coproduction is successful. Such a theory would provide scope for accumulating knowledge over time and across settings (Eccles et al. 2009). This will enhance understanding of what has worked in the past. Moreover, it will help prospectively to establish and sustain meaningful, impactful research coproduction initiatives. There is no overarching, dominant, or grand *theory of research coproduction* at this time (Nguyen et al. 2020), but there is valuable work *theorizing about research coproduction*.

In this chapter, we begin with a more detailed look at meaningful participation and research partnerships. We distinguish between theory and theorizing, and then provide examples of theorizing in the field. These examples are mostly based on our combined interests in participatory health research, community-based participatory research, social network analysis, participatory spaces and participatory learning, and action research from European and North American research. Throughout, we consider the implications of this work for the practice of research coproduction. We highlight how findings from these examples can be used to guide project partnership development and sustainability, project development, implementation, evaluation, etc. We end with a close look at how theorizing about research coproduction can have complementary benefits for theories of implementation.

MEANINGFUL PARTICIPATION

In the broad and diverse literature around coproduction, there are frequent references to "meaningful participation." What does this look like exactly? Jagosh et al. (2012) found that, at a minimum, it involved the empowerment of partners in identifying the project goal, its governance, and interpretation and dissemination of its results. This sustained involvement and power-sharing, from project start to end, was found to create resilience, sustained health-related goals, and extended program infrastructure; and, further, new and unexpected ideas and outcomes.

Given the centrality of meaningful partnerships for research coproduction, it is important that we do not regard them or the processes they involve as a "black boxes." We need to fully understand what these partnerships are and how they work. This is beneficial for understanding the successes and failures of completed work and, more importantly, to develop and nurture effective partnerships for planned work. The literature on research coproduction is expanding all the time; there are new journals and more and more examples of projects that describe and reflect on what has been done, what worked, the lessons learned, and so on. These are important additions to our knowledge but, at the same time, they can be overwhelming. The expanding amount of information about different projects, in different settings, with different processes and outcomes, can be challenging to navigate. Are the lessons learned comparable, given the differences in context, process, and outcome? Can we synthesize key messages from across projects? Sometimes, researchers use emerging ideas from grounded theory research and/or established concepts, typologies, models, and theories as a conceptual lens through which to view the issues they are exploring in a new way and to synthesize key messages. This is where theory and theorizing come in.

THEORY AND THEORIZING

Put simply, a theory is a set of ideas that are linked together to explain and predict a phenomenon. Theories can be used to provide a picture of how things "fit together" and be tested empirically to see if that is accurate or not in real world settings (Creswell and Creswell 2017; Hammond 2018). Brazil et al. (2005) highlight the specific value of theory in health research: a theory provides a heuristic to understand the relationship between program inputs (resources), program activities (how the program is implemented), and their outputs or *outcomes*. This is a process of identifying the *mechanisms* by which programs are effective

(Astbury and Leeuw 2010). Theory also offers the opportunity to examine the *context* and its influence on the effectiveness of an intervention (Pawson 2003). As mentioned, the use of theory in different studies over time leads to an accumulation of more generalizable knowledge that can be used to "alert" researchers to factors that are relevant to their study (Eccles et al. 2009).

The process of thinking theoretically, or building theory, is known as theorizing (Hammond 2018; Silver 2019) and this involves four iterative processes (Silver 2019). First, it involves identifying ideas that need to be clearer or critically appraised and "unpacked." This means that we question things that we take for granted. Second, it involves identifying where there is ambiguity in the ideas, perhaps because the terminology used is complicated or contested, or because there is confusion between ideas that look the same but are actually different. Third, it encourages us to "think through" how ideas could be organized in relation to each other – do they all have the same "weight" or are some subcomponents of others? Typologies and conceptual logic models may be developed at this stage. Finally, theorizing encourages us to think about relationships between ideas and to start to develop hypotheses about the mechanisms between them or what the outcomes are likely to be. Through this, we may identify gaps and weaknesses, and refine and recommend further adaptations to improve theoretical knowledge. As mentioned earlier, at present there is no established "grand theory" of research coproduction but there are important examples of theorizing, to which we now turn.

THEORIZING ABOUT RESEARCH COPRODUCTION

As we have seen, theorizing about research coproduction involves different layers of inter-related work. Here we describe some work by researchers that has focused on (i) enhancing conceptual clarity and model building and (ii) utilizing existing concepts for new and deeper understanding.

Enhancing Conceptual Clarity and Model Building

One of the well known features and challenges in the field of research coproduction is that there are different traditions, approaches, and terminologies in use (Nguyen et al. 2020). There has been some work done *within* traditions to enhance conceptual clarity. In a critical comparative analysis of community-based participatory research, for example, eight core principles were identified, including genuine partnership and co-learning, capacity building of community members in research, applying findings to benefit all partners, and long-term partnership commitments (Israel et al. 1998, 2017). See Chapters 2.3, 3.3, and 3.5 for more on principles. There has also been work done to enhance conceptual clarity *across* traditions – integrated knowledge translation, engaged scholarship, mode 2 research, coproduction, and participatory research. A comparison of their disciplinary origins, primary motivation, and so on highlighted that there are core principles and values across them. These are power-sharing, cocreation, reciprocity, trust, fostering relationships, collaboration, respect, colearning, active participation, and democratization of knowledge (Nguyen et al. 2020).

Enhanced conceptual clarity will allow us to synthesize lengthy detail in descriptive, empirical accounts into a smaller number of more meaningful, abstract key concepts and processes. This allows us to organize our thinking further. For example, a conceptual logic model for community-based participatory research (CBPR) has been developed and adapted (Wallerstein et al. 2008, 2017). This provides a useful framework for understanding CBPR processes and the contextual and process-related factors that affect the partnership process, as well as the project goals and outcomes. Further, highlighting the iterative nature of theorizing mentioned earlier, the CBPR model highlights where there is a need for more critical investigation. The centrality of trust in partnerships, for example, is well recognized in the CBPR model and other literature (Jagosh et al. 2012; Nguyen et al. 2020; Wallerstein et al. 2017) but this has not been "unpacked" to determine its internal dimensions and processes (Gilfoyle et al. 2020).

Utilizing Existing Concepts for New and Deeper Understanding

There are many existing concepts in the literature that can be used to bring a new and deeper way of thinking to research coproduction. The aforementioned analysis of the internal dimensions and processes involved in trust is an example of this (Gilfoyle et al. 2020). This analysis was taken forward by combining knowledge about the literature on CBPR, trust and social network theory (Gilfoyle et al. 2020). This is a novel analysis because although existing literature discusses trust and CBPR, or trust and social networks, *none had linked all three concepts*. The analysis revealed important findings about the multidimensionality of trust in each of the conceptual domains in which it operates as context, mechanism, *and* outcome. This kind of deeper understanding of trust will move us past "taken for granted" assumptions about what it is and how it features in, and shapes, partnerships for research coproduction. This knowledge can be used for building and sustaining partnerships by, for example, having methods to measure trust to alert stakeholders if they would benefit from an intervention to improve trust during a project's lifetime (Gilfoyle et al. 2020).

Another example relates to research about inclusivity and feelings of belonging. Like trust, these are important for coproduction because they strengthen stakeholders' engagement with the process. This, in turn, strengthens the scope for implementation of co-generated knowledge into practice (Rycroft-Malone et al. 2013). "Inclusivity," again like trust, is something we can have taken for granted knowledge about; but, in fact, we need to know much more about its internal dimensions and processes. Clarke et al. (2019) became interested in how inclusivity is realized through rituals and drew on sociologist Erving Goffman's 1967 *ritual theory* to empirically examine this further (Goffman 1967). Their analysis of rituals in meetings for collaborative health partnerships in the UK revealed that the common ritual of inviting *and* using stakeholders' feedback developed coherence and an affective sense of belonging among stakeholders to the goals of their projects. This enhanced ownership and the success of collaborations (Clarke et al. 2019). We can use this knowledge about meeting rituals and the mechanisms of inclusivity to design communication and governance plans in new research partnerships.

Other scholars have drawn on the writings of social scientists in geography and development studies, such as Massey (2005) and Cornwall (2002), about *spaces for participation*. This concept encourages critical thinking about the physical, social, and temporal dimensions of public participation. Following this conceptualization, questions arise, such as: Where does research coproduction take place (physical dimension)? de Freitas and Martin (2015) found that the involvement of migrants in the coproduction of mental health services in Portugal benefited from holding the meetings *in community settings*. Unlike statutory initiated spaces, representatives of the state were invited into a space designed to empower people from a marginalized community and the statutory stakeholders had to adapt to *their* norms for sharing voice and knowledge. There was equitable discussion and examples of changes to mental health service policy and services as a result. This finding can be used to guide project planning in terms of the *symbolic* and *practical* impact that arises from the location of meetings.

What power dynamics are at play within research coproduction teams (social dimension)? Think about how to *operationalize* power-sharing in diverse stakeholder groups. In an Irish project, designed to develop a national guideline for communication in cross-cultural consultations between migrants and general practitioners, meaningful participation was enacted by using a participatory approach: Participatory Learning and Action (PLA) research (described further below). In this project, the use of PLA meant that migrants, general practitioners, service planners, and interpreters in Ireland had an equal say in the development of the guideline because specific visual and analytic tools and techniques (see Table 2.1.1) were used to give everyone an equal opportunity to share perspectives and to vote on the content of the guideline (O'Reilly-de Brun et al. 2015). This work highlights that it pays to take time to identify participatory approaches that *explicitly* and *practically* attend to power asymmetries (see Chapter 2.2). This will help to counteract established socio-cultural norms and practices about who is (or is not) an expert in the room.

TABLE 2.1.1 PLA techniques

PLA Technique	Purpose
Flexible Brainstorming	Fast and creative approach of using materials, such as pictures or objects, to generate information and ideas about the topic
Card sort	An interactive method for facilitating, recording and thematically analyzing brainstorming around topics
Direct ranking	A transparent and democratic process that enables a group of stakeholders to indicate priorities or preference
Seasonal calendar	A grid-based diagram used for co-operative planning and democratic. Decision-making and can be used as a "running record" of stakeholders' planning over time
Speed evaluation	Short verbal or written evaluations to indicate what key positive, negative and/or neutral experiences have occurred during a PLA session

How does the timeframe of a partnership impact on its functioning and outcomes? Some studies of participatory spaces have found that community stakeholders' resources and capacities in terms of knowledge and confidence, and their feelings of power, are not fixed; they can strengthen and grow in *empowering* participatory spaces *over time* (de Freitas and Martin 2015). The implications of this are that the more empowering the space is, and the more resources there are for it to continue over a long period of time, the more the likelihood that stakeholders and decision-makers can engage in dialogues and co-learning in equitable ways. This, in turn, is associated with *transformational learning* among decision-makers to inform their thinking about changes to policy and practice (de Freitas and Martin 2015; MacFarlane et al. 2021).

Across these examples, we can see how theorizing about *a research coproduction approach can enhance the implementation of knowledge.* In this final part of the chapter, we consider work that has focused explicitly on participatory implementation in healthcare.

PARTICIPATORY IMPLEMENTATION RESEARCH

Scholars from the field of research coproduction and implementation science are fundamentally concerned with the same thing: multiple failures of implementation in health care which diminish the development and delivery of policy and practice to improve people's health and wellbeing (de Brun et al. 2016). Yet, research coproduction is not usually guided by knowledge from implementation theory, and implementation theory does not usually attend to coproduction processes. For example, there is a wide variety of implementation theories from different disciplines (see Nilsen (2015) for an overview) but few focus on coproduction with stakeholders from healthcare settings. In terms of attention to coproduction processes, Greenhalgh et al. (2004), in their review of the diffusion of innovations in service organizations, did emphasize that implementation research should be participatory, engaging "on the ground" *practitioners* as partners in the research process. Greenhalgh's more recent work considers the ethics of participatory implementation research with community stakeholders (Goodyear-Smith et al. 2015). Normalization Process Theory (NPT) (described in more detail further down) and its application have been critiqued for lacking consideration to patient and service user perspectives (see May et al. 2018; McEvoy et al. 2014), even though the originators of NPT do not restrict its focus to professional activity. May et al. (2018) consider that the exclusion of patients and carers from NPT-informed analysis may arise because they are not usually centrally involved as stakeholders in implementation processes. Overall, however, attention to how partnerships and research coproduction are relevant to understanding implementation *is under explored* and *warrants further investigation*. Here we present a detailed case study of a novel European Union (EU) funded participatory implementation project known as the RESTORE project (2011–2015).

Case Study: Blending Implementation Theory with Research Coproduction Practice

MacFarlane et al. (2012) were concerned with adapting primary care services to improve communication between migrants and their primary care providers. The research question was "Does the combination of a participatory research approach and implementation theory improve implementation of guidelines and training initiatives in daily practice?" RESTORE established participatory spaces to support partnership development and co-learning between diverse stakeholders: migrants, primary care clinicians and practice staff, health service planners, interpreters, and researchers. These stakeholders were invited to work collaboratively to implement communication guidelines and training initiatives in real-world primary care settings in Austria, England, Greece, Ireland, and the Netherlands.[1]

The research was based on an exploratory combination of concepts from participatory learning and action, which has roots in Freire's (1970) and Chambers' (1994) work in the Global South (Chambers 1994; Freire 1970), with NPT,

---

[1] The sixth RESTORE country partner was Scotland where the focus was on policy analysis.

which is a contemporary sociological theory of implementation developed in the UK by May and Finch (2009). Participatory Learning and Action research is a practical, adaptive research strategy that enables diverse groups and individuals to *participate*, *learn*, work and *act* together in a co-operative manner. Stakeholders focus on issues of joint concern, identify challenges and generate positive responses in a collaborative and democratic manner. The great strength of PLA lies in the democratic inclusion of locals as "experts in their own right" – the reconfiguring of locals as stakeholders capable of providing unique insights to the issue. PLA researchers have a specific role to adopt a participatory *mode of engagement* and, as mentioned previously, can utilize an extensive *tool kit of techniques* that can be used in sequential ways to create meaningful partnerships via dialogues and co-learning processes (de Brun et al. 2017; O'Reilly-de Brun et al. 2018) – see Table 2.1.1.

Normalization Process Theory (May and Finch 2009) was developed from a grounded theory process, based on over a decade of research about change and innovation in the UK health system. It provides a heuristic to think through the work that stakeholders have to do in order to make a new intervention part of routine and normalized practice. NPT describes four different kinds of inter-related implementation work (see Table 2.1.2).

The rationale for combining PLA and NPT (see de Brun et al. (2016)) was that both had been developed in response to multiple failures to implement innovations and both are located within the broad frame of social constructionism, which acknowledges that reality is defined and conveyed through a range of socio-cultural means. There were differences; NPT has focused on the perspectives of "professionals" (service providers, planners, policy-makers) and does not explicitly address power dynamics. PLA does pay attention to power but may "miss" implementation processes that NPT has identified through systematic theory building processes.

The challenge for RESTORE researchers was twofold. First, they had to think about *how* to combine PLA and NPT in a way that would investigate and support the implementation of guidelines and training initiatives.

TABLE 2.1.2 Normalization Process Theory: Four Constructs describing implementation work

Construct	Implementation work
Sense making	Can stakeholders make sense of the intervention?
Engagement	Can stakeholders get others involved in implementing the intervention?
Enactment	What needs to be done to make the intervention work in practice?
Appraisal	Can the intervention be evaluated and re-configured to make it more workable in practice?

Figure 2.1 shows that there were three stages to RESTORE and how PLA and NPT were operationalized in each stage. In the first stage, the emphasis was on using the concepts, mode of engagement and tools and techniques from PLA to create a welcoming participatory space for stakeholders from diverse backgrounds. In parallel with this, the research team completed a mapping exercise to identify guidelines and training initiatives and used NPT to "think through" how implementable they would be in each country setting based on policy, practice organization and the migration context.

In Stage 2, research teams in each country used PLA to create partnerships between themselves and all the other stakeholders and to support them to have meaningful dialogues about the guidelines and training initiatives. The goal was to reach a consensus decision in each setting about one to take forward as their local implementation project. This was achieved in all sites following a period of dialogue and a PLA direct ranking exercise and fostered ownership of the implementation process.

In Stage 3, stakeholders became the "champions" of their selected guideline/training initiative and worked together to get it working in daily practice. This involved ongoing dialogues, sharing of expertise, and co-learning to understand all the work required to get resources in place, to develop skills for and confidence in the new ways of working, and to explore if it helped them reach their goals of enhanced communication. The importance of appraising the new way of working, which NPT emphasizes, was not something that all stakeholder groups thought of themselves. In this case, the research teams alerted them to the fact that this was missing from their implementation work and it was then

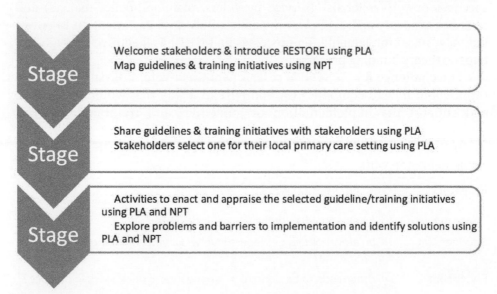

FIGURE 2.1   Summary of using PLA and NPT in each stage of RESTORE.

incorporated into stakeholders' implementation plans. NPT was also used to guide a comprehensive conceptual qualitative analysis of all the PLA-informed focus groups to synthesize knowledge about levers and barriers to stakeholders' implementation work.

Second, the researchers had to explore if PLA and NPT provided a stronger heuristic device combined as opposed to individually. An extensive participatory qualitative evaluation of stakeholders' experiences during RESTORE revealed that they felt PLA had provided tools and techniques to create meaningful partnerships between all the stakeholders involved (migrants, primary care clinicians and practice staff, health service planners, interpreters, and researchers) (de Brun et al. 2017; O'Reilly-de Brun et al. 2018). They also reported that PLA addressed power dynamics within stakeholder groups where there were asymmetries of power (de Brun et al. 2017; O'Reilly-de Brun et al. 2018). The use of PLA created a safe and enjoyable participatory space for dialogue, deliberation, co-learning and transformational or "aha" moments, all of which helped to support the implementation: stakeholders learned to see things from each other's perspective and could combine knowledge to think through solutions to many arising problems. It became clear that this was helping the implementation work. In NPT terms, the evaluation found that PLA enabled implementation work strengthening *engagement* (buy-in) and supporting *enactment* (problem solving) (Lionis et al. 2016; Teunissen et al. 2017). In terms of impact, a follow-up study (van den Muijsenbergh et al. 2020) found that many positive changes in knowledge, attitude, and behavior among reception staff, primary care nurses, and doctors documented during RESTORE were sustained in clinical settings four years later. There were also examples of unanticipated positive "ripple effects," such as enhanced confidence and opportunities for advocacy among migrants, and new inter-sectoral collaborations between researchers, migrants, and service planners to improve access to healthcare for migrants.

The implementation work was not, however, problem-free (Teunissen et al. 2017). Some stakeholders from clinical backgrounds were concerned about time commitment involved in PLA (PLA focus groups were usually two to three hours in length). There were structural influences, such as funding mechanisms for primary care, that limited the scope to advertise and embed a new interpreting service, as well as policies and budget allocations that undermined the scope to introduce or sustain healthcare adaptations through RESTORE. It became clear that, when stakeholders had resources *themselves* to progress problems and remove barriers to implementation, they were largely successful, but when their ideas and efforts were thwarted by structural factors this was not the case (MacFarlane et al. 2021).

It is also important to ask whether RESTORE could have been more participatory. A critical analysis of this with primary care academics and community partners, two of whom were RESTORE stakeholders, (see Acknowledgements) revealed important insights in this regard:

1. History and composition of partnerships: while some of the researchers involved had longstanding partnerships with migrants and health sector stakeholders, some did not and the governance of RESTORE was solely by a consortium of researchers. Having partners at the consortium meetings may have changed the understanding and decision-making about the project and its deliverables.

2. Deeper involvement in the NPT process: while the follow-up study documented examples of positive impact there are, of course, many aspects of service delivery that had, and have not been, adapted or improved. There is a persistent lack of interpreting services in Ireland and Greece, in particular. It is important to acknowledge that for this project, and many others, change is a function of *evolution* rather than "intervention." Many stakeholders "on the ground" in community and clinical settings are frustrated that significant change is so slow and incremental *even after investing time and effort in a meaningful participatory process*. If they had been more involved in the NPT analysis of their implementation work, they might have been able to provide insight into the reasons for their slow progress. Further, stakeholders' perspective on the accuracy and relevance of NPT as a conceptual lens would have been valuable.

3. Losing the relational "magic ingredients" at project end: the RESTORE project created unique groups of diverse stakeholders who had been through the implementation and co-learning process together. They understood the participatory process and what it would take to succeed. When a project ends like this, the issue "goes off" into practice / policy to other stakeholders who do not have a real understanding of the partnership, what made it work, and what will be required to progress the implementation work further. This relates to the "wicked" problem of scalability. Indeed, this is where the concept of participatory space is really valuable for analyzing RESTORE because *space is always open* (Massey 2005). Thus, it is worth thinking about *inter-connected webs of participatory spaces* and how stakeholders can *move between them* and shape dialogues with other relevant stakeholders who may have power over specific decisions of interest (MacFarlane et al. 2021). This is particularly important in the area of migrant health in the European context where many decision-makers are white people from the ethnic majority in the host country with, sometimes, limited understanding of institutional racism and the importance of healthcare adaptations for migrants. So, scalability might be more about *networks of participatory action* rather than a large project or network per se. For example, migrants who partic-

ipated in the Irish fieldwork in RESTORE have sustained their partnership and involvement with the researchers and have participated in national and regional policy working groups to further support the implementation of trained interpreters in the Irish healthcare setting. In this way, their participation in dissemination and implementation activities is ongoing.

Notwithstanding these points, overall NPT and PLA were found to be compatible in RESTORE to investigate and support implementation of guidelines and training initiatives. Combined, they did provide a stronger heuristic device than either one on their own may have provided. The main advice from RESTORE about how to use a research coproduction approach with an implementation theory would be to *start as early as possible with principles of partnership building* and *centralize attention to the partnership* throughout the project, particularly with regard to project governance. Find ways to operationalize partnership by, for example, the use of a PLA mode of engagement and PLA tools and techniques that shape and support inter-stakeholder dialogue and decision-making. These actions are an investment in the scope for co-learning and transformative learning between stakeholders about the implementation work at hand. Implementation theory can be used to alert stakeholders to the range of levers and barriers that shape the likelihood that the intervention involved can be introduced, embedded, and sustained as a new practice. Equally, implementation theory can be adapted and advanced by involving community and health sector partnerships in co-analyzing how it is being used and what impact it is having on the implementation work. Participatory evaluations are essential from project start to completion to monitor the partnership process and to evaluate how the process is working, for whom, and so on. This provides a "feedback loop" to support and strengthen meaningful participation. Finally, seek to establish a formal structure for partnership that will endure beyond the lifetime of a specific project to support community members to drive the work forward. It is also important that the partnership report to partners and other stakeholders what the process and outcomes are as the partnership continues.

There are, of course, many other participatory approaches and other implementation theories that could be combined, which brings us to the final part of our chapter where we explore knowledge gaps and directions for future research.

FUTURE RESEARCH

Drawing from the RESTORE case study and other examples provided in this chapter, we argue that we are missing an opportunity by not paying attention to research coproduction in implementation theory. If we take this opportunity, we can *harness the wealth of knowledge in each field to create a broader base for investigating and supporting knowledge generation, implementation, and sustainability.* Some ideas for future research include the value of:

- Systematically analyzing the attention to coproduction in implementation frameworks and theories
- Exploring the utility and impact of other combinations of participatory approaches and implementation theories to augment the evidence and learning generated from combining PLA and NPT
- Exploring the role of *participatory spaces* in implementation
- Increasing the participatory elements of such studies.

CONCLUSION

Progress is being made to develop research coproduction models and theories but there is more work to be done. There are many mechanisms (e.g., trust, belonging, dialogue) that are known to be relevant but are poorly conceptualized, operationalized, and measured (see Chapter 3.3). We need to investigate these further because this theorizing presents building blocks for theory, leading to more conceptually robust understanding, and scope to accumulate a generalizable knowledge base. Further, given that theories of implementation have underplayed the value of equal and meaningful participation of stakeholders from community and healthcare settings, and that research coproduction can benefit from implementation theory, we also need to "close the gap" between these fields. This will help to illuminate each other's blind spots with the former's attention to issues of power, equity, and self-determination, and the latter's attention to knowledge utilization and outcomes. Thus, there is potential for conceptual and practical gains for research coproduction and its impact on health care settings.

ACKNOWLEDGEMENTS

Thanks to the following who participated in an online workshop and provided critical insights about ways to enhance participatory aspects of the EU RESTORE project: Community partners – Maria Manuela de Almeida Silva (Ireland), Ekaterina Okonkwo (Ireland), Robina Mir (England), Graham Prestwich (England); Primary care academic clinicians – Jess Drinkwater (England), Lara Nixon (Canada), and Vivian R. Ramsden (Canada).

We acknowledge the work of the entire RESTORE consortium and all stake-holders who participated in the research. The RESTORE project was funded by EU Seventh Framework Programme (FP7/2007–2013) under Grant Agreement No. 257258. RESTORE: Research into Implementation STrategies to support patients of different ORigins and language background in a variety of European primary care settings

REFERENCES

1. Astbury, B. and Leeuw, F.L. (2010). Unpacking black boxes: mechanisms and theory building in evaluation. *American Journal of Evaluation* 31: 363–381. doi: 10.1177/1098214010371972.

2. Boyer, E.L. (1996). The scholarship of engagement. *Bulletin of the American Academy of Arts and Sciences* 49: 18–33. doi: 10.2307/3824459.

3. Brazil, K., Ozer, E., Cloutier, M.M., Levine, R., and Stryer, D. (2005). From the-ory to practice: improving the impact of health services research. *BMC Health Services Research* 5: 1. doi: 10.1186/1472-6963-5-1.

4. Chambers, R. (1994). The origins and practice of participatory rural appraisal. *World Development* 22: 953–969. doi: 10.1016/0305-750X(94)90141-4.

5. Clarke, J., Waring, J., and Timmons, S. (2019). The challenge of inclusive copro-duction: the importance of situated rituals and emotional inclusivity in the coproduction of health research projects. *Social Policy and Administration* 53: 233–248. doi: 10.1111/spol.12459.

6. Cornwall, A. (2002). Making Spaces, Changing Places: Situating Participation in Development, IDS Working Paper 170. Brighton, UK: Institute of Development Studies.

7. Creswell, J.W. and Creswell, J.D. (2017). *Research Design: Qualitative, Quantitative, and Mixed Methods Approaches*. Thousand Oaks, CA: Sage.

8. de Brun, T., O'Reilly-de Brun, M., O'Donnell, C.A., and MacFarlane, A. (2016). Learning from doing: the case for combining normalisation process theory and participatory learning and action research methodology for primary healthcare implementation research. *BMC Health Services Research* 16: 346. doi: 10.1186/s12913-016-1587-z.

9. de Brun, T., O'Reilly-de Brun, M., Van Weel-Baumgarten, E., Burns, N., Dowrick, C., Lionis, C., O'Donnell, C., Mair, F.S., Papadakaki, M., Saridaki, A., Spiegel, W., Van Weel, C., Van den Muijsenbergh, M., and MacFarlane, A. (2017). Using Participatory Learning & Action (PLA) research techniques for inter-stake-holder dialogue in primary healthcare: an analysis of stakeholders' experiences. *Research Involvement and Engagement* 3: 28. doi: 10.1186/s40900-017-0077-8.

10. de Freitas, C. and Martin, G. (2015). Inclusive public participation in health: policy, practice and theoretical contributions to promote the involvement of marginalised groups in healthcare. *Social Science & Medicine* 135: 31–39. doi: 10.1016/j.socscimed.2015.04.019.

11. Duran, E. and Duran, B. (1995). *Native American Postcolonial Psychology*. Albany, NY: SUNY Press.

12. Eccles, M.P., Armstrong, D., Baker, R., Cleary, K., Davies, H., Davies, S., Glasziou, P., Ilott, I., Kinmonth, A.L., Leng, G., Logan, S., Marteau, T., Michie, S., Rogers, H., Rycroft-Malone, J., and Sibbald, B. (2009). An implementation research agenda. *Implementation Science: IS* 4: 18. doi: 10.1186/1748-5908-4-18.

13. Freire, P. (1970). *Pedagogy of the Oppressed*. New York: Herder & Herder.

14. Gilfoyle, M., MacFarlane, A., and Salsberg, J. (2020). Conceptualising, operationalising and measuring trust in participatory health research networks: a scoping review protocol. *BMJ Open* 10: e038840. doi: 10.1136/bmjopen-2020-038840.

15. Goffman, E. (ed.) (1967). *Interaction Ritual: Essays in Face-to-Face Behavior*. Garden City, NY: Doubleday.

16. Goodyear-Smith, F., Jackson, C., and Greenhalgh, T. (2015). Co-design and implementation research: challenges and solutions for ethics committees. *BMC Medical Ethics* 16: 78. doi: 10.1186/s12910-015-0072-2.

17. Greenhalgh, T., Robert, G., Macfarlane, F., Bate, P., and Kyriakidou, O. (2004). Diffusion of innovations in service organizations: systematic review and recommendations. *The Milbank Quarterly* 82: 581–629. doi: 10.1111/j.0887-378x.2004.00325.x.

18. Hammond, M. (2018). "An interesting paper but not sufficiently theoretical": what does theorising in social research look like? *Methodological Innovations* 11: 1–10. doi: 10.1177/2059799118787756.

19. Israel, B.A., Schulz, A.J., Parker, E.A., and Becker, A.B. (1998). Review of community-based research: assessing partnership approaches to improve public health. *Annual Review of Public Health* 19: 173–202. doi: 10.1146/annurev.publhealth.19.1.173.

20. Israel, B.A., Schulz, A.J., Parker, E.A., Becker, A.B., Allen, A.J., Guzman, J.R., and Lichtenstein, R. (2017). Critical issues in developing and following community-based participatory research principles. In: *Community-Based Participatory Research for Health: Advancing Social and Health Equity*, 3e (ed. N. Wallerstein, B. Duran, J.G. Oetzel, and M. Minkler), 32–35. New York: Wiley.

21. Jagosh, J., Macaulay, A.C., Pluye, P., Salsberg, J., Bush, P.L., Henderson, J., Sirett, E., Wong, G., Cargo, M., Herbert, C.P., Seifer, S.D., Green, L.W., and Greenhalgh, T. (2012). Uncovering the benefits of participatory research: implications of a realist review for health research and practice. *The Milbank Quarterly* 90: 311–346. doi: 10.1111/j.1468-0009.2012.00665.x.

22. Lewin, K. (1946). Action research and minority problems. *Journal of Social Issues* 2: 34–46. doi: 10.1111/j.1540-4560.1946.tb02295.x.

23. Lionis, C., Papadakaki, M., Saridaki, A., Dowrick, C., O'Donnell, C.A., Mair, F.S., van den Muijsenbergh, M., Burns, N., de Brun, T., O'Reilly de Brun, M., van Weel-Baumgarten, E., Spiegel, W., and MacFarlane, A. (2016). Engaging migrants and other stakeholders to improve communication in cross-cultural consultation in primary care: a theoretically informed participatory study. *BMJ Open* 6: e010822. doi: 10.1136/bmjopen-2015-010822.

24. Macaulay, A.C. (2017). Participatory research: what is the history? Has the purpose changed? *Family Practice* 34: 256–258. doi: 10.1093/fampra/cmw117.

25. Macaulay, A.C., Commanda, L.E., Freeman, W.L., Gibson, N., McCabe, M.L., Robbins, C.M., and Twohig, P.L. (1999). Participatory research maximises community and lay involvement. North American Primary Care Research Group. *BMJ* 319: 774–778. doi: 10.1136/bmj.319.7212.774.

26. MacFarlane, A., Dowrick, C., Gravenhorst, K., O'Reilly-de Brun, M., de Brun, T., van den Muijsenbergh, M., van Weel Baumgarten, E., Lionis, C., and Papadakaki, M. (2021). Involving migrants in the adaptation of primary care services in a "newly" diverse urban area in Ireland: the tension between agency and structure. *Health & Place* 70: 102556. doi: 10.1016/j.healthplace.2021.102556.

27. MacFarlane, A., O'Donnell, C., Mair, F., O'Reilly-de Brun, M., de Brun, T., Spiegel, W., van den Muijsenbergh, M., van Weel Baumgarten, E., Lionis, C., Burns, N., Gravenhorst, K., Princz, C., Teunissen, E., van den Driessen Mareeuw, F., Saridaki, A., Papadakaki, M., Vlahadi, M., and Dowrick, C. (2012). REsearch into implementation STrategies to support patients of different ORigins and language background in a variety of European primary care settings (RESTORE): study protocol. *Implementation Science: IS* 7: 111. doi: 10.1186/1748-5908-7-111.

28. Massey, D. (2005). *For Space*. London: Sage.

29. May, C. and Finch, T. (2009). Implementing, embedding, and integrating practices: an outline of Normalization Process Theory. *Sociology* 43: 535–554. doi: 10.1177/0038038509103208.

30. May, C.R., Cummings, A., Girling, M., Bracher, M., Mair, F.S., May, C.M., Murray, E., Myall, M., Rapley, T., and Finch, T. (2018). Using Normalization Process Theory in feasibility studies and process evaluations of complex healthcare interventions: a systematic review. *Implementation Science: IS* 13: 80. doi: 10.1186/s13012-018-0758-1.

31. McEvoy, R., Ballini, L., Maltoni, S., O'Donnell, C.A., Mair, F.S., and Macfarlane, A. (2014). A qualitative systematic review of studies using the normalization process theory to research implementation processes. *Implementation Science: IS* 9: 2. doi: 10.1186/1748-5908-9-2.

32. Nguyen, T., Graham, I.D., Mrklas, K.J., Bowen, S., Cargo, M., Estabrooks, C.A., Kothari, A., Lavis, J., Macaulay, A.C., MacLeod, M., Phipps, D., Ramsden, V.R., Renfrew, M.J., Salsberg, J., and Wallerstein, N. (2020). How does integrated knowledge translation (IKT) compare to other collaborative research approaches to generating and translating knowledge? Learning from experts in the field. *Health Research Policy and Systems / BioMed Central* 18: 35. doi: 10.1186/s12961-020-0539-6.

33. Nilsen, P. (2015). Making sense of implementation theories, models and frameworks. *Implementation Science: IS* 10: 53. doi: 10.1186/s13012-015-0242-0.

34. O'Reilly-de Brun, M., de Brun, T., O'Donnell, C.A., Papadakaki, M., Saridaki, A., Lionis, C., Burns, N., Dowrick, C., Gravenhorst, K., Spiegel, W., Van Weel, C., Van Weel-Baumgarten, E., Van den Muijsenbergh, M., and MacFarlane, A. (2018). Material practices for meaningful engagement: an analysis of participatory learning and action research techniques for data generation and analysis in a health research partnership. *Health Expectations* 21: 159–170. doi: 10.1111/hex.12598.

35. O'Reilly-de Brun, M., MacFarlane, A., de Brun, T., Okonkwo, E., Bonsenge Bokanga, J.S., Manuela De Almeida Silva, M., Ogbebor, F., Mierzejewska, A., Nnadi, L., van den Muijsenbergh, M., van Weel-Baumgarten, E., and van Weel, C. (2015). Involving migrants in the development of guidelines for communication in cross-cultural general practice consultations: a participatory learning and action research project. *BMJ Open* 5: e007092. doi: 10.1136/bmjopen-2014-007092.

36. Ostrom, E. (1996). Crossing the great divide: coproduction, synergy, and development. *World Development* 24: 1073–1087. doi: 10.1016/0305-750X(96)00023-X.

37. Pawson, R. (2003). Nothing as practical as a good theory. *Evaluation* 9: 471–490. doi: 10.1177/135638900300900407.

38. Rycroft-Malone, J., Wilkinson, J., Burton, C.R., Harvey, G., McCormack, B., Graham, I., and Staniszewska, S. (2013). Collaborative action around implementation in Collaborations for Leadership in Applied Health Research and Care: towards a programme theory. *Journal of Health Services Research and Policy* 18: 13–26. doi: 10.1177/1355819613498859.

39. Silver, D. (2019). Theorizing is a practice, you can teach it. *Canadian Review of Sociology = Revue Canadienne de Sociologie* 56: 130–133. doi: 10.1111/cars.12236.

40. Teunissen, E., Gravenhorst, K., Dowrick, C., Van Weel-Baumgarten, E., Van den Driessen Mareeuw, F., de Brun, T., Burns, N., Lionis, C., Mair, F.S., O'Donnell, C., O'Reilly-de Brun, M., Papadakaki, M., Saridaki, A., Spiegel, W., Van Weel, C., Van den Muijsenbergh, M., and MacFarlane, A. (2017). Implementing guidelines and training initiatives to improve cross-cultural communication in primary care consultations: a qualitative participatory European study. *International Journal for Equity in Health* 16: 32. doi: 10.1186/s12939-017-0525-y.

41. van den Muijsenbergh, M., LeMaster, J.W., Shahiri, P., Brouwer, M., Hussain, M., Dowrick, C., Papadakaki, M., Lionis, C., and MacFarlane, A. (2020). Participatory implementation research in the field of migrant health: sustainable changes and ripple effects over time. *Health Expectations* 23: 306–317. doi: 10.1111/hex.13034.

42. Wallerstein, N. and Duran, B. (2010). Community-based participatory research contributions to intervention research: the intersection of science and practice to improve health equity. *American Journal of Public Health* 100 (Suppl 1): S40–S46. doi: 10.2105/ajph.2009.184036.

43. Wallerstein, N., Duran, B., Oetzel, J.G., and Minkler, M. (eds.)(2017). *Community-Based Participatory Research for Health: Advancing Social and Health Equity*. New York: Wiley.

44. Wallerstein, N., Oetzel, J., Duran, B., Tafoya, G., Belone, L., and Rae, R. (2008). What predicts outcomes in CBPR? In: *Community-Based Participatory Research for Health: Process to Outcomes*, 2e (ed. M. Minkler and N. Wallerstein), 371–392. San Francisco, CA: Jossey-Bass.

2.2 Equity, Power, and Transformative Research Coproduction

Katrina Plamondon, Sume Ndumbe-Eyoh, and Sana Shahram

Key Learning Points

- All social systems, structures, and human interactions within them are inextricably shaped by equity and power.
- Research coproduction is therefore also inherently shaped by issues of equity and power within these contexts.
- Understanding how power works to produce inequitable representation, voice, and benefits is foundational to equity-informed coproduction practices.

Knowledge rooted in experience shapes what we value and as a consequence how we know what we know as well as how we use what we know.

bell hooks

INTRODUCTION

As scholars who explicitly seek to advance health equity, we are constantly attentive to power in our work: from our interactions, our priorities, and practices. An important part of this attentiveness is our acknowledgement of how legacies of the formal colonial period shape contemporary power relationships and wealth distribution of societies both within and between countries. Populations with histories of various forms of colonization, displacement, or disenfranchisement experience consistent, systematic inequalities in virtually every measurable health outcome, including life expectancy (Came and Griffith 2018; Commission of the Pan American Health Organization on Equity and Inequalities in the Americas 2019). Depoliticized narratives that naturalize poverty while elevating the interests and perspectives of particular (dominant, privileged) groups over others have contributed to the maintenance, justification, and seemingly invisible nature of these structures over time (Brisbois et al. 2019; Came and Griffith 2018; Escobar 2012). Social, historical, economic, and environmental conditions – collectively referred to as the social and structural determinants of health (SSDH) – shape people's life trajectories and health outcomes more than their lifestyle, behavior, or biology combined (Commission of the Pan American Health Organization on Equity and Inequalities in the Americas 2019). Interventions that focus solely on behavior, lifestyle, or specific diseases are therefore unlikely to lead to meaningful improvements in health and/or progress in promoting health equity. Interrupting health inequities instead requires action on social and structural inequities to redistribute power, resources, and wealth as a critical pathway to improving virtually *any* health outcome. Efforts to promote health equity and reduce health inequities through attention to issues of power are therefore essential for advancing health, well-being, and happiness.

As critical equity scholars, our work focuses on illuminating or interrupting social and structural inequities to advance health equity action. We do research and knowledge translation *with* people who use it, aiming to position our skills and resources as researchers and boundary spanners to bring people together to examine or generate knowledge (including that generated through research) to create more equitable futures together. Our thinking is guided by decolonizing (Escobar 2012; Smith 1999) and other critical theorists such as Paolo Freire (1997) and bell hooks (2010), both of whom describe the transformative potential of people coming together in dialogue to deepen mutual understanding and examine issues of power and equity (Freire 1997; hooks 2010). We engage in doing and using research as a means for transformative change for a more equitable future. Our work includes a wide range of groups, populations, communities, organizations, and systems – on a diverse range of global and public health topics – to collaboratively and strategically align equity intentions, evidence, and action.

If coproduction is understood to be about the *way* research is done and used, **transformative coproduction** extends this commitment to advancing health equity through *both the content and processes* of research. Rather than directing attention to a particular research method or study design, it directs its gaze toward who is engaged, how questions are asked and research problems and designs framed, what is prioritized, what is produced, how coproduced knowledge is worked with, how positionalities are attended to, and how environments of curiosity, learning, and listening are created. Methodologies are then able to be responsive to diverse teams, using mixed methods that always involve dialogue as either a tool for generating research data, facilitating knowledge translation, or supporting their processes. All of these research practices should involve an active and continuous commitment to examining and intervening on systems power, using inclusive, decolonizing, antiracist, and dialogue-based practices to unsettle inequities and leverage the positionalities of all involved.

In this chapter, we unpack our assumptions and language, sharing our reflexive insights and grappling with questions about how we engage in transformative research coproduction. We begin by exploring power – *the central* coproduction problem, arguing it is always present and productive, and that we ought to strive to leverage and shift it toward equity. We offer readers a high-level summary of literature on health equity, suggesting equity- and evidence-informed coproduction plays an important role in shaping more equitable futures. We use examples to demonstrate the scope and scale of equity work, pointing to the relationship between coproduction and systems transformations. We offer examples from our own practice, featuring the transformative potential of coproduction at organizational, network/communities, and systems levels. In naming specific examples and practices for transformative coproduction, our attention to language is deliberate, because definitions "can reflect deep divides in values and beliefs that can be used to justify and promote very different policies and practices" (Braveman et al. 2017, p. 1). When research efforts strive to be transformative, they *must* involve coproduction and therefore *must* involve a continuous attentiveness to issues of power. We are also deliberatively provocative in our suggestion that *any* kind of health research has the potential to be transformative, regardless of whether it involves basic or clinical sciences, health systems or services research, or population and public health research.

POWER IS THE CENTRAL RESEARCH COPRODUCTION PROBLEM

Coproduction is a process of generating new understandings, insights, knowledge, or constructing futures in relationship with others. Power is the overarching and essential problem of research coproduction. Though dynamic, changeable, and productive, power is always at play, in every relationship.

Research involves relationships between people, ideas, contexts, findings and interpretations, results and impacts, processes and outcomes, etc. As a systematic pursuit of inquiry involving relationships, research is therefore intrinsically and essentially about power and positionality. Returning to Weber's definition of power, power is about the possibility of being able to assert will – as individuals or collectives – even in the face of resistance (Wallimann et al. 1977). Power and positionalities shape who and what is seen, privileged, and legitimized as worthy of research and implementation attention and resources.

Research is therefore never benign and always political – even (and especially) if those leading the research do not themselves consider it so. Indeed, power lies even in the degree to which we require ourselves to afford it attention, with the dominant positivist scientific worldview adopting a positionality of absoluteness, correctness, and self-reinforcing assertion of objectivity that often denies the role of power. Whether and how we examine our systems of thinking and the assumptions that shape what is privileged and legitimized as science, data, evidence, or knowledge are existentially about power and positionality. Accepting the inevitable and unavoidable presence of power extends the concept of positionality to knowledge systems themselves.

Box 2.2.1 Clarifying our language (key terms)

Systematic inequalities in health that are associated with modifiable and unfair social disadvantages are called *"health inequities"* (National Collaborating Centre for Determinants of Health 2015). Health inequities vary systematically with social positionality (see below), with those holding greater access to power, resources, and wealth experiencing unfair and unearned advantage and with those holding less experiencing unfair and unearned disadvantage (CSDH 2008; Nixon 2019).

Health equity means that "all people (individuals, groups, and communities) are able to reach their full potential and are not disadvantaged by social, economic or environmental conditions" (National Collaborating Centre for Determinants of Health 2015). It "requires removing obstacles to health, including poverty, discrimination and their consequences, including powerlessness, lack of access to good jobs with fair pay, quality education and housing, safe environments, and health care" (Braveman et al. 2017, p. 2).

Positionality is the complex social location that any person, group, or community occupies in relationship to others, characterized by intersecting identities and factors (both ascribed to by themselves, or assigned by others) that directly shapes the ways in which they navigate society and their access

(continued)

(*continued*)

to power, resources, and wealth. It is fluid – can change over time. It may be more or less taken for granted, depending on the degree of advantage afforded a particular positionality, wherein those holding greater access to power, resources, and wealth may not be afforded the need or opportunity to be attentive to their own positionality (Cousins 2010; Crenshaw 1997; Nixon 2019).

Power exists in any relationship between people, organizations, systems, ideas, and action. One of the most commonly cited theorists on power, Max Weber, argued that: "within a social relationship, power means any chance, (no matter whereon this chance is based) to carry through one's own [individual or collective] will (even against resistance)" (Wallimann et al. 1977, p. 234). It is complex, always productive, and exerted through different means, such as concepts of justice, rights, and social structures (Linares-Péreza and López-Arellanob 2008). Power is not a problem in and of itself, but *how* it is used, distributed, and/or shared has important consequences for equity.

Power-privileged people, ideas (ways of knowing; bodies of knowledge), and institutions are those that experience less resistance in carrying through their individual or collective will, and therefore experience greater advantage in their navigation and influence in society. *Power privilege* relies on often taken-for-granted assumptions that ideas from these sources are non-contestable and above reproach, effectively imposed on society as "natural," "logical," or "correct." The collective impact of power privilege is an assertion of rarely contested systems, structures, and norms that impact our worldviews and approaches to research.

Praxis and reflexivity go hand-in-hand. Praxis is about connecting what we know with what we do, through deep self-awareness and attentiveness to one's own positionality, as it is related to the broader contexts in which we are situated and as it relates to what we (think) we know, what we do, and how we do it (Finlay and Gough 2003; Kowal et al. 2013).

Transformative, in the context of this chapter, is effort that aims to shift or change power in ways that enable or advance health equity. Transformative research coproduction is aspirational and achievable through public and private decisions (and actions).

Transformative research coproduction challenges notions of knowledge, redefines research roles and relationships, and elevates issues of equity. As a process of generating knowledge, the first and most foundational assumptions for us to unpack are about how we understand knowledge and knowing. Knowing, acting, and being, in the dominant, Western-Eurocentric worldview tend to privilege linear, reductionistic conceptualizations of the world and things within it as discrete and separate (e.g., biomedical, behavioral, neoliberal, capitalist, racist, White supremacist). This conceptual separation of knowledge, knowing, and action stretches back to the influential 17th century theories of Descartes and Newton, who advanced a reductionist view of the world that broke phenomenon, experience, and living things into constituent parts with hierarchical, linear relationships that lead from input to output (Jayasinghe 2011). Their theories advanced one way of thinking about reality, what "counts" as real and what constitutes legitimate and (purportedly) objective ways of describing, measuring, and reporting what is real. Dominance of this thought system since that time is a signal of power more than a signal of correctness. Indigenous ways of thinking about the world, though diverse and unique to each nation, tend to weave these verbs into interdependent co-existence, as one and the same (Smylie et al. 2014). When we consider equity and power in what "counts" as knowledge, what we know and how we come to know are fluid, and socially constructed – as are who we determine to be legitimate knowledge holders (Escobar 1988; Freire 1997; hooks 2010; Smith 1999; Smylie et al. 2014).

Research systems are complex and multi-institutional, made up of a complex network of people, agencies, and governments. They include funding and peer review mechanisms, research ethics boards, healthcare organizations, universities, researchers, students, staff, knowledge brokers, knowledge translation platforms, and all of the communities they serve. These systems are power-privileged, wielding influence in determining what and who is funded, what approaches are judged as feasible and scientifically sound. They serve to reinforce conditions that normalize *in*attention to issues of power. Research priorities and the distribution of research resources through funding agencies and university investments in graduate education are all part of the systems that serve to uphold particular knowledge systems and positionalities. Despite the intention of contributing to public good (by virtue of the public investment in academic pursuits), these systems often miss the mark by not being afforded the need or opportunity to examine power in a meaningful way.

As researchers we are often positioned as experts with authority over knowledge and knowing. We are privileged to be the definers of research problems, legitimizing our work by situating it within an academic literature that, itself, is reflective of power-privileged bodies of knowledge (Croom 2017; Gair et al. 2015; Ramirez-Castaneda 2020). The academic enterprise is constructed by power systems that make coproduction challenging and transformative coproduction even more so, declaring some knowledge systems as more relevant than others (Ratima et al. 2019). Even when research priorities to motivate and incentivize partnered, impactful research are articulated, systems of power shape assumptions of what counts as a legitimate scholarly record in ways that privilege individual excellence and productivity. As such, transformative research coproduction affords attentiveness to issues of power *across research systems themselves* and not just within a particular project. (See the example of the xaȼqanaⱡ ʔitkiniⱡ project, described in the *Experiential Knowledge* section below.)

Recognizing health inequities as embedded in SSDH, themselves shaped by historical legacies of colonialism, another central assumption of transformative research coproduction is that power dynamics are never neutral. Genuine engagement in coproduction requires actively engaging in examining power, both within the research team and as part of framing and understanding research problems. Issues of inclusion, representation, and voice are inevitably prone to inequity. If we wish to advance a more equitable future, we must be deeply attentive to epistemological (in)justice and the ways in which research has historically reinforced particular systems of power by elevating particular systems of knowing and knowledge (Greenwood et al. 2018; Rowe et al. 2015; Shahram no date). And we must be willing to prioritize research content and process that offers the possibility of a more equitable future, wherein research is designed to actively redistribute power and actually improve the lives of marginalized, colonized peoples. The purpose and problem of transformative research coproduction is not research for research's sake, but rather to be responsive to known health inequities and focused on impacts that promote health equity, be it through theory, research, practice, or policy.

WHAT IS KNOWN FROM THE LITERATURE?

The literature on health inequities, health equity, and the SSDH has evolved over time. In 2008, the World Health Organization released an influential report summarizing years of findings from nine knowledge networks around the world. In "*Closing the Gap in a Generation*," leaders from around the world provided irrefutably clear evidence about the relationship between health and the social and structural conditions of living. They argued that "social injustice is killing people on a grand scale" (CSDH 2008, p. 1) and showed that health inequities were directly related to the unfair (and changeable) distribution of resources, power, and health in societies. Though the report provided specific recommendations for policy and research, it fell short of naming the sociopolitical and historical legacies of colonialism as deterministic of contemporary distribution of power, resources, and wealth within and between countries. Though the report served to amplify the attention on SSDH, it avoided critical power analysis. When the Pan American Health Organization opened the table to include diverse perspectives in its Commission on Equity and Health Inequalities in the Americas, this action shifted the dialogue, advancing an evidence- and equity-informed process that was explicitly attentive to the role of power (Commission of the Pan American Health Organization on Equity and Inequalities in the Americas 2019). In essence, *what* questions are asked, *who* is represented, and *how* the process unfolds matters.

We can examine what the literature reveals in a living example where transformative research coproduction *could* be playing a role in shaping a more equitable future. In 2020, a pandemic surged around the world, revealing the interconnectedness of our collective global health. Also revealed were the depths of social, economic, and racial divides that positioned Black, Indigenous, and people of colour in greater economic and health hardship (Bhala et al. 2020; Oppel Jr et al. 2020; Tai et al. 2021). Though initially described as a "great equalizer," dramatic inequities in the burden and impact of COVID-19 mirror patterns exposed by previous pandemics in ways that provided a substantive knowledge base that *should* have drawn research, practice, and policy attention to SSDH (Gaynor and Wilson 2020; Mein 2020). Despite the strength of evidence, responses to the pandemic focused predominantly on public health interventions that make power-privileged assumptions about basic health, living, and working conditions – made by people positioned with enough privilege to assume the SSDH didn't factor into the epidemiology of an infectious disease. It would be laughable for researchers to overlook the pandemic as involving a virus, yet many responded with surprise when epidemiological data demonstrated it involves inequities. There is no legitimate scientific, ethical, or practical justification for this surprise or for *not* understanding the pandemic as inextricable from SSDH. The strength of evidence about the ubiquity and impacts of SSDH on health is irrefutable. Absence of critical and equity-centered power analysis is harmful for everyone.

Transformative research coproduction draws systems to task. It invites creative consideration of how people, environments, behaviors, and practices work to restrict or share power. Most health professions and health science researchers are not sensitized to the importance (or even presence) of power, let alone hold capacity to identify and analyze its role in society or in their work settings. Absence of the attentiveness to the power is self-reinforcing, regardless of how seemingly good or sincere the intention, and serves to maintain or entrench inequities in the distribution of power. Further, even when efforts in global and public health are described as doing *something* to address health inequities or promote health equity, evidence about the causes of health inequities is overlooked as often as not (Plamondon et al. 2020). When efforts to connect knowledge with action focus on issues of health equity, much of it tends to problematize the disparities or inequities – with the bulk of interventions aimed at the behaviors, lifestyles, or living conditions of those who are navigating positionalities of disadvantage. The problem is defined as belonging to the populations experiencing inequities, rather than those experiencing advantage. In order to dismantle the systems and structures that uphold inequitable SSDH, our gaze needs to turn to dismantling systems of unfair unearned advantage. When attentiveness to positionality and power is low, the likelihood of a thorough and honest examination of the ways in which power is shaping a particular health outcome is also low.

Research aimed at examining *how* to connect knowledge with action for health equity showed that *how* we think about health equity is in constant relationship with *how* we engage in efforts to act. Civil society movements and scholars alike are pushing boundaries of action on SSDH. Evidence-informed practices for connecting knowledge with action for health equity challenge the core structures and functions of relationships between power-privileged and others in society. Given the ubiquitous role of SSDH in shaping health outcomes and life trajectories, we argue that these practices have much to offer *any* effort to use or do research – and are essential to transformative research coproduction. Several tools and strategies are also available to support critical engagement in power analysis and attentiveness to issues of equity. Offered by a Canada-based network of people interested in using and doing research to address issues of equity in global health settings, the Canadian Coalition for Global Health Research (CCGHR) Principles for Global Health Research offer a platform for critically reflective dialogue that can be used in any effort to center equity (https://www.ccghr.ca/resources/principles-global-health-research). The six principles include partnering authentically, fostering inclusion, creating shared benefits, planning with a commitment to the future, responding to the causes of inequities, and practicing humility (Plamondon and Bisung 2019). With their deeply relational focus, the principles and accompanying tools provide people with a mechanism to support conversations about equity implications, emphasizing that there are always choices in what and how we approach research or knowledge translation – with some choices more equity-centered than others.

The World Health Organization's health equity assessment tools are used by governments to provide a mechanism for elevating equity considerations in municipal, regional, national and international policy, monitoring and evaluation efforts. Political economy frameworks, such as that described by Raphael and colleagues, provide another useful tool to engage in critical power analysis of context and players connected to the SSDH (Raphael and Bryant 2019). The Systems Health Equity Lens (SHEL), developed in partnership with health system partners, is a dual lens that focuses on recognizing health inequities as well as promoting health equity. The lens necessarily shifts attention away from identifying "at-risk" or "vulnerable" populations toward the root causes of inequities: the systems, structures, and processes that create disadvantage and vulnerability in the first place. Guided by intersectionality and complexity, the SHEL incorporates health system actions across all levels of the health system through application of a socio-ecological model (Pauly et al. 2018). Both the SHEL and the CCGHR Principles for Global Health Research are useful tools for people involved in coproduction to think through the equity implications and choices they navigate in any given endeavor.

The National Collaborating Centre for Determinants of Health, a Canadian knowledge translation organization, moves forward equity-oriented knowledge translation by attending to multiple ways of knowing, explicitly centering equity and naming systems of power, taking a problem-solving approach, drawing on and working with affected communities (particularly outsiders-within), learning from multisectoral and multidisciplinary perspectives, and understanding the context within which knowledge is generated and applied (Davison et al. 2015). With these considerations in mind, resources on key health equity, structural and social determinants of health issues are developed in partnership with researchers and practitioners. These resources take up issues of power and how it influences health, contributing to the normalization of a power analysis in public health. For example, through the Let's Talk series the NCCDH has explored health equity, racism, and Whiteness and provides questions to support reflection and dialogue within organizations. The resources and tools articulate roles for public health to contribute to reducing health inequities through policy advocacy, community engagement, collaborative practice, and partnerships with non-health sectors.

EXPERIENTIAL KNOWLEDGE

Research coproduction that transforms includes and facilitates power analysis to eliminate echo chamber research, redistributes power, and empowers people who are not typically given the opportunity to analyze power to engage in the power analysis (because they are usually the subject of study). Below, we offer three examples of transformative coproduction from our own experience within organizations, networks and communities, and systems.

Coproduction to Transform Organizations (Sume)

My engagement in transformative research coproduction sits at the intersection of research and practice. I have chosen to work at the margins of public health and through knowledge translation, collaboratively develop tools and resources to support policy and practice change to improve health equity. I actively bring in perspectives that have the potential to transform health inequities into the consciousness of public health practitioners and decision-makers. I position SSDH, such as racism and Whiteness, as being pertinent to public health practice, research, and education (National Collaborating Centre for Determinants of Health 2015; Ndumbe-Eyoh et al. 2020). I pay thoughtful attention to who is invited to provide open peer review of publications and aim to draw on an inclusive pool of reviewers with expertise and lived experience. I actively privilege outsiders-within, those who have lived experience of structural marginalization and resistance, who practice or research in health equity. This consideration extends to who I invite to provide advice on the knowledge translation resources I develop. Through webinars and workshops, I regularly profile the knowledge of researchers and practitioners from health and other sectors (Ndumbe-Eyoh et al. 2020). My transformative coproduction practice centers co-learning on individuals and organizations, positioning practitioners as legitimate knowledge-holders and working collaboratively to capture their experiences. This invites different ways of knowing that are rooted in issues that matter to the field. I strive to be a critical friend to public health practitioners and organizations, inviting learning and curiosity while always moving dialogue and action in the service of reducing social and health inequities.

Coproduction to Transform Networks/Communities (Katrina)

I engage in transformative research coproduction with the broad and dispersed academic fields of global and public health, advancing health equity action by working with those in positions of influence. I do research with people who use it, collaboratively designing research that examines the determinants of uptake and integration of equity-centered approaches among those individuals and collectives that constitute health research systems such that transformative coproduction is unfolding from *within* our own practice community. I do this by constructing my role as an academic around advancing health equity action, such that my teaching, service, and research are all incremental contributions to transforming practices in global and public health. I confront scholarly and research practices that restrict our collective capacity to align equity intentions with action (Plamondon et al. 2020). I contribute to theoretical and methodological debate that contributes to sparking dialogue about *how* we strive for transformative coproduction (Plamondon 2021; Plamondon and Caxaj 2018). I build long-term relationships with networks and communities over time, listening for direction and positioning my time, skills, and resources in service. Transformative research coproduction is a career commitment to working with this community of influence, catalyzing the potential for change by strengthening attentiveness to issues of power and equity among networks and practice communities whose work is influential in shaping (and re-shaping) the SSDH.

Coproduction for Systems Transformation: The xa¢qanaɬ ʔitkiniɬ Project (Sana)

The xa¢qanaɬ ʔitkiniɬ (Many Ways of Doing the Same Thing) research project is a long-term partnership between Ktunaxa Nation Council, Interior Health, the University of British Columbia, and the University of Victoria to coproduce solutions for promoting equitable health outcomes for people within Ktunaxa territory. The research team includes scholars, leaders, and Elders from the Nation, with oversight and guidance from the xaȼqanaɬ ʔitkiniɬ Advisory Group, composed of Ktunaxa Elders, knowledge holders and language experts. There are several examples of practically implementing coproduction practices that are attentive to power and transformative in application from this project (Shahram et al., in progress). One example is the allocation of over 80% of all research funds directly into communities through hosting local research events, contracting local vendors, appropriate compensation of Knowledge Holders and team members, and purposefully supporting the training and capacity of Ktunaxa citizens. Another is the team's collaboration with Ktunaxa Nation Council to cofund three local Ktunaxa artists to capture themes from research findings and community wellness concepts to display in the Ktunaxa Nation Governance Building. Finally, in a departure from academic traditions that claim data and knowledge as "owned" by researchers, our team's refusal to publish or share community data that is contextualized, and for the sole purpose and gain of the Nation and community, is an important act of honoring the spirit of coproduction. Instead, we publish only the insights gained about transformative *processes* as a means of informing anti-colonial actions in broader systems (e.g., healthcare and health research systems). While this project has importantly generated useful data and products for Ktunaxa Nation to support health and wellness, as well as contributed to the refinement of methods, policies, and resources that are being applied in many sectors, a major contribution has been the process of doing this work in the first place. By creating space for different ways of knowing and doing, our project demonstrates how coproduction, that is equitable in process as well as purpose, can confront systems-level barriers with community-driven solutions, create shared and mutual benefits for all partners and transform broad systems alongside local and context-rich efforts to engage with and balance issues of power and privilege (Shahram et al., in progress).

PRACTICE IMPLICATIONS

Practice is a word comfortably used by the health professions, often with clinical implications. As critical equity scholars, we understand practice as the daily, habitual actions people or collectives engage in as routine ways of doing, working, and interacting in *any* setting. All people engage in practices relevant to their own lives and interactions. Practices exist in a constant relationship with what and how individuals and collectives think, and are therefore acts of asserting power. Returning to our definition of *transformative*, we focus our energy on research and knowledge translation topics that we believe can shift or change power in ways that enable or advance health equity – and also on practices that can do the same. Transformative research coproduction is aspirational, future-facing, and achievable. What we do with power on a daily, routine basis is foundational to achieving transformation for a more equitable future.

What we do with power in our routine practices is, indeed, precisely the point at which individuals or collectives generate the conditions that determine the distribution of power and resources. Far from trite, and regardless of the degree of attentiveness afforded them, practices *are* enactments of power and agency. They can be more or less responsive to issues of equity, more or less transformative. The relationship between practice and transformative potential is circular and mutually reinforcing, such that adopting a practice of identifying and examining practices themselves *is* transformative. It turns a critical, analytical gaze upon the role of individual or collective practices in shaping power relationships, and it requires deep attentiveness to positionality. This analysis must extend to the systems, structures, and social narratives that serve to construct particular ideas about "truth" and "knowledge."

Because power is inescapable, and because all people and ideas are embedded in social contexts, no individual or collective is immune from its effects. Power-privileged narratives elevate particular ideas and priorities while silencing others – bell hooks describes how the power dynamics of patriarchy are constantly and actively constructed by both men and women:

> We need to highlight the role women play in perpetuating and sustaining patriarchal culture so that we will recognize patriarchy as a system women and men support equally, even if men receive more rewards from that system. Dismantling and changing patriarchal culture is work that men and women must do together.
>
> (hooks 2004)

The practice implication for those pursuing transformative research coproduction is a call to reflexivity and power-aware praxis. It is intense, demanding head and heart work. It is a call to stay in conversation and embrace a willingness not only to change but also to teach. It is an everybody problem, inviting individuals and collectives (research teams and research systems) to take up our autonomy and exert our agency to be part of a transformative solution.

One of the paradoxes of engagement that we grapple with in the ever-expanding scholarly field of "coproduction" stems from the use of language that assigns a code and positionality to different kinds of knowledge user or team member. Terms like "patient-oriented" can sound like good ways to open transformative possibilities, but they often require particular team members to legitimize their presence or foreground their status through an illness or some kind of diversity or inclusion quota, while others foreground their professional qualifications or formal titles. Researchers are commonly assigned leadership roles or authority in research processes, even in teams or on projects that explicitly center themselves around an intention of coproduction. Risk of tokenism, or worse – of diminishing the multiplicities of our humanity – arises, however, when assumptions about language and positionality are left unquestioned. In any interaction there is power. Coproduction teams must prioritize and engage in dialogue about power. Being aware of our own power and positionality, in our own complex social position, allows us to leverage, share, and redistribute it. The more power we hold, the greater our responsibility to be aware and the greater our accountability to redistribute it.

Box 2.2.2   Ten basic practices for transformative coproduction

1. Engage in a personal reflective practice to understand your own positionality. Commit to routine practices that draw upon your own creativity, using art, poetry, journaling, or dialogue to advance your reflective practice. Do some work on your own, and other work in safe places where you can be vulnerable. For each of the following points, engage in dialogue with others, balancing talking, listening, and reflecting as a foundation.

2. Intentionally articulate assumptions, values, theories, and philosophies that influence your worldview. Invite others with different perspectives to be part of identifying these things, because it can be hard to do in isolation. Challenge each other. Engage in working through all of these practices together.

3. Do difficult, deep reading of critical authors whose writing invites reflection on issues of power and privilege. For example, visit the NCCDH website for resources on Whiteness (http://nccdh.ca/resources/glossary), or use tools to support reflective dialogue (e.g., https://toolsforchange.org/wp-content/uploads/2014/03/to%20equalize%20power.pdf). Many of the authors we cite in this chapter are a great starting place, as are the many incredible Indigenous, anti-racism, and anti-White Supremacy scholars whose works can easily be found by searching your local or online bookstore for these topics.

4. Practice humility, approaching from a position of listening and learning rather than knowing.

5. Don't assume that your perspective is neutral. Acknowledge that you bring a perspective and experiences into the space that will create biases and taken-for-granted assumptions. Invite dialogue that interrogates these perspectives.

(continued)

(continued)

6. Locate health in the broader political historical contexts that are known to shape inequities and imbalances in the distribution of wealth, resources, and power. Extending consideration of these broader contexts to your research design, approaches, questions, and knowledge translation plans.

7. Embrace theoretical research approaches that allow space for and honor different ways of knowing.

8. Center the purpose of coproduction on the benefits it will produce for the groups, communities, or populations it is supposed to serve.

9. Ask critical questions about the benefits of research: where does the money go? Is the community building capacity in ways that transform? Are communities sharing the benefits and burdens of research?

10. Observe your own emotional response to challenges to power. Recognize when you are feeling uncertain, vulnerable, bold, or confident. Use this observation to support a practice of power-sharing, power redistribution, and transformation.

Reprinted with permission from: CCGHR Principles for Global Health Research, Figure and questions (for which Katrina Plamondon was the lead author and concept designer of the figure). Agreed and accepted by Christina Zarowsky and Susan Elliott, Co-Chairs CAGH Interim Board.

FUTURE RESEARCH

Transformative research coproduction is evolving, iterative, and full of future potential. It builds on a deep and diverse tradition that strives for more equitable societies in which all communities thrive. Each of us is actively involved in knowledge translation science that examines questions of how to achieve health equity action. We believe future research can extend to explore the impact of training on the capacity, confidence, and competence of people engaging in coproduction. There may be spaces where it is more likely to be taken up, or more needed – and there may not be space for transformative research in all settings. Future efforts should include ongoing monitoring and research on the long-term impacts of working in more equity-informed and transformative ways to promote health equity and reduce inequity.

CONCLUSION

Transformative research coproduction may be more comfortably embraced by people who have an explicit equity intention; however, because of the ubiquity and influence of issues of power in shaping virtually *any* health outcome, we argue that all research could more or less be equity-informed; therefore any effort to use or do research could be more or less transformative. Both between and within countries, vast inequities shape dramatically different life trajectories among people who either benefit or are harmed by the persistent legacies of colonialism. Legacies of power inequities directly shape the SSDH today, and have for centuries. In the twenty-first century, waves of critical public dialogue demonstrate an increasing intolerance for inattention to issues of power and privilege. There is growing desire and interest to do better. Activist and poet, Maya Angelou famously said *"...when you know better, you do better."* We know that there is a need to strengthen collective capacity to identify, understand, and transform inequitable power structures and relationships in society. Inviting power-privileged perspectives and populations into brave and productive dialogue, with accountability and responsibility, is central to transformative coproduction. Doing so requires compassion, advanced facilitative skills (that can be learned and developed), researchers, and facilitators who invest in the deep critical thinking work required to unpack complex issues of power and understand their own positionality and its embeddedness in broader social narratives. Health equity work is everyone's work, and the more we see each other as connected to our collective futures, the more likely we are to be accepting in the process of learning how to engage in power analysis and transformation.

Transformative potential is fluid, with coproduction serving to favorably shift research efforts toward advancing equity. It can be applied to research questions that seek to analyze the powerful, or to setting priorities for discovery-driven research by, for example, examining issues of equity in what benefits are imagined and established, and for whom. When we engage in coproduction for transformation, we commit to building knowledge and knowing together, we create space for honoring many ways of knowing, and we approach everything we do from a position of listening and learning, rather than authority. We embrace optimism for our collective capacity to create more equitable futures. We take risks of disruption, unlearning, and re-creating relationships. When we authentically engage in transformative coproduction, we make ourselves vulnerable, examining our own positionalities in the context of broader societal narratives and inviting critical conversations with others. We build our individual and collective capacity to engage in uncomfortable, unsettling learning because we believe in the creative and amazing capacity of humanity. We hold optimism and hope with reverence, and acknowledge our role in service to a greater public good, as one voice among the many needed to create a more equitable future.

REFERENCES

1. Bhala, N., Curry, G., Martineau, A.R., Agyemang, C., and Bhopal, R. (2020). Sharpening the global focus on ethnicity and race in the time of COVID-19. *Lancet* 395: 1673–1676. doi: 10.1016/S0140-6736(20)31102-8.

2. Braveman, P., Arkin, E., Orleans, T., Proctor, D., and Plough, A. (2017). *What Is Health Equity? And What Difference Does a Definition Make?* Princeton, NJ: Robert Wood Johnson Foundation. https://nccdh.ca/resources/entry/what-is-health-equity-and-what-difference-does-a-definition-make.

3. Brisbois, B.W., Spiegel, J.M., and Harris, L. (2019). Health, environment and colonial legacies: situating the science of pesticides, bananas and bodies in Ecuador. *Social Science & Medicine* 239: 112529. doi: 10.1016/j.socscimed.2019.112529.

4. Came, H. and Griffith, D. (2018). Tackling racism as a "wicked" public health problem: enabling allies in anti-racism praxis. *Social Science & Medicine* 199: 181–188. doi: 10.1016/j.socscimed.2017.03.028.

5. Commission of the Pan American Health Organization on Equity and Inequalities in the Americas. (2019). *Just Societies: Health Equity and Dignified Lives. Report of the Commission of the Pan American Health Organization on Equity and Health Inequalities in the Americas.* Washington, DC: PAHO. https://iris.paho.org/handle/10665.2/51571.

6. Cousins, G. (2010). Positioning positionality: the reflexive turn. In: *New Approaches to Qualitative Research: Wisdom and Uncertainty*, 1e (ed. M. Savin-Baden and C. Howell Major). London and New York: Routledge.

7. Crenshaw, K. (1997). Demarginalizing the intersection of race and sex: a Black feminist critique of antidiscrimination doctrine, feminist theory and antiracist politics. In: *Feminist Legal Theories* (ed. K. Maschke), 35–64. Routledge.

8. Croom, N.N. (2017). Promotion beyond tenure: unpacking racism and sexism in the experiences of Black womyn professors. *The Review of Higher Education* 40: 557–583. doi: 10.1353/rhe.2017.0022.

9. CSDH. (2008). *Closing the Gap in A Generation: Health Equity through Action on the Social Determinants of Health. Final Report of the Commission on Social Determinants of Health.* Geneva: World Health Organization. http://www.who.int/social_determinants/final_report/csdh_finalreport_2008.pdf.

10. Davison, C.M., Ndumbe-Eyoh, S., and Clement, C. (2015). Critical examination of knowledge to action models and implications for promoting health equity. *International Journal for Equity in Health* 14: 49. doi: 10.1186/s12939-015-0178-7.

11. Escobar, A. (1988). Power and visibility: development and the invention and management of the Third World. *Cultural Anthropology* 3: 428–443. http://www.jstor.org/stable/656487.

12. Escobar, A. (2012). The problematization of poverty: the tale of three worlds and development. In: *Encountering Development: The Making and Unmaking of the Third World*, 21–54. New Jersey: Princeton University Press.

13. Finlay, L. and Gough, B. (2003). *Reflexivity: A Practical Guide for Researchers in Health and Social Sciences*. Hoboken, NJ: Wiley-Blackwell.

14. Freire, P. (1997). *Pedagogy of the Oppressed*. New York: Continuum.

15. Gair, S., Miles, D., Savage, D., and Zuchowski, I. (2015). Racism unmasked: the experiences of Aboriginal and Torres Strait Islander students in social work field placements. *Australian Social Work* 68: 32–48. doi:10.1080/0312407X.2014.928335.

16. Gaynor, T.S. and Wilson, M.E. (2020). Social vulnerability and equity: the disproportionate impact of COVID-19. *Public Administration Review*. doi: 10.1111/puar.13264.

17. Greenwood, M., de Leeuw, S., and Lindsay, N. (2018). Challenges in health equity for Indigenous peoples in Canada. *Lancet* 391: 1645–1648. doi: 10.1016/S0140-6736(18)30177-6.

18. hooks, b. (2004). *The Will to Change: Men, Masculinity, and Love*. New York: Atria Books.

19. hooks, b. (2010). *Teaching Critical Thinking: Practical Wisdom*. New York: Routledge.

20. Jayasinghe, S. (2011). Conceptualising population health: from mechanistic thinking to complexity science. *Emerging Themes in Epidemiology* 8: 2. doi: 10.1186/1742-7622-8-2.

21. Kowal, E., Franklin, H., and Paradies, Y. (2013). Reflexive antiracism: a novel approach to diversity training. *Ethnicities* 13: 316–337. doi: 10.1177/1468 796812472885.

22. Linares-Péreza, N. and López-Arellanob, O. (2008). Health equity: conceptual models, essential aspects, and the perspective of collective health. *Social Medicine* 3: 194–206.

23. Mein, S.A. (2020). COVID-19 and health disparities: the reality of "the Great Equalizer." *Journal of General Internal Medicine* 35: 2439–2440. doi: 10.1007/s11606-020-05880-5.

24. National Collaborating Centre for Determinants of Health. (2015). *Glossary of Essential Health Equity Terms*. [Online]. http://nccdh.ca/resources/glossary (accessed 31 August 2021).

25. Ndumbe-Eyoh, S., Massaquoi, N., Yanful, N., and Watson-Creed, G. (2020). *Webinar: actionable ways to address anti-Black racism & police violence through public health practice*. [Online]. https://nccdh.ca/workshops-events/entry/webinar-antiBlackracism-policeviolence-public-health (accessed 31 August 2021).

26. Nixon, S.A. (2019). The coin model of privilege and critical allyship: implications for health. *BMC Public Health* 19: 1637. doi: 10.1186/s12889-019-7884-9.

27. Oppel, R.A.O., Jr, Gebeloff, R., Lai, K.K.R., Wright, W., and Smith, M. (2020). The fullest look yet at the racial inequity of coronavirus. https://www.nytimes.com/interactive/2020/07/05/us/coronavirus-latinos-african-americans-cdc-data.html.

28. Pauly, B., Shahram, S.Z., van Roode, T., Strosher, H.W., and MacDonald, M. (2018). *Reorienting Health Systems Towards Health Equity: The Systems Health Equity Lens (SHEL)*. Victoria, BC: The Equity Lens in Public Health (ELPH) Research Project. https://www.uvic.ca/research/projects/elph/assets/docs/kte-resource-6---systems-health-equity-lens.pdf.

29. Plamondon, K. and Caxaj, S. (2018). Toward relational practices for enabling knowledge-to-action in health systems: the example of deliberative dialogue. *ANS. Advances in Nursing Science* 41: 18–29. doi: 10.1097/ANS.0000000000000168.

30. Plamondon, K.M. (2021). Reimagining researchers in health research comment on "experience of health leadership in partnering with university-based researchers in Canada: a call to "re-imagine" research." *International Journal of Health Policy and Management* 10: 86–89. doi: 10.15171/ijhpm.2020.05.

31. Plamondon, K.M. and Bisung, E. (2019). The CCGHR principles for global health research: centering equity in research, knowledge translation, and practice. *Social Science & Medicine* 239: 112530. doi: 10.1016/j.socscimed.2019.112530.

32. Plamondon, K.M., Bottorff, J.L., Caxaj, C.S., and Graham, I.D. (2020). The integration of evidence from the Commission on Social Determinants of Health in the field of health equity: a scoping review. *Critical Public Health* 30 (4): 415–428. doi: 10.1080/09581596.2018.1551613.

33. Ramirez-Castaneda, V. (2020). Disadvantages in preparing and publishing scientific papers caused by the dominance of the English language in science: the case of Colombian researchers in biological sciences. *PLoS One* 15: e0238372. doi: 10.1371/journal.pone.0238372.

34. Raphael, D. and Bryant, T. (2019). Political economy perspectives on health and health care. In: *Staying Alive: Critical Perspectives on Health, Illness, and Health Care*, 3e (ed. T. Bryant, D. Raphael, and M.H. Rioux), 61–83. Toronto, ON: Canadian Scholars' Press Inc.

35. Ratima, M., Martin, D., Castleden, H., and Delormier, T. (2019). Indigenous voices and knowledge systems – promoting planetary health, health equity, and sustainable development now and for future generations. *Global Health Promotion* 26: 3–5. doi: 10.1177/1757975919838487.

36. Rowe, S., Baldry, E., and Earles, W. (2015). Decolonising social work research: learning from critical Indigenous approaches. *Australian Social Work* 68: 296–308. doi: 10.1080/0312407X.2015.1024264.

37. Shahram, S.Z. (no date). *What's in a Name? The Story of xaǥqanaɬ ʔitkiniɬ (Many Ways of Working Together)*.

38. Smith, L.T. (1999). *Decolonizing Methodologies*. London: Zed Books.

39. Smylie, J., Olding, M., and Ziegler, C. (2014). Sharing what we know about living a good life: indigenous approaches to knowledge translation. *The Journal of the Canadian Health Libraries Association / CHLA = Journal de l'Association des Bibliothèques de la Santé du Canada / ABSC* 35: 16–23. doi: 10.5596/c14-009.

40. Tai, D.B.G., Shah, A., Doubeni, C.A., Sia, I.G., and Wieland, M.L. (2021). The disproportionate impact of COVID-19 on racial and ethnic minorities in the United States. *Clinical Infectious Diseases: An Official Publication of the Infectious Diseases Society of America* 72: 703–706. doi: 10.1093/cid/ciaa815.

41. Wallimann, I., Tatsis, N.C., and Zito, G.V. (1977). On Max Weber's definition of power. *The Australian and New Zealand Journal of Sociology* 13: 231–235. doi: 10.1177/144078337701300308.

2.3 Effects, Facilitators, and Barriers of Research Coproduction Reported in Peer-Reviewed Literature

Katheryn M. Sibley, Femke Hoekstra, Anita Kothari, and Kelly Mrklas

Key Learning Points

- Research coproduction reporting and evaluation design practices should be strengthened.
- Many types of effects have been identified, although the strategies or mechanisms to produce them are not clear.
- Many facilitators and barriers are also effects of coproduction, suggesting a need for further study to identify a causal pathway.
- Outcomes and impacts are not well defined in coproduction research.

Research Coproduction in Healthcare, First Edition. Edited by
Ian D. Graham, Jo Rycroft-Malone, Anita Kothari, and Chris McCutcheon.
© 2022 John Wiley & Sons Ltd. Published 2022 by John Wiley & Sons Ltd.

INTRODUCTION

Previous chapters have explored what research coproduction in healthcare is, relevant theories and theorizing about research coproduction. This chapter provides an overview of the effects of, and facilitators and barriers to, coproduction as reported in peer-reviewed academic literature. While acknowledging that there are many ways to gain insight about research coproduction, peer-reviewed literature is an important source of evidence because the review process provides a measure of quality that ensures a minimum standard. Understanding the effects of research coproduction is important for building knowledge about how research coproduction works, making the decisions easier to engage in coproduction, planning a coproduction approach, and its evaluation. Understanding facilitators and barriers to research coproduction – what helps or hinders it – is critical for optimizing coproduction.

What Are Effects? What Are Facilitators and Barriers?

While there is no universally accepted definition of effects of coproduction, they have been described as intended and/or unintended changes due directly or indirectly to an intervention (Belcher and Palenberg 2018) (i.e., the coproduction strategy). Short- or medium-term effects are often referred to as "outcomes," which are measured or assessed as a component of a study (Hoekstra et al. 2018). Impacts are often considered long-term or secondary effects with "an identifiable benefit to, or positive influence on, the economy, society, public services, health, the environment, quality of life, or academia" (Higher Education Funding Council for England 2014). Outcomes and impacts are not well-differentiated in published literature on research partnerships, suggesting that these terms may be used interchangeably (Hoekstra et al. 2020). For this reason, in this chapter we use the term "effects" to cover both and do not distinguish between the two.

Facilitators and barriers can be considered factors that influence research coproduction. In this chapter we define facilitators as single or multilevel factors that are positively associated with, or enhance, research coproduction effects (Hoekstra et al. 2018). We define barriers as single or multilevel factors that are negatively associated with, or hinder, the effects of research coproduction (Hoekstra et al. 2018).

Understanding Research Coproduction – an Evolving Area of Study

Explicit studies exploring and evaluating research coproduction in healthcare have grown steadily over time, particularly in the early decades of the twenty-first century (Gagliardi et al. 2016; Mitton et al. 2007). The nature of these publications has evolved and expanded as coproduction paradigms mature. For example, integrated knowledge translation emerged from the broader field of knowledge translation and implementation science, and patient and public involvement in research has grown with mandated and expanded acceptance. However, three limitations of coproduction evidence persist: many publications on coproduction are based on case study descriptions of partnerships in individual projects or research networks; much of the synthesized partnership evidence to date is "sliced" into discrete foci on specific knowledge user groups, paradigms, or approaches; and, a lack of evaluation remains prominent.

Numerous examples illustrate both the shifts and consistencies in coproduction research. Mitton et al.'s (2007) review of studies published between 1997 and 2005 included both knowledge transfer and exchange literature in a reflection of the developing field of integrated knowledge translation (Mitton et al. 2007). The majority of papers included in that review were opinion pieces, reviews, or surveys of knowledge user perspectives, and just 20% of articles reported on the application of a knowledge transfer or exchange strategy. The few large cross-sectional studies of research coproduction are based on data that is more than a decade old (Sibbald et al. 2019). Sibbald et al. (2019) reported the results of their survey conducted in 2010 with 216 researchers and knowledge users who received Canadian funding for coproduction research projects between 2005 and 2009. Most syntheses of coproduction are restricted to one type of knowledge user. For example, the Gagliardi et al. (2016) review focused solely on policy makers and administrators. Camden et al. (2015) included all types of research users in their analysis but restricted their scope to rehabilitation research. Many systematic analyses of patient and public involvement in research do not include other users (e.g., Camden et al. 2015; Domecq et al. 2014). With regards to challenges with evaluation, Kislov et al. (2018) systematically reviewed published evaluations of funded Collaborations for Leadership in Applied Health Research and Care (CLAHRCs) in the United Kingdom and determined that much of the focus was on organizational arrangements and processes, with minimal evaluation exploring evidence of impact (Kislov et al. 2018). These issues persist in newer studies as well. A 2019 scoping review of integrated knowledge translation studies published between 2005 and 2017, which involved public health policy makers, reported that only one of the 20 included studies evaluated the coproduction process and only one examined knowledge use (Lawrence et al. 2019).

Identifying Effects, Facilitators, and Barriers – Our Approach

We used a rapid review approach (Khangura et al. 2012) to identify the effects, facilitators, and barriers to research coproduction, relying on published or ongoing evidence syntheses of research partnerships. Rapid reviews are based on rigorous systematic review methodologies but simplify or restrict the scope of a review to produce information in a timely manner (Tricco et al. 2015). In our review we included a review of reviews published in 2020 (Hoekstra et al. 2020) as well as eight systematic or scoping reviews of health research partnerships published between 2016 and 2020 that were general in focus and not confined to a specific population or sub-area of research identified from an established search strategy (Bird et al. 2020; Brush et al. 2020; Bush et al. 2017; Drahota et al. 2016; Gagliardi et al. 2016; Lawrence et al. 2019; Tricco et al. 2018; Vat et al. 2020) (Table 2.3.1). These were supplemented with incoming information from two ongoing reviews conducted by chapter co-authors (Kothari, work in preparation; Mrklas, work in preparation). We identified all effects, facilitators, and barriers reported in each review, then organized the information into categories over multiple rounds of team discussion. Methodological details are available on the Open Science Framework (OSF) (Sibley et al. 2021).

EFFECTS OF RESEARCH COPRODUCTION

Many positive and negative effects of research coproduction have been reported. We grouped these effects into seven broad categories: effects on the research process, on relationships among those involved in coproduction, on the individuals involved in coproduction, on the results or output of research, on practices and programs, on communities, and effects on policies and systems (Table 2.3.2).

Effects on the Research Process

There are a number of documented effects of research coproduction relating to the conduct of research. Research coproduction can influence decision-making in the research process, such as setting priorities for the overall direction of research (Gagliardi et al. 2016; Hoekstra et al. 2020; Lawrence et al. 2019), establishing research questions, selecting methods (such as recruitment and data collection approaches), choosing interventions, and determining study outcomes (Bird et al. 2020; Vat et al. 2020). Research coproduction can also affect the feasibility (Lawrence et al. 2019), efficiency, and/or quality of conducting research. For example, it can help improve enrolment and retention of participants (Bird et al. 2020; Vat et al. 2020). It can also facilitate the development of inclusive, accessible, and appropriate study procedures (Vat et al. 2020), improve protocol adherence, assessment quality, and speed of study completion (Vat et al. 2020). Partnerships can also facilitate the ability to develop funding applications (Bird et al. 2020) and in some cases improve the fundability of research proposals (Vat et al. 2020). In turn, these effects can influence the number of collaborative projects undertaken (Gagliardi et al. 2016) and have an effect on subsequent stages of research (Bird et al. 2020).

TABLE 2.3.1 Characteristics of the included reviews.

Reference	Title	Type of review	Partnership approach	Knowledge user type	# of included papers	Date range	Indicators reported
Hoekstra et al. 2020	A review of reviews on principles, strategies, outcomes and impacts of research partnerships approaches: a first step in synthesizing the research partnership literature	Review of reviews	Research partnership	All types	86 reviews	Inception – Apr 2018	Effects
Brush et al. 2020	Success in Long-Standing Community-Based Participatory Research (CBPR) Partnerships: A Scoping Literature Review	Scoping review	CBPR	Not specified	26 studies	2007–2017	Effects Facilitators and barriers

Reference	Title	Type of review	Partnership approach	Knowledge user type	# of included papers	Date range	Indicators reported
Bird et al. 2020	Preparing for patient partnership: A scoping review of patient partner engagement and evaluation in research	Scoping review	Patient engagement	Patients, family members and caregivers	14 studies	Inception – Oct 2019	Effects Facilitators and barriers
Vat et al. 2020	Evaluating the "return on patient engagement initiatives" in medicines research and development: A literature review	Scoping review	Patient engagement	Patients, patient advocates, patient representatives and/ or caregivers	91 studies	Inception – Jul 2018	Effects
Lawrence et al. 2019	Integrated Knowledge Translation with Public Health Policy Makers: A Scoping Review	Scoping review	Integrated KT	Public health policy makers	20 studies	2005–2017	Effects Facilitators and barriers

(Continued)

TABLE 2.3.1 (Continued)

Reference	Title	Type of review	Partnership approach	Knowledge user type	# of included papers	Date range	Indicators reported
Tricco et al. 2018	Engaging policy makers, health system managers, and policy analysts in the knowledge synthesis process: a scoping review	Scoping review	Knowledge user engagement	Policy makers, health system managers, policy analysts	91 studies	1996 – Aug 2016	Effects Facilitators and barriers
Bush et al. 2017	Organizational participatory research: a systematic mixed studies review exposing its extra benefits and the key factors associated with them	Systematic review	Participatory research	Health organization members	107 studies	Inception – Nov 2012	Effects Facilitators and barriers

Reference	Title	Type of review	Partnership approach	Knowledge user type	# of included papers	Date range	Indicators reported
Drahota et al. 2016	Community-Academic Partnerships: A Systematic Review of the State of the Literature and Recommendations for Future Research	Systematic review	Community-academic partnership	Community stakeholders	50 studies	Inception – May 2015	Effects Facilitators and barriers
Gagliardi et al. 2016	Integrated knowledge translation (IKT) in healthcare: a scoping review	Scoping review	Integrated KT	Organizational or policy-level decision-makers	13 studies	2005–2014	Effects Facilitators and barriers

Abbreviations: CBPR = community-based partnership research; KT = knowledge translation

TABLE 2.3.2   Summary of reported effects of research coproduction (full list reported at OSF (Sibley et al. 2021)).

Category	Positive effects	Negative effects
Research Process	Setting priorities for research Establishing research questions Determining research methods Developing interventions Choosing research outcomes Improved participant enrollment & retention Inclusive accessible and appropriate study procedures Improved protocol adherence, assessment quality Faster study completion Facilitating funding applications & fundability	
Relationships	Strengthened relationships Trust Communication Synergy Power sharing Mutual understanding Continued willingness to partner Sustainable partnership infrastructure	Conflict Feelings of frustration, dissatisfaction, lack of respect Temporary partnerships
Individuals	Knowledge users: Personal growth in knowledge & skills Empowerment & confidence Continued involvement in partnerships Compensation Researchers: Increased knowledge, capacity, skills Motivation Additional academic work	Feelings of overburden Feelings of frustration, dissatisfaction, lack of respect Discomfort Additional time and financial commitments
Research results or outputs	Enhanced relevance of results Tangible research products	Little or no research being produced Biased data Tokenism

Category	Positive effects	Negative effects
Practices/ programs	Influences on service delivery Influences on practice recommendations	
Communities	Clear, concrete, sustainable community benefits Changed community context Improved community care Emergence of community leaders Community empowerment Community acceptance and trust in research	Time burden Financial burden Stigmatization of groups Negative findings
Policies/ Systems	System or policy change Improved services and health outcomes More appropriate resource allocation Uptake of evidence by regulators	Research produced not used in policy-making

Effects on Relationships

Coproduction has effects on relationships between those involved in coproduction (typically academic researchers and knowledge users as individuals or as organizations). These effects are primarily related to the establishment or maintenance of ongoing interactions. Many reported effects are positive and generally relate to strengthened relationships (Brush et al. 2020; Gagliardi et al. 2016). Specific positive effects include trust (Gagliardi et al. 2016), communication (Bush et al. 2017), synergy (Drahota et al. 2016; Gagliardi et al. 2016; Hoekstra et al. 2020), power sharing (Brush et al. 2020), and mutual understanding (Gagliardi et al. 2016; Hoekstra et al. 2020; Lawrence et al. 2019). Other positive relationship effects include continued willingness (Brush et al. 2020; Lawrence et al. 2019) to partner and a sustainable infrastructure (Drahota et al. 2016) for partnership. Negative relationship effects have also been reported, including conflict (Hoekstra et al. 2020), feelings of frustration, dissatisfaction, not being listened to or respected (Hoekstra et al. 2020), as well as a failure to overcome differences resulting in temporary partnerships (Gagliardi et al. 2016).

Effects on Individuals

Research partnerships have many effects on the individuals involved (both researchers and knowledge users) at a personal level. Knowledge users can experience personal growth in terms of knowledge, skills (Bird et al. 2020;

Bush et al. 2017; Hoekstra et al. 2020), empowerment (Bird et al. 2020; Bush et al. 2017), and confidence (Bird et al. 2020; Bush et al. 2017; Hoekstra et al. 2020). Knowledge users may also continue to stay involved in research and engage in additional research partnerships (Bird et al. 2020), which can contribute to them experiencing increasingly positive perceptions of the value of research (Gagliardi et al. 2016), as well as the practical benefits of earning money (Bird et al. 2020). However, knowledge users can also feel overburdened by tasks and responsibilities (Hoekstra et al. 2020) and not respected or empowered, which can lead to frustration and/or dissatisfaction with the research process (Hoekstra et al. 2020).

Researchers can experience increased capacity, knowledge, and skills for working in partnership, as well as the area of study (Hoekstra et al. 2020), increased motivation (Hoekstra et al. 2020), and in some cases may go on to pursue additional research or academic work as a result of a partnership (Bird et al. 2020). Negative effects experienced by some researchers include discomfort about power sharing and the pressures associated with additional time and financial commitments required by a partnership approach (Hoekstra et al. 2020).

Effects on Research Results or Outputs

To date, relatively few effects of research partnerships on research findings generated through research coproduction have been identified. The most commonly reported effect on research results is an enhanced authenticity or relevance of the findings (Bird et al. 2020; Gagliardi et al. 2016; Hoekstra et al. 2020; Lawrence et al. 2019; Vat et al. 2020). Others have described the production of tangible research products as a result of research partnerships (Drahota et al. 2016). Negative effects on research partnerships include poor or failed partnerships that produce little to no research (Gagliardi et al. 2016), biased data (Hoekstra et al. 2020), and tokenism (Hoekstra et al. 2020).

Effects on Practices or Programs

Few effects on practices or programs have been identified, but can include influencing service delivery (Gagliardi et al. 2016) and incorporating patient partner concerns into practice recommendations (Bird et al. 2020).

Effects on Communities

A community is defined here as "a group of people with diverse characteristics who are linked by social ties, share common perspectives, and engage in joint action in geographical locations or settings" (MacQueen et al. 2001) and can be affected by research partnerships. General effects include clear, concrete, sustainable community benefits (Brush et al. 2020) and changed community context (Drahota et al. 2016). Specific beneficial effects include improved community care (Lawrence et al. 2019), the emergence of community leaders (Gagliardi et al. 2016), community empowerment and ownership of research (Hoekstra et al. 2020) as well as community acceptance and trust in research (Hoekstra et al. 2020). Conversely, time and financial burdens, further stigmatization of groups, as well as negative research findings (Hoekstra et al. 2020) can negatively impact communities.

Effects on Policies and Systems

System or policy change (Bush et al. 2017; Gagliardi et al. 2016), sometimes beyond the initial target setting or intended time frame (Bush et al. 2017), is an important policy and system effect. Other benefits include improved community services and health outcomes (Hoekstra et al. 2020), more appropriate resource allocation (Vat et al. 2020), and uptake of evidence by regulators (Vat et al. 2020). It is also important to note that one review reported the research produced in partnerships has not been used in policy-making (Gagliardi et al. 2016).

FACILITATORS AND BARRIERS TO RESEARCH COPRODUCTION

We identified many facilitators and barriers to research partnerships, which we placed in four primary groups: individual-level factors, relationship factors, process factors, and system factors (Table 2.3.3).

TABLE 2.3.3 A summary of the reported facilitators and barriers to research coproduction (full list available at OSF (Sibley et al. 2021)).

Category	Facilitator	Barrier
Individual level	Commitment Willingness to share power, risk, accountability, responsibility Able to make decisions Having research skills and topic expertise	Lack of skill Lack of understanding about partnership processes Negative attitudes about researchers or research Life challenges related to living situation, trauma, poverty Aspects of research may be upsetting

(Continued)

TABLE 2.3.3   (Continued)

Category	Facilitator	Barrier
Relationships	Trust Mutual respect Openness Transparency Established relationship Shared goals and values Cultural diversity Differing values Attention to power imbalance Effective conflict resolution	Persisting power imbalances Lack of shared mission and goals
Process	Establishing clear expectations and goals Formal structures to support processes Providing background information Developing shared governance structures Regular evaluations Dedicated funds and resources Compensating partners Hiring dedicated staff Flexible and tailored approaches Space, equipment, technology	Time requirements
System level		Readiness of health system for applying findings Frequent turnover of policy makers and managers

Individual-Level Factors

The personal characteristics of the individuals involved in research partnership play a key role in the outcomes of research coproduction. Facilitating factors of coproduction include involving those who have an appropriate role relative to the project (Brush et al. 2020); commitment; willingness to share power, risk, accountability, and responsibility (Brush et al. 2020); and those who by role and/ or through organizational support are able to make meaningful decisions (Brush et al. 2020; Gagliardi et al. 2016). Among knowledge users, research skills and topic expertise facilitate partnership (Tricco et al. 2018). Conversely, lack of skill and understanding of the process of research partnerships can be a barrier to individuals (Gagliardi et al. 2016). Certainly, individuals' negative attitudes to researchers or the value of research (Gagliardi et al. 2016), or an unwillingness to get involved (Tricco et al. 2018), are also identified barriers. It is important to recognize the realities of life challenges that patients or community partners may experience that can serve as barriers to engaging in research partnerships, such as health issues, living situations, poverty, trauma (Bird et al. 2020), and subsequently, that aspects of the research process may be upsetting to partners (Bird et al. 2020).

Relationship Factors

The nature of the relationship among partners can serve as facilitators or as barriers to research coproduction (Bird et al. 2020; Drahota et al. 2016; Lawrence et al. 2019; Tricco et al. 2018). For example, trust (Bird et al. 2020; Brush et al. 2020; Lawrence et al. 2019), mutual respect (Brush et al. 2020; Drahota et al. 2016), openness (Brush et al. 2020; Gagliardi et al. 2016), and transparency (Brush et al. 2020) are all documented facilitators of partnership relationships, while their absence are known barriers (Drahota et al. 2016). An established relationship can be a facilitator (Bird et al. 2020; Gagliardi et al. 2016; Lawrence et al. 2019). While shared goals and values are known facilitators (Drahota et al. 2016; Gagliardi et al. 2016; Lawrence et al. 2019), effective partnerships do not all necessarily need to be homogenous, as cultural diversity (Brush et al. 2020) and even differing values (Tricco et al. 2018) can be facilitators in some situations. It is important to recognize, though, that a lack of shared mission and goals (Drahota et al. 2016) can be a barrier in some partnerships. In this regard, attention to power imbalances (Brush et al. 2020) and effective conflict resolution (Brush et al. 2020; Drahota et al. 2016) are important facilitators to prevent the negative influence of a persistent power imbalance (Bird et al. 2020).

Process Factors

Most facilitators and barriers we identified are related to processes associated with managing and operating research partnerships – both early on in the establishment or development of the partnership, and in an ongoing manner throughout the partnership. Facilitators early in the partnership process include the establishment of clear expectations and roles for partners (Bird et al. 2020; Brush et al. 2020; Drahota et al. 2016; Lawrence et al. 2019; Tricco et al. 2018), formal structures to support processes (Bird et al. 2020; Brush et al. 2020; Gagliardi et al. 2016) – such as providing background information in writing or through a workshop (Bird et al. 2020; Lawrence et al. 2019) or development of shared governance structures (Bird et al. 2020; Gagliardi et al. 2016). In this regard, regular evaluations can also serve as facilitators (Brush et al. 2020; Gagliardi et al. 2016). Practically speaking, dedicated funding and resources, typically through direct compensation to community and patient partners (Bird et al. 2020; Brush et al. 2020; Lawrence et al. 2019), are important facilitators. Among public, community, and patient partners, flexible and tailored approaches are important facilitators (Bird et al. 2020; Brush et al. 2020). Other facilitators include dedicated staff (Bird et al. 2020; Lawrence et al. 2019) and access to resources, such as space, equipment, or technology to support the work and conduct of the partnership (Bird et al. 2020; Lawrence et al. 2019). Given the importance of resources as a facilitator, their absence is an unsurprising barrier (Bird et al. 2020; Tricco et al. 2018). Lastly, it is important to acknowledge that the time requirements associated with partnerships (Bird et al. 2020; Lawrence et al. 2019) can be a barrier for some.

System-Level Factors

System-level factors have been consistently identified as barriers to partnership. These relate to readiness of the health system for research findings (Bird et al. 2020) and frequent turnover of policy makers and managers that affect partnership continuity (Bird et al. 2020; Gagliardi et al. 2016).

CONNECTING OUTCOMES, IMPACTS, FACILITATORS, AND BARRIERS TO RESEARCH COPRODUCTION

It is noteworthy that several categories of facilitators and barriers (individual-level factors, relationship factors, and process factors) are also reported effects of coproduction (Figure 2.3.1). While additional study is warranted, we propose as a working hypothesis that these overlapping facilitators, barriers, and effects may represent mediating factors or mechanisms that could influence the direct effects (outcomes) of coproduction (the research results) and, in turn, more distal effects (outcomes and impacts, practice change, community effects, and policy and systems effects). Although at this point we can only reflect on the potential significance of this overlap, additional study could help identify a causal pathway for more directly influencing beneficial outcomes and impacts of research partnerships. We also note that system factors may be overarching contextual influences on a potential research partnership pathway, but on the other hand, may also be considered external or secondary if they are not within the direct control of a partnership.

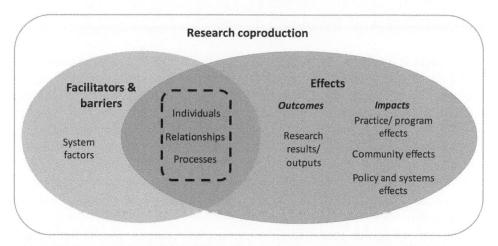

FIGURE 2.3.1   Interacting facilitators, barriers, and effects in research coproduction.

IMPLICATIONS FOR THE PRACTICE OF RESEARCH COPRODUCTION

Synthesizing the reported effects, facilitators, and barriers to research coproduction in healthcare can help inform the practice of research coproduction by highlighting potential key ingredients which can optimize the strategies used in coproduction and enhance positive effects. For example, the characteristics of individuals identified as both facilitators and barriers to research coproduction can be considered when identifying potential team members for a partnership. Strategies can also be undertaken to foster productive relationships, such as building trust and mutual respect, as well as identifying shared values or goals around which to build partnerships and coproduce research. For example, in 2005, Bowen et al. discussed using both formal and informal strategies for building mutual trust, such as shared decision-making in selecting research deliverables and team dinners (Bowen et al. 2005). Process factors may be particularly actionable for the practice of research coproduction. For example, verbal or written discussions about expectations can clarify roles and responsibilities, describing protocols and processes in writing can help to establish formal structures, and written forms or workshops can facilitate processes. The importance of dedicated funds is clear: coproduction teams need them to establish and nurture relationships. Depending on funding regulations, there may be the opportunity to allocate coproduction funds to existing research grants, as well as emerging funding opportunities which are dedicated to engagement costs.

LIMITATIONS AND EVIDENCE GAPS

While there is a growing body of work on research coproduction in healthcare and the synthesis presented here provides useful insights, it is also important to recognize its limitations. We recognize that others may have grouped effects, facilitators, and barriers into different categories, and that there may be some overlap. For example, we coded tokenism as a negative effect on research outputs as it was reported in reviews in this way, but we also recognize that tokenism could be experienced by individuals and affect relationships. We also recognize that some system factors may be intractable with other types of factor – such as the frequent turnover of health system staff, which would necessarily affect relationships.

We also recognize that, like all syntheses, our summary is limited by the existing evidence on effects, facilitators, and barriers to research coproduction. First, the literature only tells us about projects reported in the peer-reviewed space, not about coproduced research projects that were absent from the literature. From our own experience, as authors and participants in unreported coproduction, the peer-reviewed literature on coproduction may just represent the proverbial "tip of the iceberg." Second, despite reporting best practice guidance for some types of coproduced research (Staniszewska et al. 2017), there is considerable variation in what is published on research coproduction in peer-reviewed literature. This affects our ability to collect and synthesize data and draw conclusions. For example, in Gagliardi et al.'s (2016) review included in this chapter, only five of the 13 included studies reported the duration and/or frequency of engagement activities, and few reported exactly how knowledge users were involved or any indicators of interim or long-term impact (Gagliardi et al. 2016). As such, the review was unable to identify characteristics that lead to beneficial outcomes. Several authors have noted the challenges associated with the overall lack of evaluation and reporting (Kislov et al. 2018) (both quantity and quality), and the majority of reported effects in this chapter pertain to proximal process outcomes, rather than more distal outcomes and impacts.

FUTURE RESEARCH

While our chapter discusses the effects of research coproduction reported in the literature, we cannot draw reliable conclusions about the frequency with which these effects occur or the specific contexts, approaches, or strategies that produce them. Furthermore, we are still unable to describe or explain how coproduction actually happens, or the social processes involved and their impacts. Realistic evaluations, which seek to answer "What works for whom, in what circumstances, and why?" (Pawson 2013), may contribute to unpacking the "black box" of coproduction. More consistent reporting will facilitate exploration of the comparative effectiveness of different coproduction strategies in future evidence syntheses on research coproduction. Large-scale primary data comparisons of coproduced research are also needed to expand generalized understanding beyond case study reports and/or specific programs. Additional study is needed to understand the specific outcomes, impacts, facilitators, and barriers to research coproduction in low- and middle-income countries. Although this review has focused on general reviews of research partnerships, none of them reported country-level characteristics, and Hoekstra's et al.'s (2020) review of 86 reviews did not identify any which focused on coproduction in low- and middle-income countries. Analysis of partnership approaches employed in global health contexts is warranted (Hoekstra et al. 2020).

CONCLUSION

Existing evidence on coproduced research in healthcare shows many potential outcomes and impacts, along with the factors that can influence their attainment. Advances in reporting standards, as well as more consistent evaluation practices, will facilitate continued study of research partnerships and a more nuanced understanding of the conditions and actions that lead to optimal, more relevant, useful, and used research findings in healthcare.

REFERENCES

1. Belcher, B. and Palenberg, M. (2018). Outcomes and impacts of development interventions: toward conceptual clarity. *American Journal of Evaluation* 39: 478–495. doi: 10.1177/1098214018765698.

2. Bird, M., Ouellette, C., Whitmore, C., Li, L., Nair, K., McGillion, M.H., Yost, J., Banfield, L., Campbell, E., and Carroll, S.L. (2020). Preparing for patient partnership: a scoping review of patient partner engagement and evaluation in research. *Health Expectations* 23: 523–539. doi: 10.1111/hex.13040.

3. Bowen, S., Martens, P., and Need to Know Team. (2005). Demystifying knowledge translation: learning from the community. *Journal of Health Services Research and Policy* 10: 203–211. doi: 10.1258/135581905774414213.

4. Brush, B.L., Mentz, G., Jensen, M., Jacobs, B., Saylor, K.M., Rowe, Z., Israel, B.A., and Lachance, L. (2020). Success in long-standing community-based participatory research (CBPR) partnerships: a scoping literature review. *Health Education & Behavior: The Official Publication of the Society for Public Health Education* 47: 556–568. doi: 10.1177/1090198119882989.

5. Bush, P.L., Pluye, P., Loignon, C., Granikov, V., Wright, M.T., Pelletier, J.F., Bartlett-Esquilant, G., Macaulay, A.C., Haggerty, J., Parry, S., and Repchinsky,

C. (2017). Organizational participatory research: a systematic mixed studies review exposing its extra benefits and the key factors associated with them. *Implementation Science: IS* 12: 119. doi: 10.1186/s13012-017-0648-y.

6. Camden, C., Shikako-Thomas, K., Nguyen, T., Graham, E., Thomas, A., Sprung, J., Morris, C., and Russell, D.J. (2015). Engaging stakeholders in rehabilitation research: a scoping review of strategies used in partnerships and evaluation of impacts. *Disability and Rehabilitation* 37: 1390–1400. doi: 10.3109/09638288.2014.963705.

7. Domecq, J.P., Prutsky, G., Elraiyah, T., Wang, Z., Nabhan, M., Shippee, N., Brito, J.P., Boehmer, K., Hasan, R., Firwana, B., Erwin, P., Eton, D., Sloan, J., Montori, V., Asi, N., Dabrh, A.M., and Murad, M.H. (2014). Patient engagement in research: a systematic review. *BMC Health Services Research* 14: 89. doi: 10.1186/1472-6963-14-89.

8. Drahota, A., Meza, R.D., Brikho, B., Naaf, M., Estabillo, J.A., Gomez, E.D., Vejnoska, S.F., Dufek, S., Stahmer, A.C., and Aarons, G.A. (2016). Community-academic partnerships: a systematic review of the state of the literature and recommendations for future research. *The Milbank Quarterly* 94: 163–214. doi: 10.1111/1468-0009.12184.

9. Gagliardi, A.R., Berta, W., Kothari, A., Boyko, J., and Urquhart, R. (2016). Integrated knowledge translation (IKT) in healthcare: a scoping review. *Implementation Science: IS* 11: 38. doi: 10.1186/s13012-016-0399-1.

10. Higher Education Funding Council for England. (2014). Research Excellence Framework: Assessment Framework and Guidance on Submissions. https://www.ref.ac.uk/2014/pubs/2011-02 (accessed 11 January 2022).

11. Hoekstra, F., Mrklas, K.J., Khan, M., McKay, R.C., Vis-Dunbar, M., Sibley, K.M., Nguyen, T., Graham, I.D., Panel, S.C.I.G.P.C., and Gainforth, H.L. (2020). A review of reviews on principles, strategies, outcomes and impacts of research partnerships approaches: a first step in synthesising the research partnership literature. *Health Research Policy and Systems / BioMed Central* 18: 51. doi: 10.1186/s12961-020-0544-9.

12. Hoekstra, F., Mrklas, K.J., Sibley, K.M., Nguyen, T., Vis-Dunbar, M., Neilson, C.J., Crockett, L.K., Gainforth, H.L., and Graham, I.D. (2018). A review protocol on research partnerships: a Coordinated Multicenter Team approach. *Systematic Reviews* 7: 217. doi: 10.1186/s13643-018-0879-2.

13. Khangura, S., Konnyu, K., Cushman, R., Grimshaw, J., and Moher, D. (2012). Evidence summaries: the evolution of a rapid review approach. *Systematic Reviews* 1: 10. doi: 10.1186/2046-4053-1-10.

14. Kislov, R., Wilson, P.M., Knowles, S., and Boaden, R. (2018). Learning from the emergence of NIHR Collaborations for Leadership in Applied Health Research and Care (CLAHRCs): a systematic review of evaluations. *Implementation Science: IS* 13: 111. doi: 10.1186/s13012-018-0805-y.

15. Lawrence, L.M., Bishop, A., and Curran, J. (2019). Integrated knowledge translation with public health policy makers: a scoping review. *Healthcare Policy = Politiques de Santé* 14: 55–77. doi: 10.12927/hcpol.2019.25792.

16. MacQueen, K.M., McLellan, E., Metzger, D.S., Kegeles, S., Strauss, R.P., Scotti, R., Blanchard, L., and Trotter, R.T., 2nd (2001). What is community? An evidence-based definition for participatory public health. *American Journal of Public Health* 91: 1929–1938. doi: 10.2105/ajph.91.12.1929.

17. Mitton, C., Adair, C.E., McKenzie, E., Patten, S.B., and Waye Perry, B. (2007). Knowledge transfer and exchange: review and synthesis of the literature. *The Milbank Quarterly* 85: 729–768. doi: 10.1111/j.1468-0009.2007.00506.x.

18. Pawson, R. (2013). *The Science of Evaluation: A Realist Manifesto*. London: SAGE Publications Ltd.

19. Sibbald, S.L., Kang, H., and Graham, I.D. (2019). Collaborative health research partnerships: a survey of researcher and knowledge-user attitudes and perceptions. *Health Research Policy and Systems/BioMed Central* 17: 92. doi: 10.1186/s12961-019-0485-3.

20. Sibley, K.M., Hoekstra, F., Mrklas, K.J., and Kothari, A. (2021). Effects, facilitators, and barriers of research co-production reported in peer-reviewed literature. [Supplementary files]. https://osf.io/z9tc5/?view_only=2bdab3da99eb4fcfa602b1536eb0ed26 (accessed 11 January 2022).

21. Staniszewska, S., Brett, J., Simera, I., Seers, K., Mockford, C., Goodlad, S., Altman, D.G., Moher, D., Barber, R., Denegri, S., Entwistle, A., Littlejohns, P., Morris, C., Suleman, R., Thomas, V., and Tysall, C. (2017). GRIPP2 reporting checklists: tools to improve reporting of patient and public involvement in research. *BMJ* 358: j3453. doi: 10.1136/bmj.j3453.

22. Tricco, A.C., Antony, J., Zarin, W., Strifler, L., Ghassemi, M., Ivory, J., Perrier, L., Hutton, B., Moher, D., and Straus, S.E. (2015). A scoping review of rapid review methods. *BMC Medicine* 13: 224. doi: 10.1186/s12916-015-0465-6.

23. Tricco, A.C., Zarin, W., Rios, P., Nincic, V., Khan, P.A., Ghassemi, M., Diaz, S., Pham, B., Straus, S.E., and Langlois, E.V. (2018). Engaging policy-makers, health system managers, and policy analysts in the knowledge synthesis process: a scoping review. *Implementation Science: IS* 13: 31. doi: 10.1186/s13012-018-0717-x.

24. Vat, L.E., Finlay, T., Jan Schuitmaker-Warnaar, T., Fahy, N., Robinson, P., Boudes, M., Diaz, A., Ferrer, E., Hivert, V., Purman, G., Kurzinger, M.L., Kroes, R.A., Hey, C., and Broerse, J.E.W. (2020). Evaluating the "return on patient engagement initiatives" in medicines research and development: a literature review. *Health Expectations* 23: 5–18. doi: 10.1111/hex.12951.

Working with Knowledge Users

3.1 Working with Knowledge Users

Jo Cooke, Susan Mawson, and Susan Hampshaw

Key Learning Points

- Focus on relationship "work" and build in time to do this. Coproduction moves by small steps and iterations and takes time to happen. Relationship activity includes identifying joint priorities and appropriate coproduction methodologies; and developing a shared vision of the project/program to ensure mutual benefit. Be prepared to be nimble, honest, and reciprocal. Listen throughout the process, and act on what you say you will do.

- Plan to develop research capacity to sustain coproduction in the research and knowledge-user workforce. Develop boundary spanning skills in both researchers and knowledge users. This is best achieved through experiential learning.

- Focus on impact from the start. Where possible plan to develop actionable outputs that are coproduced using local embedded knowledge, and include a budget to develop these.

Research Coproduction in Healthcare, First Edition. Edited by
Ian D. Graham, Jo Rycroft-Malone, Anita Kothari, and Chris McCutcheon.
© 2022 John Wiley & Sons Ltd. Published 2022 by John Wiley & Sons Ltd.

- You may need to think of developing formal agreements, particularly when working with industry partners, and confirm intellectual property (IP) issues where appropriate at the beginning of the project.

INTRODUCTION: STARTING THE COPRODUCTION JOURNEY

This chapter sets out advice on how to get started in the coproduction journey. It is drawn from our experiences working within a CLAHRC (Collaboration and Leadership in Applied Health and Care) partnership program as both researchers and knowledge users. CLAHRCs were funded in the UK by the National Institute for Health Research (NIHR) to address the research practice gap through developing collaborations between academia and knowledge users across the health and care system. Knowledge users came from a variety of contexts including primary and secondary healthcare, local government, and industry. The CLAHRC partnership architecture was planned to enable coproduction where appropriate. Our "getting started" advice is distilled from this experience and draws upon recent literature.

WHAT IS THE FOCUS OF THIS CHAPTER?

This chapter focusses on how to plan coproduction at two levels: research program and research project. Firstly, we describe how to set up a large collaboration that, we hope, offers insight into other research programs in terms of engendering a supportive environment for coproduction. We then provide two vignettes which describe project work underpinned by coproduction with different knowledge users: one based in local government, working with a design team; and the second describes an international collaboration between healthcare partners, CLAHRC academics, and a medical-tech company. Although different, some common themes can be drawn out to help plan the coproduction journey; these were distilled into the key points at the beginning of this chapter.

SOME POINTS FROM THE LITERATURE

First of all, consider whether coproduction is the right approach. This question can be answered by exploring and recognizing partners' motivation, agreeing expectations, and setting mutually beneficial agendas with an eye to impact from the outset (Boaz et al. 2018). This includes the importance of focusing on the right topic and acceptable methodologies by setting priorities (Cooke et al.

2015). Knowledge users often have different expectations, experiences, and views on the meaning and usefulness of research, including what constitutes knowledge and research priorities, and how research questions should be answered (Pawson et al. 2003). Policy makers and researchers are considered to be from different cultures (Oliver and Cairney 2019). Lorenc et al. (2014) conducted a systematic review of cultures of evidence use across policy sectors and found that non-health sector policy makers valued evidence that informed their practice and felt that research evidence did not meet their needs. So unearthing knowledge views and assumptions should be part of the initial steps in any new coproduction partnership, which can then inform the development of shared values and objectives (Buick et al. 2016). If this is not done tensions in research partnerships can persist (Oliver et al. 2019). Having such conversations at the beginning of the partnership can establish that all partners agree to a coproduction approach which aligns with their beliefs.

The heart of coproduction is equity, power-sharing, and inclusiveness, which gives all project team members an opportunity to develop and express their knowledge (Langley et al. 2018). This requires that researchers move out of their academic "ivory towers" and become creative about the methods they use (Greenhalgh et al. 2016; Langley et al. 2018). Project plans should include the facilitation of the process, support for relationship building, and democratic governance in order to maximize synergy and impact (Greenhalgh et al. 2016; Jagosh et al. 2015). Time spent on developing relationships can create a partnership that has a ripple effect, creating more value than the sum of parts (Jagosh et al. 2015). But undertaking this approach can produce tension between productivity and inclusion (Boaz et al. 2018). Both the funding bodies and researchers need to feel prepared and able to accept this trade-off to gain these benefits. It takes time. Such flexibility can impede a focus on more "academic" research (Buick et al. 2016). Importantly, project plans need to reflect time scales for relationship work and inclusion activity.

Resource allocation is an important consideration at the start of the coproduction journey. Many authors state that coproduction projects should be adequately resourced (Boaz et al. 2018; Cooke et al. 2015). This does not only mean financial resources. The experience of the CLAHRCs is that matched or "in kind" funding can be very useful in coproduction partnerships, where partners' time on project work is agreed at senior levels in partner organizations. This provides legitimacy of time spent on projects and can ensure some partners adopt roles that cross organizational boundaries (Cooke et al. 2015). It might be useful to support boundary-spanning or "hybrid" roles (Kislov et al. 2018; Rycroft-Malone et al. 2016) within any coproduction partnership. These roles include practitioners working in the academic sector, and researchers embedded in services, usually on a part-time basis. They can include "joint posts" or be developed as a temporary secondment opportunity. These roles should be resourced adequately, including providing support as they can be challenging to enact (Kislov et al. 2018).

Understanding and recognizing the context and motivations of different knowledge users is important to inform the process, but it also ensures impact (Rycroft-Malone et al. 2016). Active conversations at the outset of a partnership can help to recognize contextual drivers, timelines, and organizational demands, priorities, and motivations. These should inform notions of "What is in this for me?" (Rycroft-Malone et al. 2016) and set realistic expectations of what can be achieved (Buick et al. 2016). Such knowledge is also a real asset to coproduction partnerships (Boyle and Harris 2009) as it activates "How to get things done" and "What will work here" in their organizational context. Such knowledge is important in the development of actionable outputs that will be useful and used in practice (Hampshaw et al. 2018; Melville-Richards et al. 2020). Impact is in the hands of knowledge users; as such, they should shape the outputs from the outset.

Many authors recognize the benefits of conducting coproduction in an ongoing and long-term relationship, with a mutual desire to make the partnership work over a long period (Buick et al. 2016). Successful collaborations should provide a physical and cognitive "space" for coproduction (Rycroft-Malone et al. 2016). So, plan protected time to build strong relationships and opportunities for reciprocity that lead to trust and mutual respect (Boyle and Harris 2009). The long-term nature also provides opportunities for "quick wins" that can build on earlier collaborative work to meet mutually beneficial goals (Cooke et al. 2015). This is illustrated by vignette two in this chapter, which builds on a long-term academic relationship and links with service providers, whilst introducing a partner from Industry to conduct a project that was considered to offer mutual benefit to all. The ability to respond quickly can support such win-win projects, and the connectivity of a large research program can provide the right partners.

EXPERIENCE FROM THE FIELD

Research Program Level: Setting up a Program Architecture that Can Enable Coproduction

We planned the CLAHRC infrastructure to enable research coproduction with diverse partners. Strategies included developing time and space for relationship building, flexibility to try new ways of working, and resources to enable this. CLAHRC included knowledge users from the National Health Service (NHS), local government, service users and carers, and industry. A requirement for participating organizations was a commitment to provide "match funding," in addition to the funds awarded to the grant. This matched funding was usually provided "in kind" through stakeholder time on projects and other activities. When working with industry the match was usually in the form of no-fee product use in exchange for impartial evaluation of these products. The

CLAHRC program of work included undertaking applied research projects, implementation or knowledge mobilization projects, and building the capacity to do both. On reflection, having a capacity-building aspect of the program was important in relation to supporting boundary-spanning activity. Table 3.1.1 describes some of these skills identified through the CLAHRC internal evaluation. CLAHRC offered "learning by doing" opportunities for knowledge users and researchers to use and develop these skills and knowledge within different contexts.

TABLE 3.1.1 Types of boundary-spanning skills developed in CLAHRC.

Boundary Skills and knowledge	Examples
• Negotiating skills	• Negotiating match funding • Developing win-win scenarios in project plans • Ensuring "buy-in" across different stakeholder groups • Agreeing on joint priorities
• Understanding culture and context – different ways of working	• Understanding different objectives of each organization • Understanding cultures of different organizations, the drivers and motivators within different contexts • Recognizing and adhering to governance and process issues within and across organizational boundaries
• Communication – translating and interpreting skills	• Learning to understand, speak and use the languages of different sectors • Interpret and use appropriate language to communicate effectively messages from your own sector
• Partnership skills. Networking and making connections	• Developing and strengthening relationships. Understanding how to sustain partnerships across different boundaries • Developing confidence and ability to cope with challenge • Using challenge positively to shape change together
• Skills in planning and developing outputs that can be impactful	• Understanding what is considered impactful in different contexts • Developing outputs that are mindful of impact

Structure, Flexible Resources, and Engagement Processes to Provide Context for Coproduction

We paid attention to collaborative structures in the partnership to provide "space" where coproduction can take place. This included project steering groups, special interest groups, and communities of practice. Such structures enabled ongoing dialogue between researchers and knowledge users. We also provided a flexible use of resources to coproduce actionable outputs. These outputs were the physical embodiment of coproduction: knowledge users could see where they had made a contribution (Cooke et al. 2015). Additional benefits included ownership of such outputs, which made them more likely to be used and provided a visible footprint of impact.

Our CLAHRC included a number of methodological and clinical themes, as well as a core team to deliver the program of work. Some methodological themes focussed on coproduction, and collaboration between themes was encouraged to increase capacity. Other themes had coproduction expertise within them (see vignette one). We adopted a distributed management structure so Theme Leads could act and use a resource allocated to them in a flexible manner. Decisions on how budgets were spent were decided at theme level and derived from priority-setting activity and expressed need from the knowledge users. Funding and matched resources contributed to research, implementation, and capacity building activities. The flexibility to exchange and interplay the resource between these three types of work meant that the immediate needs of clinical practice, delivered through implementation projects, could be balanced by the longer timeframe of research activity and outputs. This helped to address time pressures for action from services and demonstrated reciprocity and building trust.

Setting Ground Rules: A Good Basis for Nurturing Productive Relationships

Paying attention to the quality of the relationships was essential to nurture a productive and resilient collaboration and promote a sense of belonging. Although formal, and sometimes legal, documentation in the form of collaborative agreements and memoranda of understanding (MoUs) were required by the funders and partners from industry, a more important contribution to the relationship included developing a set of "ground rules" – what we called "principles of working together." Our principles were agreed to at an initial "time out" and included: enabling coproduction; supporting partner engagement; addressing inequalities, and building research capacity across the whole collaboration. Coproduction was described as "activity that engages the right people (service users, practitioners, NHS and care managers, and academics from a range of disciplines) to make decisions and support the conduct of projects and activities on issues that are important and matter to them" (Cooke et al. 2015, p. 3). These principles were "hardwired" into theme-reporting frameworks to ascertain progress and provide examples of how they were being put into practice. A three-monthly reporting schedule acted as a reminder of the collaboration's aspirations and provided excellent learning and sharing opportunities. Newcomers to the CLAHRC were introduced to the principles through workshops and induction materials.

Planning Priority-setting, Action, and Impact from the Start and Throughout

Priority-setting was an important aspect of coproduction from the outset. We considered this a marker of authenticity when it led to visible action (Cooke et al. 2017). How priorities were set varied between themes. A large collaboration will have a wide range of skills and abilities to undertake coproduction, and approaches were often influenced by the expertise, research disciplines, and epistemologies within themes. For example, themes that included researchers more familiar with positivist approaches might use a Delphi technique to identify priorities, whereas other themes used design workshops and creative design approaches. Sometimes a funding call would be made, asking service partners to identify projects based on their needs (see vignette one). The CLAHRC included a diverse range of researchers and knowledge users, and we worked on the strengths and assets of each theme and supported their interpretation of coproduction based on these strengths. Other themes demonstrated collaboration but not necessarily coproduction. By this we mean that knowledge users might contribute to steering groups and partnership working to make decisions on what should be researched, but more traditional methods were executed, with little power-sharing in the research process. This reflected the leadership style and expertise of the researchers. But it also reflected whether a coproduction approach could address the research questions being asked.

Thinking of the Impact from the Beginning

Impact matters to all stakeholders and is the reason they get involved. It energizes a collaboration and promotes engagement. On reflection, a number of factors supported impact planning. Firstly, spend time to set up platforms for ongoing dialogue. These can support joint priority-setting, which can help to focus project work where it matters. Secondly, projects should aim to develop actionable outputs that are visible and attributable to the project. Examples are given in the vignettes below but others can be found at (http://clahrc-yh.nihr.

ac.uk/resources/e-repository). They include: the development of decision aids; training packs for knowledge users; and, outcome measures for practice. Funding for such outputs needs to have a budget line. Thirdly, develop impact stories and share these. Investing in good communication methods is important and should be adequately resourced. Finally, plan to develop skills in the research and knowledge user workforces to make coproduction happen in a sustainable and flexible manner (see Table 3.1.1). We have found this is best achieved through experiential learning, combined with reflection through supervision, mentorship, or action learning sets/communities of practice.

VIGNETTE ONE: THE CO-DESIGN OF AN INTERVENTION TO INCREASE PHYSICAL ACTIVITY IN DONCASTER. COPRODUCTION IN LOCAL GOVERNMENT.

The Doncaster Council Public Health team worked with colleagues in the Regeneration and Environment Directorate, and with Doncaster Rovers Football Club (FC) to develop an asset around Doncaster Lakeside. The Lakeside area of Doncaster is a mix of recreation, housing, and shopping built around a man-made lake. Colleagues in environment and recreation were keen to expand its use and foresaw opportunities to develop the area for visitors. The Public Health team wanted to find a way to increase physical activity. The World Health Organization recommends that adults should accumulate at least 150 minutes of moderate aerobic exercise each week, 75 minutes of vigorous activity, or an equivalent combination of the two (World Health Organization 2010). At the time of the project, 55% of Doncaster's residents (60% of females) stated they had done no physical exercise in the previous four weeks. Inactivity was estimated (a conservative estimate at the time) to result in health costs of £5 million. Some stakeholders wanted to use Lakeside for recreational and retail activities, while others favored improving the environment and conserving wildlife.

At the same time as the work in Doncaster was being developed, the User Centre Design Theme within the then CLAHRC was extending its methods to different sectors and advertised for partners to take part in a final case study of an approach called Better Services by Design (BSBD). One of the members of the Doncaster Public Health team (chapter co-author) was also part of the CLAHRC matched funded service partners. Two things encouraged the Doncaster team to apply for a co-design project. First, the application process was straightforward: an expression of interest which simply outlined the area of interest based on need and relevance to the service. Second, due to various knowledge exchange events and seminars – a regular feature of the CLAHRC – the public were aware of the theme and its approach. The BSBD ran workshops to promote their final case study and attendance at these cemented the interest in Doncaster. We have observed throughout the CLAHRC there were easier beginnings when there was some form of existing relationships between organizations and individuals. Events such as research seminars offer opportunities for practitioners and academics to meet and find common ground or at least recognize common interests. Within the workshops to advertise the BSBD project, consideration was given to timescales and permissions/governance to get going in any project. The local service improvement activity was assessed not to require full NHS Ethics approval. Nevertheless, there were still approvals to go through within the council's decision-making structures. It is useful to understand these issues at the beginning of the project and anticipate that this may not be a one-off process. For example, as the project develops, there may be a need to formalize the relationship with a memorandum of understanding or a formal collaboration agreement. This agreement should result from discussions about outputs (and the different products for different audiences), as well as authorship, and are worth signposting at the beginning of the relationship.

This vignette is written from a unique perspective and reflects the experience of a local government officer whose role spans the boundary between academic and public health practice, who was also a participant in this BSBD coproduction case study. Broader reflections on all the projects that were part of the Better Service by Design case study can be found here https://bsbd.org.uk/bsbd. Wolstenholme et al. (2017) identifies that their co-design methods resulted in the teams exhibiting characteristics that supported innovation. They also highlight how the design research team offered both practical and intellectual support throughout the project. The design team was able to create props – for example, such as mocked-up QR code boards linked to a working website – to support a pilot of the Lakeside trail. These resources could not have been created in a timely manner without the coproduction partnership and helped to promote credibility of the lakeside project internally in the later stages of the project. They also helped to debunk the idea that academics might not be able to offer practical solutions to service and policy issues.

This vignette describes the early stages of the project and reflects on what helped at the beginning of the journey. It attempts to isolate the magic ingredients which led to a successful coproduction research project and the installation of the Discover Doncaster trail. The project was underpinned by use of the Design Council's Double Diamond design process which has four phases to guide the coproduction process (Design Council 2004). These are: Discover, Define, Develop, and Deliver (see Figure 3.1.1). We have identified above how the introductory workshops and ease of application and early discussion regarding outputs helped in establishing the coproductive research project. Here we focus on the discovery phase, which involves opening up and questioning and naturally coincides with the beginnings of the coproduction journey.

Each phase in the Double Diamond process either Opens up or Focuses the project. This both directs activity and suggests the types of activity that will get the 'most' out of a particular phase (see example 'walk and talk' at Lakeside as an activity during the Discover phase).

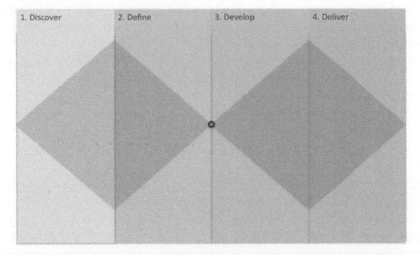

1. Discover   2. Define   3. Develop   4. Deliver

1. Open up and question what it is your improvement/innovation project should focus on. This is the Discover phase, where you might explore and understand service-users' needs, for example;
2. Focus on the important issues to tackle in your project, based on what you've discovered. This is the Define phase, where you define problems and begin to interpret them;
3. Open up again to explore different ways of tackling the problem by designing things. This is the Develop phase, where you design and test potential solutions; and
4. Focus on producing practical, working solutions and implementing them. This is the Deliver phase, where you concentrate on the final specification and production of the service.

Adapted from https://bsbd.org.uk/bsbd/double-diamond-design-process/

FIGURE 3.1.1 The Double Diamond Design Process.

The lakeside project team consisted of Public Health colleagues and colleagues from the CLAHRC research theme. The team of knowledge users from Doncaster Council included a physical activity public health specialist, the public health research lead (and chapter author) and the Assistant Director of Public Health. The project also worked with a broader group of stakeholders including other local government officers (from regeneration and environment, including colleagues with enforcement and tourism roles), a local wildlife action group, Doncaster Rovers FC, and retail representatives.

Once the Doncaster team had successfully completed the funding application stage, they were invited to an introductory workshop to meet other project teams that were part of the BSBD program. This workshop was designed to introduce and use the Double Diamond Design Process with all the projects in the BSBD program. Service project teams were asked to share their project idea by each producing a collage. A variety of materials, photographs, and magazines were made available. The resulting collages acted as an icebreaker and also helped to develop a useful visual language around desired outcomes that identified different expectations from members of each project team. For example, the tension in the Doncaster project – between the desire of some stakeholders to increase the use of Lakeside for recreation and of those who wanted to increase and protect the wildlife – was revealed by the visual imagery.

Following on from these introductory workshops the Doncaster-based project team concentrated on the first phase of the Double Diamond – i.e., the Discover phase. The principle of opening up and questioning can be used to facilitate the beginning of a coproduction journey. It is underpinned by the notion of openness, of nothing being off the table or irrelevant to the discussion. This principle, together with some of the creative methods the academics brought, helped to mitigate power differentials.

Some of the project team meetings took place in rooms at the football ground, adjacent to Lakeside. This presented opportunities to walk through the environment to observe and build consensus as we walked and talked. Working in a different place also helped with democratizing ownership of the work and helped to focus on the partnership. Trust is crucial in the beginning, and indeed throughout any coproductive journey. What worked well, in this example, is the use of the Double Diamond Process – once explained we could all see the steps of our project. It was also simple to understand and did not require us to (at an early stage) agree on a complex protocol (in researcher terms) or project initiation document (in knowledge user terms). It meant we could simply begin to think of solutions together. The ability of the design academics to produce prototypes at a subsequent meeting was also an aid, and reinforced trust within the team as it showed progress and action based on our joint vision (see Figure 3.1.2). At the beginning of the journey considerable effort was made to listen to knowledge users, and this was aided within the Discover phase of the project, underpinned by friendly, pragmatic, and respectful approaches.

VIGNETTE TWO: RESEARCH COPRODUCTION WITH INDUSTRY: DIGITAL TECHNOLOGY TO TRANSFORM END OF LIFE CARE

This vignette provides an example from the telehealth and care technology (TaCT) theme based in the CLAHRC. The aim of this theme was to produce a change in knowledge and practice in the design and use of telehealth and care technologies within services. This example helps to illustrate the time spent on developing a productive partnership and the gatekeeping role of knowledge users in setting up/"allowing" a coproduction research project to take place, and ensuring momentum and impact continues throughout, and importantly after the project has finished. This vignette focusses on the adaptation, implementation, and evaluation of a technology into a UK setting that was shown to

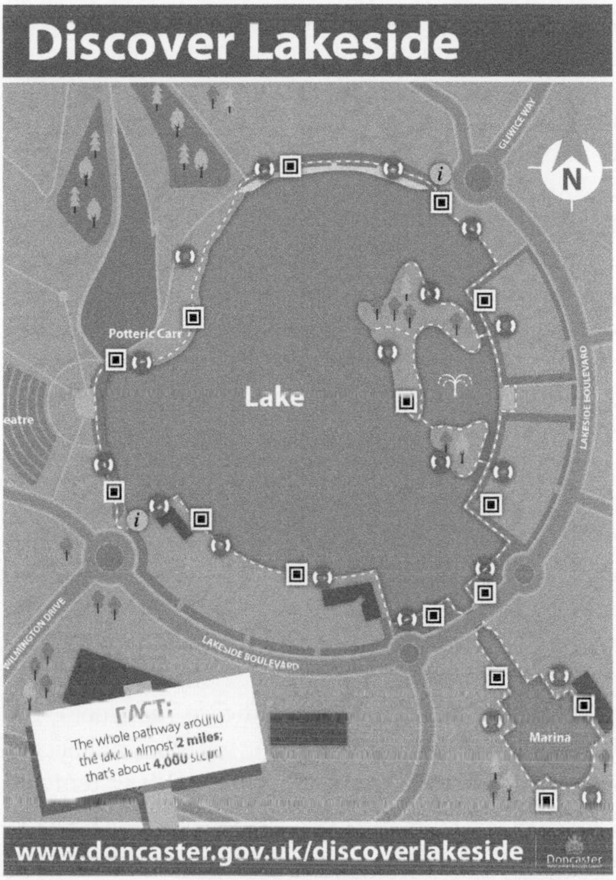

FIGURE 3.1.2 Doncaster Lakeside.

be effective in Canada. This technology is a digital platform, called "eshift," that enables communication and decision-making to take place between experts in palliative care and community nurses delivering end of life care to people in their own home. This technology is delivered using a hand-held device held by community nurses whilst caring for patients in their home. The project aimed to adapt the digital platform and coproduce a care pathway that had eshift embedded into it. This was developed along with an ongoing and embedded evaluation to assess the clinical and cost effectiveness of the technology. The project resulted in community nurses being able to provide care to multiple patients in their own homes and extended the reach of expertise from the hospice. Both specialist and community nurses were able to review data via an online dashboard, thereby improving communication and the quality of shared information across the service. The evaluation of this project, known as the Enhanced Community Palliative Support Service (EnComPaSS) (Arris et al. 2015), found that during the evaluation period the number of hospice patients admitted to acute hospital care reduced by 6.6%. Total hospital time per acute patient fell by 5.6 days, or 19.5%. These changes contributed to estimated savings of £2.4m per year to the NHS and an increase in patient and carer satisfaction.

This project became part of the CLAHRC program through dialogue in the wider network of the theme and was an outcome of the "horizon scanning" objective of the theme, which looked for new technologies and how they might be helpful in problem-solving in NHS services. This horizon-scanning activity marked the beginning of the coproduction journey. The academic working on the evaluation of the platform in Canada had once worked in the TaCT theme and believed that the technology offered an ideal solution to meeting patients' needs. The context of this project is that many end-of-life care patients would prefer to die at home, but a lack of specialist palliative support leads to poor symptom control, use of emergency services and hospital admission.

The possibilities of adapting and using this technology in the UK was explored with theme partners from hospital and hospice providers. Once this was agreed the project moved to a planning phase and partnership work. Key stakeholders were brought together to assess whether the technology could meet the service demand and could be introduced into an adapted care pathway. International consultation meetings were held with those who had implemented the system in Canada, the multi-professional team from Sheffield, and TaCT theme members. Knowledge users included senior healthcare managers, the medical director, nurses and patients, technologist from Sensory Technology the company producing eshift, senior managers from the Ontario health system and evaluators from the university. The purpose of these virtual meetings was to understand the end-of-life pathway in the UK. They also helped to develop a shared vision of the project, which was to develop a new platform that could enhance the pathway and delivery of care and enable patients to be well cared for in their own homes. Differences in culture and language were also identified. Further visits and workshops were developed between the company, the evaluation team, and services to build foundations for the project and adaptation of both services and the technology. Workshops included process mapping of existing pathways, with technology "touch points" to explore how eshift integrated into the UK pathway. We have undertaken a similar process using eshift in a stroke patient pathway too (see Figure 3.1.3) and recommend including designers to do this from the start. The next phase was to introduce the adapted technology through testing prototypes and making modifications based on feedback from services. In order to do this the company needed to listen, be nimble, agile, and responsive to requests for change, and the services needed to understand that you don't always get it right the first time. When problems arose in the clinical field, solutions needed to be swift. A failure to respond in this manner would have a significant impact on the user experience, the quality of the product, and its implementation. The journey from concept through to final live implementation took over three years, with frequent modification and iterations.

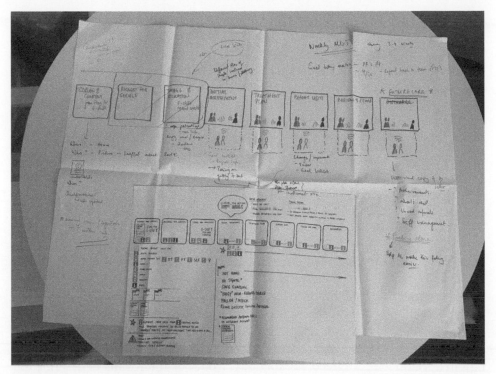

FIGURE 3.1.3   Pathway Model.

It became apparent that we needed to have a clear understanding of IP issues from the start of the journey, as the new model of care was coproduced with services and industry partners. Both used their knowledge to customize eshift to a UK setting. Intellectual property (IP) issues were clarified by developing a collaborative agreement and a MOU. In hindsight this should have been approved before the coproduction started. The MOU detailed collaborators, project scope, financial arrangements, and information governance plans together with an agreement on IP. The Lambert tool kit (https://www.gov.uk/guidance/univer sity-and-business-collaboration-agreements-lambert-toolkit) may be a helpful resource if you need to develop a MoU with knowledge users.

IMPLICATIONS FOR PRACTICE WHEN BEGINNING THE COPRODUCTION JOURNEY

This chapter has offered advice on what might be important to consider when planning coproduction at research program and research project levels. Both programs and projects need to ensure there is time and adequate resources to work together, to consider spending time and effort to learn skills together, and to focus on impact from the outset. Paying attention to relationships and enabling trust-building is the most precious resource in coproduction.

Developing coproduction partnership with industry needs some thoughtful consideration. Try and identify companies willing to share, change, and adapt their technology or product. We have found that smaller companies are more willing to work this way. Issues of IP also need to be agreed and discussed. This includes clarifying what belongs to the company before the partnership work (background IP) and what is developed together (foreground IP). Funding bodies should recognize resources, time requirements, and the flexibility needed when commissioning coproduced research.

FUTURE RESEARCH

Our experience is that coproduction takes time and needs to be adequately resourced. Budgets and funding arrangements should be flexible based on emerging needs and priorities. It may be fruitful to examine how funding bodies resource coproduction, identify how resources are used, and link patterns of resource with sustainable impact. It could also be possible this may vary with different combinations of stakeholders. For example, would impact be more sustainable with industry partners?

Similarly, we consider that setting priorities with all stakeholders is important to develop jointly agreed workplans. It would be interesting to describe the different methods of priority-setting, identify which stakeholders are involved and how, and whether this leads to impact and change.

CONCLUSION

This chapter has focussed on how to get started on the coproduction journey and offered learning from our experience as knowledge users and researchers. We have explored how to develop an environment in which coproduction can flourish, how to support capacity-building, create innovative boundary-spanning, and promote leadership that will enhance and support coproduction in the workplace. We hope this will encourage others to plan their journey, as the benefits in relation to sustainable partnerships and impact on practice is worth this careful planning.

REFERENCES

1. Arris, S.M., Fitzsimmons, D.A., and Mawson, S. (2015). Moving towards an enhanced community palliative support service (EnComPaSS): protocol for a mixed method study. *BMC Palliative Care* 14: 17. doi: 10.1186/s12904-015-0012-4.
2. Boaz, A., Hanney, S., Borst, R., O'Shea, A., and Kok, M. (2018). How to engage stakeholders in research: design principles to support improvement. *Health Research Policy and Systems / BioMed Central* 16: 60. doi: 10.1186/s12961-018-0337-6.

3. Boyle, D. and Harris, M. (2009). *The Challenge of Co-production*. London: New Economics Foundation.

4. Buick, F., Blackman, D., O'Flynn, J., O'Donnell, M., and West, D. (2016). Effective practitioner–scholar relationships: lessons from a coproduction partnership. *Public Administration* 76: 35–47. doi: 10.1111/puar.12481.

5. Cooke, J., Ariss, S., Smith, C., and Read, J. (2015). On-going collaborative priority-setting for research activity: a method of capacity building to reduce the research-practice translational gap. *Health Research Policy and Systems / BioMed Central* 13: 25. doi: 10.1186/s12961-015-0014-y.

6. Cooke, J., Langley, J., Wolstenholme, D., and Hampshaw, S. (2017). "Seeing" the difference: the importance of visibility and action as a mark of "authenticity" in co-production comment on "collaboration and co-production of knowledge in healthcare: opportunities and challenges. *International Journal of Health Policy and Management* 6: 345–348. doi: 10.15171/ijhpm.2016.136.

7. Design Council. (2004). *What is the framework for innovation? Design council's evolved Double Diamond.* [Online]. https://www.designcouncil.org.uk/news-opinion/what-framework-innovation-design-councils-evolved-double-diamond (accessed 31 August 2021).

8. Greenhalgh, T., Jackson, C., Shaw, S., and Janamian, T. (2016). Achieving research impact through co-creation in community-based health services: literature review and case study. *The Milbank Quarterly* 94: 392–429. doi: 10.1111/1468-0009.12197.

9. Hampshaw, S., Cooke, J., and Mott, L. (2018). What is a research derived actionable tool, and what factors should be considered in their development? A Delphi study. *BMC Health Services Research* 18: 740. doi: 10.1186/s12913-018-3551-6.

10. Jagosh, J., Bush, P.L., Salsberg, J., Macaulay, A.C., Greenhalgh, T., Wong, G., Cargo, M., Green, L.W., Herbert, C.P., and Pluye, P. (2015). A realist evaluation of community-based participatory research: partnership synergy, trust building and related ripple effects. *BMC Public Health* 15: 725. doi: 10.1186/s12889-015-1949-1.

11. Kislov, R., Wilson, P.M., Knowles, S., and Boaden, R. (2018). Learning from the emergence of NIHR Collaborations for Leadership in Applied Health Research and Care (CLAHRCs): a systematic review of evaluations. *Implementation Science: IS* 13: 111. doi: 10.1186/s13012-018-0805-y.

12. Langley, J., Wolstenholme, D., and Cooke, J. (2018). "Collective making' as knowledge mobilisation: the contribution of participatory design in the co-creation of knowledge in healthcare. *BMC Health Services Research* 18: 585. doi: 10.1186/s12913-018-3397-y.

13. Lorenc, T., Tyner, E.F., Petticrew, M., Duffy, S., Martineau, F.P., Phillips, G., and Lock, K. (2014). Cultures of evidence across policy sectors: systematic review of qualitative evidence. *European Journal of Public Health* 24: 1041–1047. doi: 10.1093/eurpub/cku038.

14. Melville-Richards, L., Rycroft-Malone, J., Burton, C., and Wilkinson, J. (2020). Making authentic: exploring boundary objects and bricolage in knowledge mobilisation through National Health Service-university partnerships. *Evidence & Policy: A Journal of Research, Debate and Practice* 16: 517–539. doi: 10.1332/17 4426419X15623134271106.

15. Oliver, K. and Cairney, P. (2019). The dos and don'ts of influencing policy: a systematic review of advice to academics. *Palgrave Communications* 5: no pagination. doi: 10.1057/s41599-019-0232-y.

16. Oliver, K., Kothari, A., and Mays, N. (2019). The dark side of coproduction: do the costs outweigh the benefits for health research? *Health Research Policy and Systems / BioMed Central* 17: 33. doi: 10.1186/s12961-019-0432-3.

17. Pawson, R., Boaz, A., Grayson, L., Long, A., and Barnes, C. (2003). *Types and Quality of Knowledge in Social Care: Knowledge Review 3*. London: SCIE.

18. Rycroft-Malone, J., Burton, C.R., Wilkinson, J., Harvey, G., McCormack, B., Baker, R., Dopson, S., Graham, I.D., Staniszewska, S., Thompson, C., Ariss, S., Melville-Richards, L., and Williams, L. (2016). Collective action for implementation: a realist evaluation of organisational collaboration in healthcare. *Implementation Science: IS* 11: 17. doi: 10.1186/s13012-016-0380-z.

19. Wolstenholme, D., Grindell, C., and Dearden, A. (2017). A co-design approach to service improvement resulted in teams exhibiting characteristics that support innovation. *Design for Health* 1: 42–58. doi: 10.1080/24735132.2017.1295531.

20. World Health Organization. (2010). *Global recommendations on physical activity for health*. https://www.who.int/dietphysicalactivity/global-PA-recs-2010.pdf. (accessed 11 January 2022).

3.2 Research Coproduction with Patients and Caregivers

Claire Ludwig and Davina Banner

Key Learning Points

- There has been a rapid increase in research coproduction with patients and caregivers over recent years.
- Research coproduction with patients and caregivers leads to more relevant and responsive research outputs.
- Multiple barriers to coproduction exist which necessitates teams working collectively to mitigate barriers and foster meaningful partnership across the research process.
- Practical supports for meaningful coproduction are essential and include orientation, training, and strategies to optimize equitable and inclusive partnerships.

Research Coproduction in Healthcare, First Edition. Edited by
Ian D. Graham, Jo Rycroft-Malone, Anita Kothari, and Chris McCutcheon.
© 2022 John Wiley & Sons Ltd. Published 2022 by John Wiley & Sons Ltd.

- The impacts of coproduction with patients and caregivers are yet to be fully understood or realized. An intentional focus on evaluating the negative and positive aspects of partnerships is urgently needed to advance the science of coproduction.

INTRODUCTION AND BACKGROUND

Hailed as a means of optimizing the relevance and impact of health research, the engagement of patients and caregivers in research has seen a rapid upsurge in popularity and has transformed the ways in which research is planned, funded, and undertaken (Domecq et al. 2014). Supported by international frameworks and strategies, including the INVOLVE initiative (INVOLVE 2012), the Patient-Centered Outcomes Research Initiative (Patient-Centered Outcomes Research Institute 2013), and the Strategy for Patient Oriented Research (SPOR) (Canadian Institutes of Health Research 2014), research coproduction with patients, caregivers, and the public has grown exponentially and has changed the landscape of health research globally. While numerous models and frameworks exist, these are underpinned by common principles that include/require: 1) authentic and meaningful partnerships across the research process, 2) clearly articulated roles and expectations, 3) mutual trust and attention to power, 4) commitment to co-creation and coproduction, and 5) access to required resources, supports, and training (Banner et al. 2019; Shippee et al. 2015).

Historically, the engagement of patients and caregivers became most entrenched in community-engaged research and evolved alongside the growing work of community activists, most notably among those living with disabilities, arthritis, and HIV (Charlton 2000). Seen as a means of enhancing democracy, ethical practice, and social responsibility within the research endeavor, patients and caregivers have become increasingly engaged in research coproduction. This has allowed for the refocusing of research to more directly address the needs, values, and priorities of patients. While these modes of research continue to grow steadily, the wider impacts have been slow to emerge and the evidence base surrounding the engagement of patients, caregivers, and the public remains somewhat limited (Brett et al. 2014). Despite this, the intrinsic value of engagement with diverse knowledge users and stakeholders, including patients and caregivers, is well accepted and recent efforts have seen the widespread transition of patient engagement from the margins to the mainstream of research. Early evidence reveals that the engagement of patients, caregivers, and the public can enhance the relevance of research, improve study planning and procedures, and facilitate generation of findings that better reflect the needs and values of those most impacted (Shippee et al. 2015). Alongside this, there has been a revival in engagement methods, focusing upon the mechanics of coproduction among diverse stakeholder groups, and demonstrating how this fosters impactful and responsive research.

Current frameworks delineating patient engagement are centered directly around the researcher-patient dyad (Canadian Institutes of Health Research 2014; Patient-Centered Outcomes Research Institute 2013); however, these frameworks complement existing research coproduction frameworks, including Integrated Knowledge Translation that advocates for meaningful partnerships with diverse knowledge users and stakeholders, and including patients and the public, to create, translate, and mobilize knowledge (Graham et al. 2006). In this chapter, we will critically examine the potential impacts of research coproduction with patients and caregivers and will identify implications for the practice of research coproduction.

WHO IS A "PATIENT?"

Diverse terminology that reflects research coproduction with patients and caregivers has emerged, but perhaps none more contentious than the term "patient." Major international health research funding organizations have widely adopted the term "patient" to denote a broad and all-encompassing group, including persons with lived experience, community members, caregivers, family, friends, and patient organizations (see Table 3.2.1), and while we adopt this terminology here, we do so cautiously noting its inherent complexity. Such latitude in definition presents both opportunities and challenges for researchers seeking to partner with patients in research coproduction. The breadth in the definition offers ease and convenience to researchers, particularly those seeking to partner with patients from groups difficult to reach due to structural vulnerabilities (e.g., populations that face intersecting challenges, such as those living with housing insecurity and immigrant and refugee populations) or those with physical or cognitive vulnerabilities (e.g., patients who are frail and seriously ill). Partnering with caregivers or representatives from community/advocacy groups invariably helps to circumvent barriers to accessing hard-to-reach patient populations. However, researchers should also exercise caution in relying solely on caregivers and community representatives to speak for patients (Largent et al. 2018). Patient and caregiver partners should reflect the characteristics, experiences, and interests of the population under study (Largent et al. 2018). Each will bring their own experiences to bear, but by using them as a proxy to speak for others, they may inadvertently lose the opportunity to voice their own unique experiences, and moreover may not truly reflect the patient experience. In considering who is best qualified to speak to the patient experience, it is imperative that research teams consider the population of interest, the research question, and the goals of the research partnership, both in the context of the overall study and with regard

TABLE 3.2.1   Major funders' definition of patients.

Major Funders' Definitions of Patients for the Purposes of Research Coproduction			
CIHR (Canada)	**PCORI (US)**	**NIHR (UK)**	**NHMRC (Australia)**
An overarching term inclusive of individuals with personal experience of a health issue and informal caregivers, including family and friends. https://cihr-irsc. gc.ca/e/48413. html#a4	Persons with current or past experience of illness or injury, family members or other unpaid caregivers of patients, or members of advocacy organizations that represent patients or caregivers. https://www.pcori. org/about-us/ our-programs/ engagement/ public-and- patient- engagement/ pcoris- stakeholders	Utilizes the INVOLVE definition of the term "public" to include patients, potential patients, carers and people who use health and social care services as well as people from organizations that represent people who use services. https://www.invo. org.uk/find-out- more/what- is-public- involvement-in- research-2	Utilizes the Australian Commission on Safety and Quality in Health Care definition: members of the public who use, or are potential users of, healthcare services – patients, consumers, families, carers and other support people. https://www.nhmrc. gov.au/about-us/ publications/ statement- consumer-and- community- involvement- health-and- medical- research#block- views-block-file- attachments- content-block-1

*Adapted from Frank et al. (2020).

to specific activities across the research cycle (Canadian Institutes of Health Research 2014). Research teams must consciously deliberate on how and where patients' contributions are situated throughout the research process and acknowledge the possibility that in privileging the voices of some, they may simultaneously be silencing the voices of others. Thus, considering issues of diversity, inclusion, and representation is essential in planning meaningful and impactful coproduced research (Banner et al. 2019). In some situations, teams may seek to include multiple perspectives, including those of the patient, caregiver, and/or community member. Each of these may contribute unique insights, but together may yield some additional sensitivities that must be considered and navigated.

WHAT DO WE KNOW ABOUT POTENTIAL BENEFITS AND IMPACTS OF RESEARCH COPRODUCTION WITH PATIENTS?

There is emerging evidence to suggest that research coproduced with patients is more relevant and responsive to patients' needs because it incorporates unique insights into living with an illness, whilst including their values and preferences (Brett et al. 2014). Patients and caregivers describe deeply personal benefits related to partnering in research, particularly with regard to validation of their illness experience and feelings of empowerment. Partnering in research can equip patients with new skills and knowledge, enhance a sense of purpose and identity, and may also serve as a transformational function for patients who have suffered debilitating loss from illness, frailty, and/or aggressive treatment regimens (Thompson et al. 2014). For elderly participants, it may potentially serve as a protective factor against loneliness or cognitive and functional decline (Bindels et al. 2014). For those with life-limiting illness, it may help to experience a sense of agency in the face of a disease over which they have little control, reducing a sense of hopelessness in the knowledge that their participation may benefit others (Cotterell et al. 2011). Patients further describe feeling emotionally supported, experiencing a sense of community with team members, and acquiring new knowledge about their disease and treatments (Brett et al. 2014; Leese et al. 2018). For caregivers, it may similarly create a welcome space to share their experiences and to highlight challenges faced when attempting to navigate the health system (Rapaport et al. 2018).

Positive experiences appear to motivate patients and caregivers to remain involved in the partnership. However, damaging effects, such as exposure to negative attitudes and perceptions, feeling undervalued or irrelevant to the project, or feeling overloaded, can discourage input and involvement from patients and caregivers, and may negatively impact the research process (Brett et al. 2014; Jørgensen et al. 2018). Patient and caregiver partners have also expressed feeling emotionally vulnerable during the research process following exposure to the suffering of others or hearing about deleterious research outcomes (Brett et al. 2014). Furthermore, patient-partners, who are dealing with significant illness and frailty, may experience additional burden on already compromised physical and cognitive stamina when participating in research activities.

Researchers and knowledge users engaged in research coproduction describe a process of mutual respect and learning that occurs as a result of their partnerships with patients and caregivers (Leese et al. 2018). Researchers report that partnerships with patients and caregivers require a different way of working, increasing their recognition of the value patients bring to the team and enhancing their interpersonal skills (Brett et al. 2014). Researchers have also described feeling motivated by the strength and resiliency that they witness in their patient-partners (Price et al. 2018). On the flip side, researchers have revealed feeling ill-prepared to deal with the emotional labor involved in partnerships with patients, including navigating partnerships which may be conflictual or challenge their assumptions (Boylan et al. 2019). Fears of delays in the research process, and feeling unprepared to deal with ethical issues of partnering with patients, have also been described as negatively impacting researchers' comfort and willingness for meaningful partnership (Belisle-Pipon et al. 2018; Ludwig et al. 2020).

Evidence examining the impacts of coproduction on the design, delivery, and uptake of research is continuing to emerge, but includes: incorporation of patients' priorities, changes to study materials to enhance accessibility to study participants (e.g., consent documents, survey tools), and increased enrolment and retention in studies (Domecq et al. 2014). Where patients have served as peer researchers there is evidence to suggest that patient partners have greater understanding and emotional connection with study participants, which in turn appears to lead to more honest and candid responses from participants and facilitate deeper analysis of the responses given by participants in focus groups and interviews (Bindels et al. 2014). Involvement of patient and caregiver partners has further contributed to more impactful and targeted dissemination activities (Brett et al. 2014).

BARRIERS AND FACILITATORS TO RESEARCH COPRODUCTION WITH PATIENTS AND CAREGIVERS

Barriers and facilitators to research coproduction have been well documented in the literature (Bethell et al. 2018; Domecq et al. 2014; Ludwig et al. 2020). At the system level, researchers have cited challenges related to culture and hierarchical power structures, lack of formal policy, insufficient governance and infrastructure, and inconsistent funding and compensation frameworks to support research coproduction (Bethell et al. 2018; Domecq et al. 2014; Ludwig et al. 2020). For example, appropriate and adequate resources continue to be cited by researchers as a key enabler of more intensive and prolonged partnerships with patients (Bethell et al. 2018). Government-based funding opportunities now encourage or mandate research coproduction with patients; in turn, this has spurred the development of infrastructure to support the process, e.g., the Strategy for Patient-Oriented Research, established by the Canadian Institutes of Health Research (Canadian Institutes of Health Research 2014). This infrastructure offers practical support and training, heightening researchers' awareness of best practices in patient engagement. However, at the operational level, researchers have continued to report barriers related to resource constraints, lack of time, funding and administrative support, and the incremental time and energy required to initiate and build meaningful relationships with patient-partners over the course of the study (Bethell et al. 2018; Domecq et al. 2014). These barriers are often amplified in coproduction with patients and caregivers from underserved populations, such as those facing intersecting structural inequities and stigma, or those who are frail and seriously ill (Heckert et al. 2020).

Relational practices remain at the heart of coproduction with patients and caregivers. Lack of familiarity with the principles and practice of coproduction amongst team members, or the lack of a primary lead for patient engagement, has left many teams without the requisite knowledge to structure practices for coproduction (Bethell et al. 2018). This can give rise to poorly defined roles and responsibilities for patient and caregiver partners, a lack of meaningful integration of patient-partners into the team, and ill-defined processes and mechanisms to support shared decision-making (Banner et al. 2019). For patients and caregivers, this can translate as tokenism and can serve as a significant barrier to meaningful partnership. Without meaningful partnership, patients and caregivers may be left wondering what their input will amount to, particularly when they are included in projects after major decisions have already been made. Lack of training, preparation, rigidity in the timing and modes of engagement, and use of complex medical or research terminology serve as a barrier to patient and caregivers' full participation (Brett et al. 2014). For those juggling with the impact of illness, aggressive treatment regimens, and/or caregiving responsibilities, partnering in research can be seen as an additional burden to an already full plate (Leese et al. 2018). Additionally, failure to evaluate or provide feedback to patient and caregiver partners about how their contributions have shaped the research process and/or the outcomes of the study contribute to feelings of uncertainty and may reduce the likelihood of their partnering in future studies.

Facilitators to successful integration of patient-partners include: providing relevant research training; providing clarity on roles and responsibilities for patient and caregiver partners that take into consideration their individual preferences, skills and abilities; maintaining flexibility in the modes and methods of contribution, including ensuring accessibility to team activities and meetings; promoting clear and jargon-free communication; offering logistical support to attend meetings; remunerating patients and caregivers for their expert contributions, or at a minimum providing compensation for out-of-pocket expenses; maintaining regular updates on study progress, results, and outcomes; acknowledging the contributions of patient and caregiver partners; and promoting a welcoming environment and relationships that are built on trust and mutual respect (Bethell et al. 2018; Brett et al. 2014; Domecq et al. 2014; Heckert et al. 2020; Ludwig et al. 2020; Shippee et al. 2015).

EXPERIENTIAL KNOWLEDGE: PATIENT AND CAREGIVER PARTNER IMPLICATIONS FOR PRACTICE

There are several practice considerations from the perspective of patient and caregiver partners involved in research coproduction. At the individual project level, patients and caregivers can adopt varied roles, ranging from advisors on project steering committees or working groups to research team members, collaborators, or peer-researchers. Despite the rapidly evolving role of patients and caregivers in research, these partnerships remain fundamentally dependent on researchers' willingness to partner and engage in coproduction. Given that most health research continues to be conceived and led by academics and clinicians, patient and caregiver involvement is contingent on both initial and ongoing invitations to partners in projects. Moreover, being an invited participant invariably influences how patients/caregivers perceive themselves in relation to the project and their overall role, including their decision-making power.

Prior to accepting the offer to partner in a study, patients and caregivers should be encouraged to think about what the research project has to offer them, what contributions they can make, what skills and experiences they bring to the table, and how they envision their role in the partnership to ensure that it aligns with their interests and abilities. Strategies to ascertain this fit and mutual interest may include ensuring that research and healthcare organizations support opportunities for knowledge exchange and networking with patients and caregivers. Examples may include Café Scientifique, community presentations, or town hall meetings that can allow participants to exchange knowledge and engage in shared learning.

Patient and caregiver partners engaged in research coproduction deserve the right to equal respect and concern. If not addressed early in the relationship, hierarchical power structures and misconceptions about the abilities of patient-partners will function as a barrier to full and meaningful partnerships. Thus, the co-creation of a safe participatory space in which the experiential knowledge of patient and caregiver partners is acknowledged and respected is essential to successful research partnerships. Expressions of tokenism have the potential to devalue the contributions of patient and caregiver partners, trigger feelings of inadequacy, and have a negative impact on the research process and outcomes (Brett et al. 2014; Price et al. 2018). Patient-partners may be particularly vulnerable to negative attitudes or indifferent behaviors, and this vulnerability may be amplified in those patients struggling with loss of self-esteem due to illness and/or aggressive or prolonged treatment regimens. Fears of being perceived as difficult, or lacking in knowledge or trust, may inadvertently force patients' compliance and acquiescence to the views of others. Tacit sentiments of paternalism and ageism can be equally detrimental to research relationships when working alongside frail and seriously ill patients, or those who are structurally vulnerable (Bindels et al. 2014).

Reciprocal communication between team members is highly valued by patients and caregivers (Leese et al. 2018). Feedback to patient and caregiver partners regarding the value and utility of their input promotes respect and serves as an impetus for patients to remain engaged and continue with their contributions (Leese et al. 2018). In particular, patients and caregivers may benefit most from feedback that is constructive, respectful, balanced, and honest, particularly in situations where their input has been perceived as not useful or relevant to the project, or is perceived as overly personal in advancing a political agenda. Failure to address both the positive and negative aspects of patient and caregiver partners' contributions may lead to feelings of tokenism, frustration, lack of trust, conciliatory behaviors, and ultimately delay research progress. Patient and caregiver partners need assurance that constructive feedback is given for the purposes of advancing the research agenda and safeguarding a productive relationship. Conversely, patient and caregiver partners have equal responsibility to provide instrumental feedback to their research team peers, particularly if the materials, conversation, or behavior of others is upsetting or offensive. Mechanisms to revisit the objectives and successes of the partnership must be securely in place throughout the research cycle to protect all members of the team (Brett et al. 2014). The results of a formal evaluation should also be shared with patients so that they can appreciate the impact of their input.

The nature of illness, frailty, and caregiving responsibilities necessitates consideration for well-being, and it is incumbent on patients not to minimize or negate these impacts as they consider partnering in research. Patient and caregiver partners may be reluctant to discuss special considerations or accommodations for fear of over-burdening busy researchers; however, failure to do so may result in additional stress and lead to inconsistent involvement in the research process. Practical considerations for patient-partners must be acknowledged, e.g., accessibility to meetings (in-person and virtual) may be difficult for those who are physically or cognitively impaired, timing of meetings should be considered against treatment or caregiving demands. Out-of-pocket expenses should be compensated in a timely manner so that patient-partners are not financially burdened. Practical considerations related to communication processes should be addressed, and patient and caregiver partners should have a consistent point of contact for the project so that special considerations can be easily addressed without needing to provide a rationale in a public forum. Finally, patient and caregiver partners also need to be aware of their right to control disclosure of their health information, such as diagnoses and prognosis. Disclosure of other information, especially financial status, can be a sensitive issue (Jørgensen et al. 2018) and discussions regarding compensation should be done privately rather than in a group setting.

EXPERIENTIAL KNOWLEDGE: RESEARCHER IMPLICATIONS FOR PRACTICE

Through research coproduction partnerships, disciplinary, and professional boundaries are minimized, as researchers, knowledge users, and stakeholders, including patients and caregivers, join forces to tackle complex healthcare problems and to support creation and mobilization of more impactful and responsive evidence. At the heart of this collaborative process is the need for researchers to partner meaningfully with patients and caregivers. Researchers hold a central responsibility and role in the creation of engagement spaces that are inclusive and allow for collaboration and shared learning (Heckert et al. 2020). In doing this, researchers are charged with the need to recognize and explicitly value the contributions of each partner, whether this be the methodological and scientific expertise of the research team members, the point of care insights and contextualized knowledge of knowledge users and stakeholders, or experiential knowledge of those with lived experience. Through the process of research coproduction, patients and caregivers are well positioned to provide essential perspectives on complex healthcare issues, contributing experiential knowledge of the healthcare system, as well as other experiences and skills based on their own personal and professional knowledge (Banner et al. 2019).

Despite offering rich contributions, patient and caregiver partners may lack the typical decision-making power afforded to other members of a team. They can be disadvantaged due to their precarious positioning, often being the only unpaid member of the team, and may experience power imbalances that result in their contributions not being valued in the same way as those of other team members. While the support of inclusive and safe engagement spaces is the responsibility of all research team members, the researcher-leads must be committed to setting the tone of the partnership by fostering collaboration and open communication. Creating safe spaces for engagement, including promoting diversity, equity, and inclusion within partnerships, is the bedrock of meaningful collaboration and is particularly important in research coproduction with patients and caregivers that face multiple barriers to engagement, including those that face complex health conditions, frailty, or structural inequities. Team leaders must spend time to build relationships with patient and caregiver partners, creating a foundation of reciprocity and trust, and promoting ways to effectively address conflicts or tensions.

Within the context of research coproduction, practical supports are also needed for patients and caregiver partners to fully contribute. Upon initiation of the partnership, this should involve a clear discussion of expectations, roles, and responsibilities, in addition to planning for compensation, training, and support. For example, research studies commonly comprise complex methodological and theoretical principles and practices. While researchers receive extensive training as part of their professional preparation, patients and caregivers may be expected to grasp the essential principles and practices with little to no training. Researchers must take time to orientate and support the patient and caregiver partners to gain a solid understanding of the focus, process, and expected outcomes of the research. This may include generating plain language summaries of key stages of the research process, delineating key terminology (e.g., plain language glossaries), providing direct training for research activities (e.g., literature screening or analysis training), and providing support for patient and community partners to contribute the development of research study and creation of proposals, grants, and study outputs.

Researchers must also successfully plan and resource projects to allow for meaningful coproduction to take place. Primarily, teams must ensure that there is sufficient time and financial resources to support intentional and purposeful engagement. This may include allocating time to build and establish relationships prior to the development of funding applications and determining project timelines that allow for ongoing engagement. As part of this, planning for appropriate and accessible remuneration and compensation is vital. Challenges in facilitating the timely payment of patient and caregiver partners has been reported, alongside a lack of flexibility in the ways in which payment can be offered. Researchers must continue to advocate enhanced options from academic institutions and funders, including flexibility in how payments are offered (e.g., cash, honorarium, gift certificates) and the ability to provide alternative payment (e.g., the opportunity to attend a conference or training classes) as determined by the patient and caregiver partner.

Care must also be taken to create inclusive and safe partnership spaces. This can include ensuring a commitment to ongoing and regular communication with patient and caregiver partners, along with the facilitation of spaces for difficult conversations to take place without endangering the broader partnership. As part of this, processes must be in place to identify and manage conflict or disparate expectations within research teams, particularly in situations where research results may not reflect or support the perspectives of patients, caregivers, or researchers. Furthermore, research teams may comprise knowledge users that span diverse disciplines and practice settings. Each may contribute different perspectives and sensitivities, meaning that teams must also navigate varied dynamics, disciplinary norms, and perspectives about the role and value of patient and caregiver engagement in research. Adopting practices that seek to minimize power imbalances is similarly important, including considering how team members are introduced, how language and jargon are used, and ensuring that dedicated time is available for patient and caregiver partners to share their insights and ideas.

Researchers must be prepared to respond to, and integrate, the insights of patient and caregiver partners. This requires researchers to be open and flexible, while balancing the methodological and scientific demands of the work. Teams must be sensitive to the perspectives of patient and caregiver partners and must be cognizant of how health issues are communicated and discussed. This should include attention to the emotional labor associated with patient and caregiver partnerships, as well as conscious efforts to avoid stigmatizing terminology or the use of inappropriate humor. For researchers, recognition of the emotional impacts of partnerships with patients and caregivers is similarly important, as team members may also be faced with emotional situations resulting from the advancing illness or potential death of a patient or caregiver partner.

When considering the process of translating and mobilizing research findings and outputs, patients and caregivers can directly inform knowledge mobilization by offering a unique and valuable perspective. Patient and caregiver partners should be supported to co-create targeted KMb products, including the creation of patient-oriented tools and resources, as well as traditional academic outputs, such as manuscripts and conference presentations. Of note, storytelling by those with lived experience can be among the most powerful forms of KMb and can inspire change, direct innovation, and support collaboration (Bourbonnais and Michaud 2018). Finally, patients may provide a valuable lens on the ongoing evaluation and sustainability of initiatives and outputs as they relate to the research outputs. Considerations related to patient and caregiver partnerships within research coproduction are summarized in Table 3.2.2.

TABLE 3.2.2   Considerations for research coproduction by research stage.

Research Stage (adapted from Shippee et al. (2015))	Researcher Perspective	Patient and Caregiver Perspective
Agenda Setting and Funding	• Identify and connect with diverse knowledge users and stakeholder partners, including patient and caregiver partners • Build and establish relationships with patient and caregiver partners • Partner with others to co-create research agendas, priorities, and proposals • Identify how patient and caregiver partners may contribute to research	• Comprehend the intention/ purpose of involvement • Contribute to the development of research agendas, priorities, and proposals • Consider how to represent or speak to the illness experience under study • Communicate with team if alternative engagement is needed • Determine and negotiate engagement and role on the team

Research Stage (adapted from Shippee et al. (2015))	Researcher Perspective	Patient and Caregiver Perspective
Study Design and Procedures	• Consider orientation and training needs of all team members • Consider roles and responsibilities of team members • Facilitate ongoing and regular communication among team members, including team meetings • Facilitate safe engagement spaces • Facilitate and promote shared learning and coproduction	• Liaise with research team leads to determine information and training needs, including orientation and access to ongoing training • Contribute to the design and execution of study activities • Negotiate and be aware of roles and responsibilities within the project • Facilitate safe engagement spaces • Participate in team activities, including team meetings
Study Participant Recruitment	• Identify and communicate potential recruitment methods • Facilitate shared decision-making to promote effective recruitment and retention of the study participants • Facilitate the creation and review of study recruitment materials • Determine how recruitment materials and processes meet required ethical criteria and standards	• Co-create recruitment plans • Provide insights around how teams might promote ongoing engagement and retention in research studies • Provide input into the development and review of advertising and recruitment materials • Identify if study materials are accessible to patients.
Data Collection and Analysis	• Support collaboration in data collection and analysis • Identify and provide training and support to optimize engagement of patient and caregiver partners • Facilitate opportunities for partners to assist with the interpretation of findings	• Determine opportunities to assist with data analysis and the interpretation of the findings • Consider training needs that may support a more active role in data collection and analysis (e.g., co-lead focus groups) • Advocate for ongoing support to bolster engagement

(Continued)

TABLE 2.3.3   (Continued)

Research Stage (adapted from Shippee et al. (2015))	Researcher Perspective	Patient and Caregiver Perspective
Dissemination	• Promote the engagement and recognition of partners in study outputs • Facilitate engagement in the planning, creation, and disseminating of KMb outputs • Communicate the impacts of multi-stakeholder partnerships in research coproduction, including partnerships with patients and caregivers	• Advocate for engagement and recognition in the intellectual and practical outputs of the study • Participate in the planning, creation, and disseminating of KMb outputs • Communicate the impacts of patient and caregiver partnerships in research coproduction
Implementation	• Obtain input into the barriers and facilitators to implementation • Facilitate opportunities for team members to work directly with stakeholders or policy makers to implement research outputs	• Provide input into the barriers and facilitators to implementation • Consider opportunities to work directly with stakeholders or policy makers to implement research outputs
Evaluation	• Facilitate open communication • Consider informal and formal means of evaluating coproduction partnerships and impacts • Report partnerships insights and impacts	• Offer honest and constructive feedback about the experience of partnerships, with recommendations for improving the process as appropriate. • Participate or lead evaluation activities • Identify partnership insights and impacts

Research Stage (adapted from Shippee et al. (2015))	Researcher Perspective	Patient and Caregiver Perspective
General considerations	• Examine perspectives around diversity, inclusion, and representation in research coproduction with patients and caregivers • Be flexible and open to new insights and new ways of approaching research problems • Remain attentive to and engaged in the prevention of actual or potential harms resulting from te partnership or research process • Consider how experiential knowledge is perceived and used in research coproduction	• Find a balance between providing input based on lived experience, whilst avoiding an overly personal or political agenda • Identify and communicate concerns, including actual or potential harms, resulting from the partnership or research process • Seek out information through research coproduction networks (locally or nationally) or from experienced patient-partners that can help support knowledge about the full extent of the role

*Phases and stages of patient and service user engagement in research adapted from Shippee et al. (2015).

FUTURE RESEARCH

Despite growing enthusiasm and uptake of coproduction with patients and caregivers, the potential impacts are yet to be fully realized (Banner et al. 2019; Shippee et al. 2015). As patient and caregiver roles in research coproduction have begun to shift away from one-off consultations to an emphasis on meaningful partnerships and shared decision-making throughout the lifecycle of a project or projects, evidence about the impacts on research, researchers, and patients/caregivers themselves continues to lag. While evidence is beginning to emerge within the patient engagement field, the nature of partnerships, along with the related costs, resources, time, and impacts require further exploration. An opportunity exists for teams to address these gaps, which in turn would advance the science of coproduction. Examples of research questions are summarized in Table 3.2.3.

An opportunity exists to systematically explore the patient and caregiver role within the context of research coproduction, and in turn investigate how

TABLE 3.2.3   Research questions to guide future coproduction scholarship.

1. How can teams engaged in coproduction foster optimal engagement among all researchers, knowledge users, stakeholders, patients, and caregivers?
2. How do patients and caregivers contribute to the process and outcomes of research coproduction?
3. How can coproduction practices foster the voices of those most often excluded from research?
4. How do clinician knowledge users and stakeholders experience research coproduction with patients and caregivers? Does this differ from non-clinician knowledge users and stakeholders?
5. How can ethical/relational practices be fostered in research coproduction?
6. How can teams identify and mitigate unintended harms for patients and caregiver partners?
7. How do research teams, and others, experience working alongside patients and caregivers that are experiencing frailty and life-limiting illness?

issues of diversity, inclusion, and safety are promoted and managed. Understanding the barriers and facilitators of engagement, along with a focus on how barriers may be overcome within the context of research, would be of particular value. Likewise, documenting and evaluating coproduction successes, along with episodes of discordance, can help to further explicate the synergies and circumstances needed to optimize engagement (Staniszewska et al. 2017). To date, there has been a tendency to over-report on the positive aspects of research coproduction. With regard to the practice of coproduction, reporting of negative outcomes is limited, particularly where strategies have been ineffective or were too time consuming to maintain (Heckert et al. 2020).

There is a need to bolster evidence on the outcomes and impacts of coproduction so that the academic community can move beyond anecdotal and intuitive support for the practice. It is imperative that we incorporate evaluation of the specific components of research coproduction which contributed to the development of the research product and determine positive and negative impacts to patients, caregivers, and researchers. The development of dedicated evaluation tools may yield valuable opportunities to understand the process and outcomes of coproduction (Staniszewska et al. 2017). Evaluation frameworks adapted for use within patient-oriented research may offer a promising opportunity to delve inside the black box of partnerships; however, further tools that address the specific context of research coproduction (including partnerships with knowledge users and other stakeholders) is needed to further deconstruct the conditions and practices inherent to meaningful and impactful coproduction.

Attention to diversity and inclusion is urgently required within the context of research coproduction, particularly with respect to the meaningful inclusion of patients and caregivers who may face multiple and intersecting barriers to engagement and may be typically excluded from research. Developing and adopting engagement methods that allow for the study of relational complexity, such as microethnography or realist methods, along with research that attends to issues of equity and social justice, may assist in achieving more inclusive modes of research coproduction. Furthermore, attending to the intended and unintended consequences of research coproduction can offer new insights. Uncovering what characteristics and environments foster and optimize coproduction amongst diverse groups, and in turn, how these partnerships drive and impact the creation and mobilization of evidence in healthcare, remains poorly understood.

There needs to be ongoing advocacy to support the documentation of coproduction within research outputs, including academic journals, along with the development of flexible financial policies. This includes lobbying high impact journals to create opportunities for teams to better share the outcomes of coproduction with patients and caregivers. For example, the small word limits of many high impact journals restrict the ability to fully document coproduction practices or fully explicate the benefits and contributions of coproduction. The use of patient and caregiver engagement evaluation tools or reporting guidelines (Staniszewska et al. 2017) may help address this gap and foster greater transparency around the nature and scope of engagement within the context of research coproduction. Likewise, ongoing lobbying of research funders to facilitate more targeted funding for coproduced research is needed. As part of this, enhanced financial flexibility for research teams to operationalize partnerships with patients and caregivers is needed. This should include an overhaul of current financial policies among health research funders and academic institutions to allow for more inclusive ways for funding to be held, accessed, and used.

Finally, given the increasing engagement of patients across the research continuum, there is heightened awareness of the need to extend recognition of the intellectual contribution of patient partners to authorship on academic papers. Although some journals have incorporated patient perspectives into their strategic direction and operations, there is a substantial number (30%) of medical journal editors-in-chief who do not view the inclusion of patient partners as authors to be appropriate (Cobey et al. 2021). In order to promote equitable inclusion, there is a need to address both the philosophical and practical barriers to the authorship of patient partners. In recognition of this tension, Richards et al. (2020) offer research teams resources and practical guidance including advice about: 1) how to open the conversation about authorship; 2) requirements for authorship and acknowledgement; and 3) the relevant commitments of all parties throughout the development and revision of a manuscript.

TABLE 3.2.4   Developing and sustaining effective partnerships.

1. Get to know each other and the project. Allocate time and resources to build relationships and trust and allow space for all team members to explore the desired nature and scope of their partnerships. Intentional relationship-building may help patients and caregivers to feel more at ease and to seek more clarity about the project.
2. Co-define the purpose of engagement, collaboratively determine the expected outcomes and contributions, along with team values.
3. Identify roles and fit, focusing on the strengths and skills of all team members.
4. Identify any barriers and facilitators to engagement prior to the initiation of the project and throughout each research stage. Re-evaluate these at regular intervals.
5. Allow opportunities for reflection and open and transparent conversation about the partnership. Creating safe spaces and addressing power imbalances can allow for meaningful connection and partnership.
6. Identify and manage conflicts of interest. Teams should have a process in place to address issues as they arise.
7. Commit to evaluating the experience and impact of coproduction partnerships and reporting these with the wider scientific community.
8. Explore the long-term goals of all team members and vision for ongoing research, paying attention to how engagement capacity and priorities may shift over time.

CONCLUSION

Research coproduction with patients and caregivers has grown rapidly over recent years and is changing the landscape of health research. Patients and caregivers have become increasingly engaged in research coproduction, allowing for a refocusing of research to more directly address the needs, values, and priorities of patients. In this chapter, practical suggestions are provided to foster curious and meaningful engagement with patients and caregivers. These strategies are summarized in Table 3.2.4. Despite widespread adoption, the impacts of research coproduction with patients and caregivers are poorly understood and are yet to be fully realized. Promoting meaningful engagement, whilst addressing barriers and research gaps, will allow for continued development in coproduction research with patients and caregivers.

REFERENCES

1. Banner, D., Bains, M., Carroll, S., Kandola, D.K., Rolfe, D.E., Wong, C., and Graham, I.D. (2019). Patient and public engagement in integrated knowledge translation research: are we there yet? *Research Involvement and Engagement* 5: 8. doi: 10.1186/s40900-019-0139-1.

2. Belisle-Pipon, J.C., Rouleau, G., and Birko, S. (2018). Early-career researchers' views on ethical dimensions of patient engagement in research. *BMC Medical Ethics* 19: 21. doi: 10.1186/s12910-018-0260-y.

3. Bethell, J., Commisso, E., Rostad, H.M., Puts, M., Babineau, J., Grinbergs-Saull, A., Wighton, M.B., Hammel, J., Doyle, E., Nadeau, S., and McGilton, K.S. (2018). Patient engagement in research related to dementia: a scoping review. *Dementia (London)* 17: 944–975. doi: 10.1177/1471301218789292.

4. Bindels, J., Baur, V., Cox, K., Heijing, S., and Abma, T. (2014). Older people as co-researchers: a collaborative journey. *Ageing and Society* 34: 951–973.

5. Bourbonnais, A. and Michaud, C. (2018). Once upon a time: storytelling as a knowledge translation strategy for qualitative researchers. *Nursing Inquiry* 25: e12249. doi: 10.1111/nin.12249.

6. Boylan, A.M., Locock, L., Thomson, R., and Staniszewska, S. (2019). "About sixty per cent I want to do it": health researchers' attitudes to, and experiences of, patient and public involvement (PPI)-a qualitative interview study. *Health Expectations* 22: 721–730. doi: 10.1111/hex.12883.

7. Brett, J., Staniszewska, S., Mockford, C., Herron-Marx, S., Hughes, J., Tysall, C., and Suleman, R. (2014). A systematic review of the impact of patient and public involvement on service users, researchers and communities. *The Patient* 7: 387–395. doi: 10.1007/s40271-014-0065-0.

8. Canadian Institutes of Health Research. (2014). *Strategy for Patient-Oriented Research – Patient Engagement Framework*. [Online]. https://cihr-irsc.gc.ca/e/45851.html (accessed 31 August 2021).

9. Charlton, J.I. (2000). *Nothing about Us without Us: Disability Oppression and Empowerment*. Berkeley, CA: University of California Press.

10. Cobey, K.D., Monfaredi, Z., Poole, E., Proulx, L., Fergusson, D., and Moher, D. (2021). Editors-in-chief perceptions of patients as (co) authors on publications and the acceptability of ICMJE authorship criteria: a cross-sectional survey. *Research Involvement and Engagement* 7: 39. doi: 10.1186/s40900-021-00290-1.

11. Cotterell, P., Harlow, G., Morris, C., Beresford, P., Hanley, B., Sargeant, A., Sitzia, J., and Staley, K. (2011). Service user involvement in cancer care: the impact on service users. *Health Expectations* 14: 159–169. doi: 10.1111/j.1369-7625.2010.00627.x.

12. Domecq, J.P., Prutsky, G., Elraiyah, T., Wang, Z., Nabhan, M., Shippee, N., Brito, J.P., Boehmer, K., Hasan, R., Firwana, B., Erwin, P., Eton, D., Sloan, J., Montori, V., Asi, N., Dabrh, A.M., and Murad, M.H. (2014). Patient engagement in research: a systematic review. *BMC Health Services Research* 14: 89. doi: 10.1186/1472-6963-14-89.

13. Frank, L., Morton, S.C., Guise, J.M., Jull, J., Concannon, T.W., Tugwell, P., and Multi Stakeholder Engagement Consortium. (2020). Engaging patients and other non-researchers in health research: defining research engagement. *Journal of General Internal Medicine* 35: 307–314. doi: 10.1007/s11606-019-05436-2.

14. Graham, I.D., Logan, J., Harrison, M.B., Straus, S.E., Tetroe, J., Caswell, W., and Robinson, N. (2006). Lost in knowledge translation: time for a map? *The Journal of Continuing Education in the Health Professions* 26: 13–24. doi: 10.1002/chp.47.

15. Heckert, A., Forsythe, L.P., Carman, K.L., Frank, L., Hemphill, R., Elstad, E.A., Esmail, L., and Lesch, J.K. (2020). Researchers, patients, and other stakeholders' perspectives on challenges to and strategies for engagement. *Research Involvement and Engagement* 6: 60. doi: 10.1186/s40900-020-00227-0.

16. INVOLVE. (2012). Briefing Notes for Researchers: Involving the Public in NHS, Public Health and Social Care Research. Eastleigh, UK: INVOLVE. https://www.invo.org.uk/wp-content/uploads/2014/11/9938_INVOLVE_Briefing_Notes_WEB.pdf.

17. Jørgensen, C.R., Eskildsen, N.B., and Johnsen, A.T. (2018). User involvement in a Danish project on the empowerment of cancer patients – experiences and early recommendations for further practice. *Research Involvement and Engagement* 4: 26. doi: 10.1186/s40900-018-0105-3.

18. Largent, E.A., Lynch, H.F., and McCoy, M.S. (2018). Patient-engaged research: choosing the "right" patients to avoid pitfalls. *The Hastings Center Report* 48: 26–34. doi: 10.1002/hast.898.

19. Leese, J., Macdonald, G., Kerr, S., Gulka, L., Hoens, A.M., Lum, W., Tran, B.C., Townsend, A.F., and Li, L.C. (2018). "Adding another spinning plate to an already busy life." Benefits and risks in patient partner-researcher relationships: a qualitative study of patient partners' experiences in a Canadian health research setting. *BMJ Open* 8: e022154. doi: 10.1136/bmjopen-2018-022154.

20. Ludwig, C., Graham, I.D., Gifford, W., Lavoie, J., and Stacey, D. (2020). Partnering with frail or seriously ill patients in research: a systematic review. *Research Involvement and Engagement* 6: 52. doi: 10.1186/s40900-020-00225-2.

21. Patient-Centered Outcomes Research Institute. (2013). *PCORI's Strategic Plan.* [Online]. https://www.pcori.org/about-us/pcoris-strategic-plan (accessed 31 August 2021).

22. Price, A., Albarqouni, L., Kirkpatrick, J., Clarke, M., Liew, S.M., Roberts, N., and Burls, A. (2018). Patient and public involvement in the design of clinical trials: an overview of systematic reviews. *Journal of Evaluation in Clinical Practice* 24: 240–253. doi: 10.1111/jep.12805.

23. Rapaport, P., Webster, L., Horsley, R., Kyle, S.D., Kinnunen, K.M., Hallam, B., Pickett, J., Cooper, C., Espie, C.A., and Livingston, G. (2018). An intervention to improve sleep for people living with dementia: reflections on the development and co-production of DREAMS:START (Dementia RElAted Manual for Sleep: STrAtegies for RelaTives). *Dementia (London)* 17: 976–989. doi: 10.1177/1471301218789559.

24. Richards, D.P., Birnie, K.A., Eubanks, K., Lane, T., Linkiewich, D., Singer, L., Stinson, J.N., and Begley, K.N. (2020). Guidance on authorship with and

acknowledgement of patient partners in patient-oriented research. *Research Involvement and Engagement* 6: 38. doi: 10.1186/s40900-020-00213-6.

25. Shippee, N.D., Domecq Garces, J.P., Prutsky Lopez, G.J., Wang, Z., Elraiyah, T.A., Nabhan, M., Brito, J.P., Boehmer, K., Hasan, R., Firwana, B., Erwin, P.J., Montori, V.M., and Murad, M.H. (2015). Patient and service user engagement in research: a systematic review and synthesized framework. *Health Expectations* 18: 1151–1166. doi: 10.1111/hex.12090.

26. Staniszewska, S., Brett, J., Simera, I., Seers, K., Mockford, C., Goodlad, S., Altman, D.G., Moher, D., Barber, R., Denegri, S., Entwistle, A., Littlejohns, P., Morris, C., Suleman, R., Thomas, V., and Tysall, C. (2017). GRIPP2 reporting checklists: tools to improve reporting of patient and public involvement in research. *BMJ* 358: j3453. doi: 10.1136/bmj.j3453.

27. Thompson, J., Bissell, P., Cooper, C.L., Armitage, C.J., and Barber, R. (2014). Exploring the impact of patient and public involvement in a cancer research setting. *Qualitative Health Research* 24: 46–54. doi: 10.1177/1049732313514482.

3.3 Conducting a Research Coproduction Project

A Principles-Based Approach

Joe Langley, Sarah E. Knowles, and Vicky Ward

Key Learning Points

- Coproduction cannot be achieved through using a specific research method. Coproduction is instead an approach to working with knowledge users.

- Researchers can adopt this approach through considering the five principles of coproduction, and through embracing open dialogue and iterative working alongside knowledge users to achieve these in practice. They are not easy tasks, and research structures and processes offer some specific challenges to achieving them in practice.

- Coproduction is not a technique you apply rightly or wrongly, but a journey of learning, and it is not a journey you make alone.

INTRODUCTION

In this chapter we aim to:

1. Illustrate why there is no research coproduction "method" through demonstrating how "traditional" and "non-traditional" methods can be more or less coproductive in action.
2. Describe the five key principles of doing research coproduction and introduce resources that can help researchers understand, plan and enact these principles.
3. Recognize that research coproduction ideals are often challenged by real world practicalities. We will describe common problems to encourage researchers to anticipate such challenges and provide suggestions for how they might be overcome.

"What does research coproduction look like?"
"How do I design a coproduction study?"
"Which is the best method to use to coproduce research?"

These are common questions we are asked by researchers looking for answers around *How* to engage in coproduction. It may disappoint readers to hear there is no "method" of coproduction. Coproduction has been described as "a way of being not a way of doing." This means that we cannot offer a toolkit to guarantee your work is coproduced, or provide a list of approved methods which would enable you to say with certainty that coproduction took place. Perhaps research coproduction could more accurately be described as "a way of **being** *with* and **doing** *with*." The crucial element is that it is a collaboration with knowledge users, rather than a method of accessing them or extracting their perspectives or insights.

Given the above, rather than list specific methods, this chapter will provide guidance and resources to help you consider how you can both embody (be) and enact (do) research coproduction. We signpost examples of tools that help to do this and offer practical suggestions to support researchers in overcoming some common challenges.

Although there are no specific methods that guarantee research coproduction, there are two common processes found across different participatory approaches; specifically dialogue and iteration (Abma and Broerse 2010). Dialogue reflects the need for interaction, for exploration of each other's views. Iteration reflects the need for this exploration to result in change, acknowledging that first attempts (such as a first set of research questions, our first study protocol, or our first design of an intervention) must be seen as beginning a process of seeking and making changes, often multiple times. Iteration reflects humility in working with others, a recognition that our own understanding is incomplete without their knowledge, that making sense of what each person brings and how all these pieces of knowledge "fit together" takes time and commitment to learning from and responding to those we coproduce with.

Underpinning or surrounding these two processes are five key principles of coproduction (Hickey et al. 2018): (a) sharing power, (b) including all perspectives, (c) valuing the knowledge of everyone, (d) reciprocity, and (e) building relationships. These are complexly interrelated, not mutually exclusive. Enacting these key principles, we propose, creates the conditions for the two common processes (dialogue and iteration), which in turn support the shared selection and application of appropriate methods. Before we get into these principles, processes, and challenges, we first want to illustrate what we mean when we say there is no coproduction method.

AIM 1. ILLUSTRATING WHY THERE IS NO RESEARCH COPRODUCTION "METHOD"

Within a coproduction research study, any number of methods, both quantitative and qualitative, may be employed. The research is considered to be coproduced if the process of choosing, applying, and analyzing the results of those methods was a process of dialogue and iteration with knowledge users themselves.

To demonstrate that dialogue and iteration do not necessarily "belong" with specific methods, we have created four descriptions of hypothetical studies (Box 3.3.1). These use two different research methods. The traditional method is a survey that involves asking a sample of respondents to answer specific questions (which can be either qualitative open-ended questions or quantitative ranking or item response questions). The non-traditional method is Lego® Serious Play® (LSP). LSP (Boaz 2016; James 2015) is a participatory method that uses Lego bricks to build metaphorical representations of thoughts, ideas, experiences, and feelings. Individuals build, explain, and combine models in response to specific questions and prompts. Our aim is to demonstrate how both methods can be examples of coproduction, and equally both can be done "about" and not "with."

For the purposes of illustrating the differences we have imagined a team of researchers tasked with understanding the views of mental health service users about a new community service...

In the survey "About, not with" example, we demonstrate how researchers can seek out knowledge user input (on the language used, and on how to promote the study) without it being coproduction. In this, support was sought but the knowledge users did not have direct influence on the process; it was the researchers who chose which feedback to include or discard. The "With, not about" survey example demonstrates how the method can be coproduction. There is collective sense-making about the research findings, with knowledge users as active contributors to analysis. The researchers consider what they can

Box 3.3.1   Coproduction of research examples.

Survey

"About, not with"
(research team
only researchers)

The researchers opt to use a survey. This is posted out to service users in a particular region. They check the language used in the survey with service users and make changes based on the feedback. The survey is sent out and local community groups are asked to promote the survey on social media. The researchers analyse the data and produce an academic paper, which includes a Plain Language Summary.

**Lego®
Serious Play®**

"About, not with"
(research team
only researchers)

The researchers opt to use LSP. They design and organise a one-day LSP workshop, checking the workshop design with service users. They send out publicity, and ask local community groups to promote it on social media. The workshop brings together eight service users and four community service staff. It uncovers views of all 12 participants including change ideas. The researchers cross reference the views with evidence from academic literature and produce an academic paper, which includes a Plain Language Summary. They go on to write an intervention development research proposal seeking funding to develop one of the ideas from the workshop.

Survey

"With, not about"
(research team
includes knowledge
users)

The researchers would like to use a survey method. Through a local trust (health authority) they consult with an established service user (SU) group about the project. The researchers talk about why they are interested in this question, and who would benefit from the research. They discuss the method as an option and why they think it is appropriate. The SU group challenge some of the language, questions and method proposed and suggest additional questions. Some members of the SU group agree to join the researchers to create a research team focused on this topic. Terms of collaboration are agreed. This new team discuss the suggestions and changes proposed and agree which ones will be made. The researchers create, send out, and ask local community groups to promote the survey. The team offer to give a talk to the groups about the study and other research they could become involved in. A collaborative analysis meeting is held, where they present early findings to some of the service users they consulted and together go through a data sense-making process. They collectively agree the priorities and different ways to disseminate the findings.
They give a talk to the wider service user group, another to the community service managers, co-author an academic paper and write a blog post on a community website. They form a wider team with representatives from the community service. Together they write a research proposal to explore themes arising from the survey in more depth.

**Lego®
Serious Play®**

"With, not about"
(research team
includes knowledge
users)

The researchers would like to use the LSP method. Through a local trust (health authority) they consult with an established service user (SU) group about the project. The researchers talk about why they are interested in this question, and who would benefit from the research and different ways they could explore the issue. The researchers discuss their interest in using LSP and why they think it is appropriate. They respond to comments and suggestions from the users about this method and other potential options. Some members of the service user group agree to join the researchers to create a research team focused on this topic. Terms of collaboration are agreed.
The researchers provide some training about the LSP method. Together, they plan, design and organise a one-day workshop. They send out publicity about the event, and ask local community groups to promote it. The workshop brings together eight service users and four community service staff. It is facilitated by one of the researchers. The workshop uncovers views and suggestions of all participants and shared change ideas.
The researcher's cross reference the views with evidence from academic literature and hold a collaborative analysis meeting with the whole team. They collectively agree priorities and different ways to disseminate these. Together they give a talk to the wider service user group, another to the community service managers, co-author an academic paper and write a blog post on a community website. They form a wider team with representatives from the community service. Together they write an intervention development research proposal to seek further funding to develop ideas from the workshop.

offer in return for community support and both analysis and dissemination decisions are made jointly.

In the LSP example version without knowledge user partners ("about, not with") we show that participatory methods can be applied by researchers in "extractive" ways, where findings are wholly "owned" and controlled by the researchers. In the coproductive variation ("with, not about"), we demonstrate that the choice of method is "up-for-debate" and decided by dialogue. We see that knowledge users are engaged in the process throughout. Training is provided to enable them to co-facilitate the chosen method and, after data are generated, they are co-owners of the process, the data, what happens to it, how it is used, and the story that is told about how the research was conducted.

These examples illustrate that it is not the method itself that leads to or constrains coproduction, but how the researchers *and* knowledge users work together. This leads to our next section, where we describe how five principles of research coproduction can help guide approaches to working with knowledge users in research.

AIM 2. FIVE PRINCIPLES OF COPRODUCTION AND RESOURCES TO ENACT THEM

Although no method can guarantee research as coproduction, some methodologies have been developed explicitly with coproduction in mind and may make it easier to enact the five principles. A rich literature exists, which describes the processes and impacts of coproduction through methodologies such as Participatory Action Research, Community Based Participatory Research, and Human-Centered Co-Design; see Vaughn and Jacquez (2020) for an overview. Rather than seeking to describe these approaches here, our goal is to identify from these methods which elements are most conducive to coproduction efforts so that we might support researchers in adopting these elements irrespective of their own methodological background. Throughout, we return to the key processes of dialogue and iteration and pose the following questions we feel researchers should consider asking themselves:

1. Does your approach explicitly elicit, recognize, and use the different kinds of knowledge and expertise that can contribute to the research? Is this done openly and transparently, with the knowledge users themselves? (Dialogue)
2. Does your approach allow "messiness?" Is the decision-making for which changes should occur a collective process where the knowledge users are in a position to change the research in unexpected ways? (Iteration)

Our hypothetical examples demonstrate that, whilst some methods are more amenable to these (e.g., LSP), the choice of method alone does not guarantee this. Researchers need to consider how dialogue and iteration are enabled and enacted in regard to the research itself, not only as approaches to working with participants or data within a study.

This brings us to wider issues around responsibility for, and ownership of, the research and about the inclusion or exclusion of different knowledge user voices; the five key principles of coproduction we mentioned earlier (Hickey et al. 2018). Here we summarize each principle and explain how each might be taken into account during a research project. We will sum up some reflective questions for researchers in Figure 3.3.1.

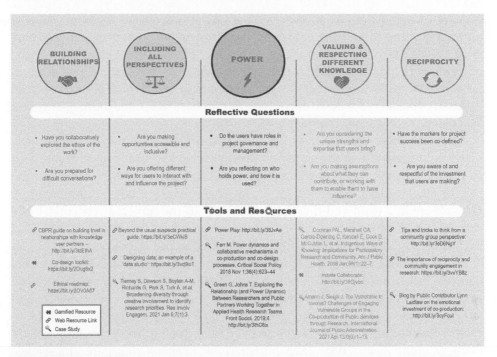

FIGURE 3.3.1   Reflective questions, tools and resources to aid the enactment of the five principles of coproduction.

Sharing Power

"... the research is jointly owned and people work together to achieve a joint understanding..."

This is the headline principle and the one from which all others follow. If coproduction is about shared ownership of, and responsibility for, a research process, then it stands to reason that this cannot happen without shared power.

Power exists in various forms, many of which we are unconscious of. Even if we do know how to hold power in a given setting so as not to deliberately wield power "over" others, there are systems of power and hierarchies, or perceptions of power, which others can see. Acknowledging power differences to begin with becomes an essential starting point. It relies on individuals reflexively assessing their own role, and exploring ownership of decisions about the research and actions within the research with knowledge users. This is best done not by researchers in isolation but with all collaborators. This enables transparency, reveals "hidden" power and considers how power might be re-distributed. It is also something that should be frequently re-visited throughout a project: power – its distribution and use – fluctuates. Continuous reflexivity throughout collaborative working is advocated by a number of authors writing from both academic and knowledge user perspectives (Farr 2018). An initial reflection on the power of the collaborators and a plan to periodically re-visit this reflection sets up a framework for transparent dialogue and iteration for the entire research coproduction project. It is rare for power to be explicitly considered, but we encourage researchers to do this more openly; see Wechsler (2017) for an example.

We recommend considering how power can be shared in research settings. This could include a researcher and knowledge user as joint project leads, with the latter, or a group of knowledge users, as the budget holder and also in the role of chair or lead facilitator. So, knowledge users are not outnumbered by researchers in a team and they have equal say in the project's reporting. They should also avoid the use of professional titles and specialist jargon, which tend to build up boundaries due to perceived knowledge and status.

Perhaps more radically, and thinking beyond the equal sharing of power, we can begin to consider models where knowledge users hold more power, and researchers work to either provide evidence to knowledge users or to advise and support knowledge users in how they might go about gathering evidence themselves. Successful examples of this already exist, such as the Parenting Science Gang (Collins et al. 2020). (See https://www.facebook.com/parentingscience gang for more details) or Heart n Soul at the Hub (see https://heartnsoulat thehub.com for more details.)

Including All Perspectives

"...make sure the research team includes all those who can make a contribution..."

The underpinning imperative of research coproduction is that those impacted by the outcome of a piece of work should have influence over it; moreover, they have a valuable contribution to make to the process. This principle relates to diversity, inclusion, exclusion, representation, access, and how we enable different knowledge users to contribute in full. Whilst practical barriers to such facilitation are easy to identify, others can be less obvious. For example, the ways that individuals process information, communicate, and share ideas can vary significantly. A dialogue (in the broadest sense of diverse forms of communication), and iteratively exploring different forms of engagement, will allow individuals to identify how, when, where, and what they can contribute.

This principle, in action, should include:

- Diversity or multiplicity of perspectives: Are we trying, for example, to present "the" patient voice, rather than engage with a variety of people with different experiences?

- Diversity in terms of inclusion and exclusion: we must move beyond the idea that some groups are "hard to reach" within research. Indeed, researchers themselves can often be immensely hard for knowledge users to reach, whilst the latter can be easy to ignore. Instead, researchers should consider the groups that are "seldom heard/involved" in research, consider why this might be the case, and whether opportunities are accessible to these groups. This can include considering whether capacity building and training is required to give knowledge users the tools they need to be research partners (evidence suggests that, with support, even very technical areas of research, such as data-linkage studies, can be made accessible to knowledge users (Jewell et al. 2019)).
- Diversity of contributions: we learn, communicate, take in and process information and express ourselves in a wide variety of ways. Some favor text or spoken word, others images, graphics, visual language, or kinesthetic and active forms of thinking and communicating. We should not make assumptions about these, nor default to those that are easy for researchers to use and apply; rather, we should embrace the opportunity to support a diversity of forms of thinking and communication (for example, Tierney et al. (2021) explored how producing artworks enabled "easy to ignore" groups to share priorities for research).

Respecting and Valuing the Research Coproduction Partners

"...everyone is of equal importance..."

Coproduction in research involves recognizing the unique expertise and insights that knowledge users can bring (which is very different from methods of research which assess users according to sampling criteria, such as whether they represent a target population). It is worth investing some resources early on into surfacing and recognizing the assets that knowledge users bring. Like power and approaches to including perspectives, some of these may be "hidden" – not obvious to individuals themselves. A variety of team-building and asset-mapping exercises provide structured formats for such dialogue and iteration to enable mutual understanding of expertise and value each person brings to the research.

Alternatively, we also suggest some team game formats which can encapsulate and combine the benefits of dialogue and iteration, a specific example being Initiate:Collaborate. This game was designed for interdisciplinary partners (initially designers and healthcare professionals) about to set out on a project together. The game takes partners through a series of exercises for collective reflection on Context, Connectivity, and Capability, in which they document

their perceptions of each other and what they will bring to the research coproduction. Themes of risk and riskiness are explored within a series of fauxjects
(fake projects) where participants are challenged by different perspectives, ultimately finishing with a greater awareness, appreciation, and respect for what
each individual brings to a partnership.

Reciprocity

"...everybody benefits from working together..."

Reciprocity can be seen as value in action – we need to make good on our claims
so that we value the labor that our partners contribute. The reciprocity principle
asks us to consider how all coproduction partners are benefiting from the coproduction. It requires us to answer that question in the here and now, rather than
consider a future hypothetical benefit which can be typical in research (for
example, the clinicians taking part will benefit in the future when our research
is published and will possibly change the training they are given). These benefits
can, for some knowledge users, be about sharing the research gains with them
– for example, providing training so they can build capacity in research, or
supporting them to be a co-author on an academic output. In other cases, we
need to think more broadly about how we can give back to our coproduction
partners; this might be through direct reimbursement, financially recognizing
their contribution. However, it can happen in other ways; for example, through
helping to promote a service, sharing content or methodological expertise with
an organization more widely, or providing opportunities that can help with
career or personal development. Dialogue is necessary here to openly explore
what will be valuable to different knowledge users.

Still more fundamentally, perhaps, reciprocity can come in the form of recognition of what people have invested. This links strongly to the previous principle
of valuing contributions but here we can be more nuanced about the types of
contribution. Specifically, the emotional labor of coproduction is only beginning
to be recognized. We do not see this effort as a reason not to engage in coproduction, but it does require us to think sensitively about what we are asking of those
involved, how we respect their time and their needs, and how we demonstrate
that we value their contribution. Recognizing the investment and contribution
beyond the practical, financial, and physical to honor their emotions, intellect,
or skills begins to frame the contributions of knowledge users in the same terms
as researchers, which also helps to address the issue of sharing power.

There has been an increased focus on the need to evaluate research coproduction, which is to be welcomed where it contributes to better understanding
the challenges of coproduction and providing learning to improve how coproduction is done. However, any such evaluations need to look beyond the perspectives of researchers and the impacts relevant to researchers (e.g., recruiting

to target more quickly, or publishable papers for the academics involved). The reciprocity principle pushes us to consider impacts and outcomes from the point of view of knowledge users themselves (see Chapter 4.3).

Building Relationships

"...an emphasis on relationships is key to sharing power. There needs to be joint understanding and consensus and clarity over roles and responsibilities. It is also important to value people and unlock their potential..."

This principle comes full circle to the first principle – the sharing of power; and it encompasses the other three principles simultaneously. When people value each other, relationships form, grow, and flourish. Evaluations of coproduced research repeatedly emphasize the importance of relationships for effective coproduction. There are ways to facilitate relationships, through encouraging partners to learn about each other, and dedicating time to do this. However, it is important to try to go beyond "managed" relationships. There needs to be a level of trust, openness to vulnerability, and recognition of imperfections on all sides.

A key part of this, in our experience, can seem like the very thing we would want to avoid: debate and dissent, even conflict. This "storming" part of a coproduction project can be essential to surface the differences between researcher perspectives and knowledge user perspectives, and to grapple with these rather than try to avoid them. In our experience, knowledge user partners reflect on these debates positively, as evidence that researchers were open to disagreement and respected differences enough to explore them. So, this demonstrates how dialogue and iteration are important in terms of relationships: the researcher must be willing to engage in open dialogue with knowledge users about the process being undertaken and to change their approach and their mind.

This can be challenging for researchers, and we do not underestimate the complexity of engaging in what can be difficult conversations. We encourage researchers to think about how they can be supported to do this. Perhaps there is a supervisor or mentor with experience of research coproduction who can help debrief afterwards? Do you have access to training or support in facilitating group discussions? Have you set ground rules for the discussions, to make sure everyone shares their perspective in constructive ways? The selection of methods can play a role in these dialogues. Methods that support richer self-expression of experiences and perspective, and externalizing these, should enable dialogue about specific experiences or perspectives rather than the person who expressed them.

We also encourage researchers to think about fostering relationships between different knowledge user groups, not just knowledge users and researchers themselves. Traditionally, separation of stakeholder groups, perhaps argued on the basis of ethics or even power, has allowed researchers to work with separate groups of patients, professionals, or other stakeholder groups. These models centralize control and power of the process with the researchers. Methods such as Experience Based Co-Design emphasize the need for all stakeholders to work together, and demonstrate how more powerful insights can be generated if researchers try to create spaces for all knowledge users to collaborate, rather than work in isolation.

AIM 3. RESEARCH COPRODUCTION IN THE REAL WORLD: CHALLENGES AND WAYS FORWARD

There are many strong champions of coproduction and occasionally dogmatic-sounding narratives on how coproduction "should" be done. From an idealistic point of view, the five principles appear incredibly challenging and potentially impossible to meet. The practical realities of the systems and cultures within which research often occurs can present many barriers. However, we are keen to support people to try and to learn. This learning itself can be a journey of mutual discovery, and is an opportunity to develop unique collaborations, inspire each other, and achieve change. We believe the very best training comes from coproduction with the humility to be open to both knowledge users' critical feedback and to the transformative possibilities that arise when working beyond the usual academic borders. We hope the following suggestions provide some reassurance that challenges are surmountable, and that learning about the best ways to address them is ongoing.

Who to Work With

Deciding who to work with when coproducing research can be complex. Stakeholder management, analysis, and mapping can potentially be Machiavellian: the people who do these activities hold the power to manipulate outcomes so that the stakeholders "selected" endorse a desired endpoint. These activities also tend to be technocratic rather than democratic by considering who will be impacted by the project and how best to mitigate (almost in an optics or public relations management sense) negative impacts.

We support a careful consideration of all stakeholders and use of the tools listed above to do this. In addition, we recommend two things: (1) this is done in dialogue and iteratively with others, as we will explain; and (2) it considers how/ when stakeholders can and would prefer to engage in the coproduction process. It is important to accommodate different preferences flexibly through multiple channels or media.

On the first issue, an evolving map of stakeholders who continuously ask the question all stakeholders ask, "Who else should be involved?" takes the selective power away from the researcher and invites wider consideration of the impact and influence of the proposed work.

On the second issue, the global COVID-19 pandemic resulted in travel restrictions and national stay-at-home orders. During this time, our experiences of socially distant co-design forced us to consider who was engaging, how they were engaging, and when they were engaging (Davis et al. 2021; Langley et al. 2021), and the dangers of excluding stakeholders when a single mode of engagement, that is easy for researchers to use, is adopted uncritically. During this time, home computer and online meeting platforms became the unchallenged default mode of engaging service users, with very little exploration of the exclusion arising from variations in digital access and literacy. An example from our exploration of these issues used local radio and social media, posted activity kits and digital co-design tools, and scheduled online workshops. Partners (staff, researchers, and local residents) were able to choose and change their mode of engagement, depending on which was most accessible to them at any given point in the process.

When to Collaborate

In some approaches, coproduction can occur at particular points within a research process and may not occur throughout. Opinions vary as to whether partial coproduction can be called coproduction at all. (Action Researchers, for example, adhere to the "stick of rock" principle, that a study has coproduction running throughout and the study viewed at any point would reveal its sticky core.) We do not have, nor seek, the authority to rule on this, but we do recommend that researchers choose their language carefully. "An evaluation of a coproduced survey tool," for example, is different to "A coproduced evaluation of a survey tool."

Figure 3.3.2 demonstrates a simplified model of the research process. Although, in an ideal world, research coproduction happens from start to finish, in a continuous research process, with the same stakeholders involved throughout, this is rarely the case. The life course of most research enquiries is fractured and fragmented, often spanning many years, with multiple attempts to secure funding for some stages, no funding for other stages, and frequent gaps, pauses, or changes of direction/emphasis within external factors (such as funders' priorities, or staff availability).

We also suggest that it is the right of research coproduction partners (including researchers) to engage and disengage from a process, without the process necessarily pausing or stopping. Examples of this could include a researcher going on parental leave whilst a coproduced research project continues, and for

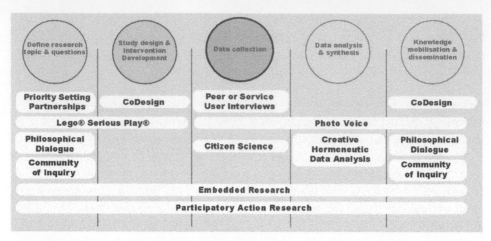

FIGURE 3.3.2   Examples of methods that facilitate coproduction at different points within a research process.

them to rejoin on their return to work. Equally, a two-year coproduced research project focused on a narrow age group (for example, adolescents aged 16–18) would require a "flow" of coproduction partners in the target age range. Similarly, a four-year medical device research program for people with Motor Neurone Disease (MND) might experience some coproduction partner deaths whilst people with newly diagnosed MND might wish to join. Applying a criterion of working with the same group throughout can inadvertently create a barrier through "membership" of coproduction becoming exclusive, closed groups. We suggest considering how to explicitly capture the learning generated by different individuals (so that knowledge is not lost when those individuals leave) but with plans that allow flexibility for new contributors to join.

Another common question we are asked regarding "when" relates to whether there are specific methods that are most appropriate for coproduction at particular stages of research. Although it may seem contrary to our argument that individual methods cannot "be" coproduction, it is true that certain methods have been adopted specifically to facilitate coproduction at particular points (for example, priority-setting partnerships are clearly intended to help collaboratively agree on research priorities). We provide further examples in Figure 3.3.2, but do not suggest these are the best or only methods appropriate, and, as illustrated earlier, do not guarantee research has been coproduced unless they are used collaboratively with researcher users.

Institutional Power

When setting out on research coproduction initiatives, we must be aware of institutional power. A common response to raising the issue of power is for researchers to respond "But I don't have power! I have to do [what my PI says/

what the funder wants/what the journals expect, etc.]" While our earlier comment about personal power asks researchers to consider the power they do have, it is still important to acknowledge wider issues that impact on how research is conducted. Research on coproduction has recognized how academic settings and structures can restrict effective coproduction. For example, research coproduction in which knowledge users can genuinely influence and change research plans can be difficult to achieve when researchers need to provide exact protocols of their work in advance, and specify intended outcomes (Madden et al. 2020). This can limit the space that researchers have to learn from the knowledge users. Production of academic papers and of further grants are the main career goals, which may come into conflict with other knowledge users' needs. In our own work, we often create templates for all individuals, including the academics and others collaborating in professional capacities, that ask people to specify their goals for, and expectations of, the project. They include prompts to consider various outputs, endpoints, or goals. These are shared with all partners and a map of shared expectations and goals is created. We are then able to collectively highlight goals or expectations that may be in tension with each other and decide on actions to amend goals or define ways to navigate and monitor these tensions. We keep the map as a work in progress, frequently revisited and updated.

EXPECTATIONS OF HEALTH SERVICES RESEARCH

Particular challenges can be encountered when applying coproduction within a health research context. These include the following three common issues:

1. The blurring of data collection and data analysis: in a research study and in research papers, typically data collection and analysis of that data are considered as distinct phases of research. In coproduction, when reporting the decisions made it may not be possible to differentiate these stages clearly. To do so would apply a framework that views the knowledge users as providing data that is then separately analyzed (with the implication that researchers needed to assess and interpret the data for results to be produced). In this scenario, the researchers have power over the data and the contributions, rather than this being shared. In practice, coproduction involves a dynamic process of concurrently generating and analyzing contributions. Different research disciplines have different levels of familiarity with this way of working. In our experience, it is welcomed as standard practice in Design journals, but typically contested in Health Services journals, where reviewers expect to see analysis "done to" the data.

2. Applying research ethics processes to coproduction practice: in the UK, Patient and Public Involvement is considered to be outside of traditional

ethical approval processes. Patients themselves have argued that completing an ethics application about a coproduction event steers the researcher to think of themselves and the knowledge users as separate, to see the activity as research on those users rather than a collaboration with them. But this, of course, does not mean that coproduction is without ethical considerations around burden and costs to those involved (see Chapter 3.2). Having formal ethics approvals (that might not cover such things) does not mean we can avoid consideration of how to manage and support partnerships in coproduced research. Careful planning is needed around issues such as confidentiality, support, and anticipation of burden, especially but not exclusively when working with service users (Pandya-Wood et al. 2017). The difference, as we have tried to illustrate throughout, is that this planning should occur with the knowledge users, not about them.

3. Debating how "representative" the knowledge users need to be: a very common perception is that knowledge users who become involved in research should be "representative" of the wider population (Maguire and Britten 2017). This applies a consideration about sampling, an important aspect of research methodology, to the coproduction process, and in doing so positions knowledge users as "participants" or sources of data, as opposed to considering them as partners or collaborators. (It is very notable that this debate tends to happen when those knowledge users are patients or service users, and not when they are different kinds of professionals.)

CONCLUSION

Many researchers are looking for answers around how to do research coproduction. But coproduction is as much a way of being as a way of doing. In this chapter we have illustrated how various methods and approaches can be more or less coproductive depending on how closely researchers relate to, and work with, knowledge users. This demonstrates the importance of the mindset that researchers need to bring to coproduction to be with people in coproduction.

We have described five key principles of research coproduction, defined by others, then introduced resources that can help researchers understand, plan, and enact these principles. These provide practical tools to support researchers in doing coproduction with people.

Finally, we have described common challenges of research coproduction and made some suggestions for how they might be overcome.

REFERENCES

1. Abma, T.A. and Broerse, J.E. (2010). Patient participation as dialogue: setting research agendas. *Health Expectations* 13: 160–173. doi: 10.1111/j.1369-7625.2009.00549.x.

2. Boaz, A. (2016). Creativity in Co-creation. *Integration and Implementation Insights*. https://i2insights.org/2016/08/04/creativity-in-co-creation (accessed 19 May 2021).

3. Collins, S., Brueton, R., Graham, T.G., Organ, S., Strother, A., West, S.E., and McKendree, J. (2020). Parenting Science Gang: radical co-creation of research projects led by parents of young children. *Research Involvement and Engagement* 6: 9. doi: 10.1186/s40900-020-0181-z.

4. Davis, A., Wallace, N., Langley, J., and Gwilt, I. (2021). Low-contact co design: considering more flexible spatiotemporal models for the co design workshop. *Strategic Design Research Journal* 14: 124–137. doi: 10.4013/sdrj.2021.141.11.

5. Farr, M. (2018). Power dynamics and collaborative mechanisms in coproduction and co-design processes. *Critical Social Policy* 38: 623–644. doi: 10.1177/0261018317747444.

6. Hickey, G., Brearley, S., Coldham, T., Denegri, S., Green, G., Staniszewska, S., Tembo, D., Torok, K., and Turner, K. (2018). *Guidance on Coproducing a Research Project*. Southampton: NIHR INVOLVE. https://www.invo.org.uk/wp-content/uploads/2019/04/Copro_Guidance_Feb19.pdf.

7. James, A. (2015). *Innovating in the Creative Arts with LEGO*. York: Higher Education Academy. https://www.advance-he.ac.uk/knowledge-hub/innovating-creative-arts-lego.

8. Jewell, A., Pritchard, M., Barrett, K., Green, P., Markham, S., McKenzie, S., Oliver, R., Wan, M., Downs, J., and Stewart, R. (2019). The Maudsley Biomedical Research Centre (BRC) data linkage service user and carer advisory group: creating and sustaining a successful patient and public involvement group to guide research in a complex area. *Research Involvement and Engagement* 5: 20. doi: 10.1186/s40900-019-0152-4.

9. Langley, J., Wallace, N., Davis, A., Gwilt, I., Knowles, S., Partridge, R., Wheeler, G., and Ankeny, U. (2021). COVID co-design does not *HAVE* to be digital! Why "which platform should we use?" should not be your first question. In: *COVID-19 and Co-production in Health and Social Care Research, Policy, and Practice: Volume 2: Co-production Methods and Working Together at a Distance* (ed. O. Williams, D. Tembo, J. Ocloo, M. Kaur, G. Hickey, M. Farr, and P. Beresford), 1e, 85–96. Bristol: Bristol University Press.

10. Madden, M., Morris, S., Ogden, M., Lewis, D., Stewart, D., and McCambridge, J. (2020). Producing co-production: reflections on the development of a complex intervention. *Health Expectations* 23: 659–669. doi: 10.1111/hex.13046.

11. Maguire, K. and Britten, N. (2017). "How can anybody be representative for those kind of people?" Forms of patient representation in health research, and why it is always contestable. *Social Science & Medicine* 183: 62–69. doi: 10.1016/j.socscimed.2017.04.049.

12. Pandya-Wood, R., Barron, D.S., and Elliott, J. (2017). A framework for public involvement at the design stage of NHS health and social care research: time to develop ethically conscious standards. *Research Involvement and Engagement* 3: 6. doi: 10.1186/s40900-017-0058-y.

13. Tierney, S., Dawson, S., Boylan, A.M., Richards, G., Park, S., Turk, A., and Babatunde, O. (2021). Broadening diversity through creative involvement to identify research priorities. *Research Involvement and Engagement* 7: 3. doi: 10.1186/s40900-020-00244-z.

14. Vaughn, L.M. and Jacquez, F. (2020). Participatory research methods – choice points in the research process. *Journal of Participatory Research Methods* 1: 13244. doi: 10.35844/001c.13244.

15. Wechsler, A.M. (2017). Overcoming the Venn diagram: learning to be a co-passionate navigator in community-based participatory research. *Research for All* 1: 147–157. doi: 10.18546/RFA.01.1.12.

3.4 The View from Within Organizational Strategies for Effective Research Partnerships

Sarah Bowen, Ian D. Graham, and Ingrid Botting

Key Learning Points

- Although appreciation of the experience and work context of organizational partners is essential for development of effective research partnerships, little attention has been directed to understanding the perspectives and needs of leaders and managers of healthcare organizations.
- There are two main approaches to increasing organizational research capacity: creating some form of "interface" with academia; developing internal embedded research capacity. Understanding the potential advantages and disadvantages of each can help organizations plan appropriate action.
- Effective initiatives within either approach require that organizations undertake key foundational activities: develop a shared understanding of

Research Coproduction in Healthcare, First Edition. Edited by
Ian D. Graham, Jo Rycroft-Malone, Anita Kothari, and Chris McCutcheon.
© 2022 John Wiley & Sons Ltd. Published 2022 by John Wiley & Sons Ltd.

the concept of research and its benefits to the organization; clarify the roles it wishes to play; and develop policy, structures, and processes to support and protect the organization.

- Healthcare organizations wishing to engage with academics in research partnerships are encouraged to focus on ongoing organization-to-organization relationships; to clearly communicate their expectations; and to build a plan to address potential pitfalls of such partnerships to their organization.

BACKGROUND/INTRODUCTION

One important evolution in the current health research landscape is re-consideration of the role of healthcare organizations in health research. This attention results both from a greater awareness that research conducted in collaboration with intended users is more likely to be relevant and used (Boaz et al. 2015; Oliver et al. 2014); and from the requirement of many health research funders for a health system partner on funding applications (McLean et al. 2018). These developments have led many health organizations to clarify their role in research and determine what research-related activities they will engage in – and how.

Because their mandate is to *deliver quality healthcare*, health organizations have historically played a marginal, and largely responsive, role in research. They have been expected to *use* research that has been produced by academics, and also to *provide access* to their data, patients, or sites in order to support university-based research projects. Only recently has there been exploration of the roles of these organizations as research *partners*, playing a meaningful (or even leadership) role in coproduction of research, and the implications of coproduction roles for researchers who wish to work with them. As a result, while much has been learned about issues related to *research use* by decision-makers (Oliver et al. 2004), less is known about effective strategies for *coproduction of research*.

We have observed that, although a number of creative models of academic-health system partnership have been reported in the literature in recent years, such examples are not widespread, and their applicability to diverse contexts is unclear. Also, although recent research has proposed "guiding principles," "mechanisms," or "features" of effective collaboration (Boaz et al. 2018; Bowen et al. 2017; Greenhalgh et al. 2016; Rycroft-Malone et al. 2016), there is little to guide an organization in developing research responses that enable it – in ways that are appropriate to the unique characteristics of their organization – to engage as an equal in the research production process (Gagliardi et al. 2017; Hoekstra et al. 2018; Hofmeyer et al. 2012). Reflecting the earlier, more passive, assumptions of the role of health organizations in research, resources focus largely on supporting researchers in developing skills in communicating research findings, or increasing the capacity of health system personnel to access and use research in planning and service delivery[1] (de Moissac et al. 2019).

In addition, while there is extensive literature on research partnerships in general, little research addresses the specific issues in partnerships between academic researchers and healthcare personnel (particularly the leaders and managers of health organizations). These partnerships have unique characteristics not necessarily found in other forms of collaborative research (e.g., patient engagement in research, community-based health research). Guidelines for health services and policy research partnership are often extrapolated from the community collaboration literature (Kothari et al. 2011). However, while many principles and characteristics identified through research with grassroots community groups are applicable to partnerships between researchers and healthcare organizations, differences in barriers, benefits, and strategies may also be expected. As one example: research with patients and community members is usually based on assumptions of a power imbalance in favor of the researcher. Some of the focus has, therefore, been on the challenges of what has been called "researching down." In contrast, much health services research involves researcher relationships with well-established power and governance structures and high-status individuals ("researching up" in the case of trainees and junior researchers; "researching across" for some senior researchers) (Marx and Treharne 2018). Ethical and logistical processes established to protect vulnerable communities may not be useful or needed in relationships with those in powerful positions.

An important gap in the current research is that, while issues faced by academics in research partnerships have been well-documented in the literature, the voices of health system leaders and health personnel are largely absent (Bartunek and Rynes 2014; Nyström et al. 2018). While academics and health system personnel often identify similar challenges to research collaboration (e.g., timelines for action), healthcare personnel often emphasize barriers not reported in the literature: the impact of organizational stress and restructuring; researchers who are unready to work in a fast-paced healthcare environment, have been identified as major barriers (Bowen et al. 2019). In addition, many within health organizations find research, as currently defined and conducted, unhelpful to their work, suggesting that health research should be redefined and promoted (Bowen et al. 2019).

Despite support of health system management for the *principles* of collaborative research (Bowen et al. 2017), in practice these collaborations commonly

---

[1] One exception to this trend is the recent release of a guide designed for health organizations, "Its time to talk about – Our Relationship with Research" (Bowen, S, Graham ID, Botting, 2021). Available at https://iktrn.ohri.ca/resources/ikt-resources.

experience many challenges (Bowen et al. 2017; Ellen et al. 2018; Jessani et al. 2018). Many are concerned about the lack of genuine collaboration on the part of some academic researchers (who may be perceived as unprepared to respond to the actual needs and priorities of healthcare organizations) (Bowen et al. 2017; Rycroft-Malone et al. 2016; Wehrens et al. 2010).

We propose that recognition of the experience and work context of health system partners is essential for development of effective partnerships: giving voice to health system perspectives and concerns will also support researchers in developing authentic partnerships. Our aim in this chapter is, therefore, to build on the emerging research which describes the experiences of health system leaders and staff with research partnerships. We suggest initial frameworks, principles, and strategies to assist organizations as they explore how they will respond to the changing expectations of their research role.

HOW SHOULD ORGANIZATIONS RESPOND TO THE EXPECTATIONS OF A RESEARCH PARTNERSHIP?

Before Beginning to Plan for "Research Partnerships": Clarifying the Concepts of "Partnership" and "Research"

Healthcare organizations are tremendously diverse, not only in size, complexity, focus, staffing, and available resources, but also in their maturity in research understanding and leadership. While there can be no "one-size-fits-all" model of organizational research engagement, all organizations can benefit from careful consideration of the issues and challenges in any action – whether to develop internal research capacity or to establish/enhance partnerships with academic researchers.

Not all organizations have an interest in research coproduction. Some feel they are not sufficiently resourced to play an active role in research production (or even to access the quality research on which organizational programs are based). Instead, they choose to focus on implementing and maintaining standards set by other bodies. Other organizations invest resources in accessing, assessing, and implementing quality research into their planning and programs.

While appropriate use of existing research is critical for any health or social care organization, we focus our discussion here on the issues facing organizations that wish to explore their role in *research production*. These may vary greatly: from responding to academic researchers' requests for access or support to researcher-initiated projects; to active engagement in all phases of a research project; to initiating research activities that address an organization's problems. It is important to recognize this diversity in types of research "partnership" activities – many participants will have different assumptions, and framing of a partnership will affect how it plays out in practice (Holmes 2020). It is often quite appropriate for an organization to select different kinds and levels of "partnership" around particular projects, though assumptions about what "partnership" means may not be shared.

There are two important distinctions that must be considered in our discussion of research partnerships. The first is whether the proposed research is driven by system needs and priorities or by researcher and/or research funder interest: Is the organizational role *reactive*, or *proactive*? For some time, healthcare organizations have been required to respond to requests for data access, and sometimes to requests for access to particular staff, programs, or sites. The increasing requirement – particularly in health services research – that researchers find a "health system partner" to support a research funding application has, however, increased both the number and types of requests a healthcare organization may receive. They may be asked to provide moral, in-kind, or even financial support for the research. They may also be asked to play a range of roles in the research itself – from helping to frame the research question, to sitting on an "advisory" body, to analyzing and interpreting data, to planning implementation. Rarely, however, are these organizations included as full partners in decision-making, including budgeting and financial management, and the demands on their organizational time and resources are rarely reimbursed, even when there is little or no benefit to the research organization. Even less common is research which addresses a problem identified by a health organization.

The second critical distinction is between *individual* and *organizational* partnerships. To date, most research partnerships are not between, for example, a particular university and a health region, but rather between one or more researchers, and a manager/director of a specific program. This arrangement creates vulnerabilities for both the organization and the researchers, as well as the research itself. While there have been extremely effective individual partnerships, organization-to-organization relationships are needed if the full benefits of research partnerships are to be achieved.

If there is confusion about the concept of "partnership," there is often even less clarity and consensus on the idea of "research" within healthcare organizations. There are often major differences – not only between organizations but within the same organization – in understanding of what "research is" and how it relates to quality improvement (QI) and other knowledge-generating activities, such as evaluation (Bowen et al. 2019). Individual staff may define research quite narrowly, limiting it to only one area (for example, basic laboratory or clinical research) or certain methods of research (e.g., randomized control trials), and may not fully appreciate the potential contributions or an expanded research role. Many confuse research with simple data analysis, while others consider a quick "internet" search on a specific topic to be research.

In addition to often limited perspectives on the scope and variety of research activities, many leaders, managers, and staff have not found research relevant to their work, or responsive to their needs (Barnes et al. 2015; Bowen et al. 2019). They may see research as limited to specific research projects, supported by research funding agencies and – often – driven by "ivory tower" interests. They may have had experience of researchers and regard them as out of touch with the realities of care provision, or they may have encountered research processes which are insensitive to the real-time demands of care delivery (Bowen et al. 2005; Jessani et al. 2018). Negative experiences range from frustration at the token roles allocated to health personnel, to feelings of being "used," to major incidents that have required legal or human resource intervention (Bowen et al. 2019).

There is also commonly a lack of consensus about how research "fits" with other knowledge-generating activities within the organization: some view activities such as QI, evaluation, and research as points on a continuum, others as distinct activities that "belong" in different places (e.g., QI as an organizational responsibility, evaluation delegated to external contractors, and research belonging to the world of academia) (Bowen et al. 2019). Many health organizations have made major commitments to QI initiatives and may feel that this removes the need for greater attention to "research."

First Things First: Preparing to Become a Research Partner

There are several important preparatory activities that allow organizations to make thoughtful decisions on how they will increase their research capacity or engage in research partnerships. These activities are often iterative in nature, and many organizations will undertake them at the same time.

Developing Shared Understanding

The common lack of clarity on the core concept of "research," and its relationship to other important organizational activities, means that many organizations may need to devote significant effort to building shared understandings before initiating any action. It is important not only to promote a definition of research that encompasses the many different types of research, but also to help staff distinguish between "*research and its potential to be useful to the organization*" and "*my personal experience of one researcher/research project*." Discussion is needed on how – if research was truly responsive – it could support and enhance the work of the organization. Research must be "re-imagined" in ways that both enable *useful* research activities within the organization, and also support and enhance other knowledge-generating activities, such as QI (Bowen et al. 2019).

Integration of "research and evaluative thinking" into discussions is one way to begin to illustrate, in practical ways, the broad scope of research and the useful roles it could play within the organization. See Table 3.4.1. for some examples of how emerging issues and questions can be used to promote in-depth discussion. Other strategies include: ensuring relevant research reports; reports from research-related committees are standing items on meeting agendas, either "for discussion" or for information; and, preparing questions to support evidence-informed discussion around agenda items.

TABLE 3.4.1   Sample discussion questions.

Presenting Problem	Sample discussion questions
How will the organization respond to the request from University X to sign on as a partner for their research proposal?	Do we have a clear research policy? What are our priorities for research involvement? Are our procedures for reviewing requests adequate to protect the organization? What will be demanded of staff time and organizational resources? What are our expectations of the research team?
Do we need to have an external evaluation/ review of Program X?	What are we hoping to learn? What skills are needed to answer this question? What questions require an external review rather an internal evaluation or original research? How often do such questions come up and what guidelines do we have for how to respond to them? What are advantages and disadvantages of internal vs. external evaluations? How do we find a research partner to help us?
We don't have the information we need to know how to respond to the crisis in our ER: what do we do?	What information do we have in-house? Are there existing systematic or scoping reviews that could guide us? Which program areas need to be involved in coming up with a solution? How do we find a research partner who can help us solve this problem?
The X Institute has just released a report on the costs of chronic disease management: what do we need to do as a health service organization?	Who can provide an analysis of the report to assess its applicability to our organization? Should we develop in-house capacity to do this? Can we find a research partner to help with this? What is current evidence on the effectiveness of our current programs and services to respond to current disease prevalence? Do we need an evaluation? What is the latest evidence of effective interventions?
Should we change Policy X in light of COVID-19?	What is the latest evidence on this question? How strong is this evidence? How do we remain current in a rapidly evolving environment? What strategies do we have for communicating policy to staff, patients and community? What skills are needed to support us in this?
How can we best design a comprehensive service to address mental health needs among the elderly?	What do we know about this population in our catchment area? Is more investigation needed? If so, what is the best way to do it? What can we learn from the literature about effective mental health services for this population? What is the evidence that these interventions would be appropriate in our context? What different forms of expertise and experience must be involved in designing our response? How do we plan for effective implementation? How do we build in evaluation activities that enables evaluation of service implementation, and promotes ongoing improvement and needed adaptation?

(Continued)

TABLE 3.4.1   (Continued)

Presenting Problem	Sample discussion questions
As we do not have the budget to continue to fund both Program X and Program Y, which one will we cancel?	On what evidence do we make this decision? Are the programs reflecting latest evidence or are changes needed? Why is the choice only between these two programs? What can we learn from the literature about most effective interventions for the issues the programs are meant to address?
Should we approve funds to hire another data analyst?	What is the purpose of this role? Do we need another analyst or are other roles to support use of evidence (knowledge dissemination, evaluation specialist) of higher importance? What can these roles do that a data analyst cannot do?

Determining Current Organizational Position

Some organizations have invested in planning processes to determine how they will engage in research, and have built concrete responses that reflect their goals and priorities. Many more organizations, however, have developed a response reactively, often to cope with demands from academic bodies seeking partnership on a specific research project. Some organizations address requests on a case-by-case basis (with decisions often varying based on who receives the request). Existing systems for evaluating requests may be based on actions taken in other organizations. As a result, current practice may not be the best fit for the particular context.

If the potential for effective, sustainable engagement in research is to be optimized, organizations must first consider how their research-related activities fit with the organization's goals, priorities, and strategic plan, and what current supports are already in place. It is useful to consider such questions as:

- Is commitment to research, or specific research-related activities, clearly identified in the organization's mission and values? In its strategic plan? Is more discussion needed?
- How committed are those in key leadership roles (board, executive, clinical lead) to research in the organization? How knowledgeable are they about the full range of research approaches and methods?
- What is the organization's current involvement in research? Is there a comprehensive inventory of research projects or collaborations with which the organization is involved? How did these come about? How are they intended to help the organization achieve its goals? How are they supported?

- What is the organization's current position on its role in research (Table 3.4.2)? What implications does this have going forward? Is there openness to revisiting this position?

TABLE 3.4.2   Organizational current position.

Description of current program/ organizational position	Current challenges	What issues should organization consider?	How can research help meet this challenge?
We depend on standards set by other bodies (e.g., provincial/ professional standards and guidelines) to ensure quality care.	Ensuring that standards are met.	Without careful attention to implementation in context, standards may not be met.	"*Knowledge translation/* implementation science" can help determine effective communication and Implementation strategies. Evaluation research expertise can inform quality assurance and improvement efforts.
We are committed to ensuring our programs reflect the latest research in order to optimize the care we provide.	Accessing and evaluating current research in a timely and ongoing manner. Ensuring findings are assessed, in collaboration with organizational leadership, for applicability to the local context Facilitating uptake of findings (including needed organizational change).	Research must be assessed for its applicability in specific organizational/ program context.	"*Knowledge translation/* implementation science" can help determine effective communication and Implementation strategies.

(Continued)

TABLE 3.4.2   (Continued)

Description of current program/ organizational position	Current challenges	What issues should organization consider?	How can research help meet this challenge?
We want to respond appropriately to requests from external sources for access to our data, patients or sites, or to partner with them on research projects.	Clarifying organizational research goals and priorities. Developing, implementing, communicating, and evaluating organizational policy, processes and structures to support consistent organizational research action.	Without organization-wide policy and associated procedures managers and clinicians may make individual decisions. This may result in a) additional stress on burdened staff/programs, b) overcommitment of organizational resources, c) unforeseen issues requiring management intervention, and d) missed opportunities to share findings with potential relevance to other areas of the organization.	Evidence-informed research policy can provide structure for consistent action in response to organizational priorities. Effective research ethics and access/ impact review processes ensure policy is followed, protect the organization, and facilitate research useful to the organization. Research coordination skills facilitate processes, positive communication, and organizational knowledge of research partners.
We would like to play an active role in research activities that could help address the major problems facing our organization	Developing a model for research participation that is feasible for the organization and supports organizational goals and priorities.	Both clarity on a) organizational priorities, and b) realistic assessment of needs/potential of in-house research expertise, or effective research partnerships is needed.	Research expertise to undertake, coordinate and oversee activities. Knowledge of research evidence on effective research partnerships.

Description of current program/ organizational position	Current challenges	What issues should organization consider?	How can research help meet this challenge?
		Strategies to ensure all program areas are supported in staying current with quality research in their areas, and to respond to external research-related requests are also needed.	

Assessing Organizational Readiness

Organizations must then ensure that there is both commitment to, and readiness to engage in, research-related activities. Pre-conditions associated with development of an effective sustainable approach to engaging in research partnerships include:

- *Commitment to the importance of research from organizational leadership* – board, CEO, executive management, and clinical leads – is essential. Recent research has identified organizational leadership as a critical factor in establishing and supporting effective research partnerships, as well as in creating a research-positive organizational culture (Bowen et al. 2019).
- *Organizational consensus on a broad definition of "research" and it's fit with other knowledge-generating activities.* It is essential to build among board, senior and middle management, and staff a shared, comprehensive understanding of research, including the diversity (in approach, field of focus, methods) of research. Discussions should begin – but not end – with the board, senior management, clinical leads, and those within the organization with research experience.
- *A shared vision of the benefits of research and research partnerships to the organization.* Building a shared understanding of the potential benefits of research involvement within the organization (the contributions it can

make to developing an effective strategic plan, to meeting organizational objectives, and to supporting the work of staff) can be a major challenge. If research partnership is viewed as just one more demand on limited time and resources, it is not likely to be prioritized – "partnerships" must fit as a "solution" to the organization meeting its goals – as an integral component of decision-making in a learning organization.

Building a Strong Foundation

As organizations move from thinking about their role in research, to developing a model appropriate for its particular context, care will be needed to ensure a) inclusion of key stakeholders in planning activities; b) effective communication of the goals of the organization's intended role and approach to research engagement; and c) development of appropriate policies, structures, and processes to support effective action.

Inclusion of Key Stakeholders in Planning

Because there are many different "kinds" of research, no one research approach (or single researcher) can bring the breadth of skills that an organization may need, either now or in the future. It may be a challenge to ensure that planning is not limited to, or dominated by, certain research areas, specific types of research question, or one or two research methods. A research team with strength in randomized control clinical trials may not appreciate the importance of, or have the expertise to conduct, multi-method community-based research. A researcher who has specialized in mental health may not have an interest in responding to organizational concern about infectious diseases.

Voices around the planning table should also include the diversity of both the catchment community, and of staff units and point-of-care providers. At a time when there is increasing recognition of the exclusion of many sectors of society from decision-making activities, it is particularly important to ensure that selection of research priorities and framing of research questions is not limited to certain research approaches, or to the perspectives and experience of those currently in decision-making roles. Research can also be an invaluable tool for integrating the voices of community and point of care to inform change. Strategies to consider include: invitations to academic centers to make presentations on types of research; integration of the expertise of staff in outreach / community development roles; and ensuring meaningful participation of clinical and program areas, as well as agencies and services outside of the organization.

Effective Communication of the Organization's Goals for Research Partnership

An organization must be clear about what it wants to achieve through its research involvement, and how such involvement will provide a strategic advantage. These objectives will need to be communicated throughout the organization, as well as to potential partners and key organizations in the community. One aspect of public communication is a clear message on what its stance will be with the research community. Is the organization happy to respond to researcher requests and assess these requests on a case-by-case basis? Will it establish criteria for research collaboration, and policies to ensure that these criteria are met? Will it contribute only to research activities that answer questions of priority to the organization, and in the time frame the organization requires it? If it develops internal research capacity (e.g., hiring evaluators, researchers, or knowledge brokers) how will these individuals or units relate to academic research bodies?

Policy, Structures, and Processes to Support a Research Response

Key policies, structures, and processes are necessary to support the organization's research activities. Without adequate and appropriate infrastructure, initiatives can easily become vulnerable to changes in leadership; to being downgraded in the face of organizational crises; and to marginalization from organizational decision-making. Even small initial efforts need the support of policy, structure, and clear processes and procedures.

Policy should address the organization's role in research: how research will be used to inform policy setting, strategic planning, and priority setting; relationships with external entities (e.g., government, university); who is responsible for research oversight; site, data, personnel, and patient access; criteria for organizational participation in research; access and ethics review processes and requirements for research reporting.

Organizational research structure is also needed: identified roles for research responsibility and accountability at the most senior level; position descriptions for responsibility areas; and, clarity on relationships with QI, evaluation, and other knowledge-generating activities.

Clear processes for decision-making around research are essential. These include processes for identifying organizational research priorities: approving researcher organizational access; approving participation in research collaborations; assessing and approving use of organizational resources; reporting research results; reviewing, updating, and amending existing research structures and processes.

FROM PRINCIPLES TO ACTION – NEXT STEPS IN DEVELOPING RESEARCH PARTNERSHIPS

While there are many actions an organization may take to build research capacity, they can be described as falling into two major approaches (Bowen et al. 2019).

The first approach is to create some form of "interface" with academic or other (e.g., provincial, national, or parent) research bodies. This interface may take many forms: joint committees, liaison offices within either the organization or another institution, discussion "tables" or planning days held in collaboration with provincial health departments, universities and other bodies, regular "research" days that showcase relevant academic and/or in-house research; or, negotiating for specialized library services. These initiatives are based on the assumption that universities (and other research institutes) are the center of research expertise: the focus of the health system should be on healthcare delivery. The most practical approach, therefore, is to collaborate with them around healthcare organizations' research needs and interests.

The second approach is to embed additional research capacity within the organization. This may include creation of some form of a "Research and Evaluation" unit, or embedding various forms of research (or expertise in accessing, assessing and communicating research), within existing departments (e.g., expanding the role of Organizational Learning). These responses are often based on the assumption that organizations can best meet their research needs if responsibility and accountability for research activity rests within the organization.

These two major approaches are not mutually exclusive – organizations may develop responses with aspects of each. There are also creative initiatives that do not fit neatly into either approach. For example, a number of health regions may collaborate to form a regional research resource, or resources may be situated within a provincial department of health or national bodies. An organization may negotiate academic appointments for senior staff, or creative arrangements for sharing research staff with academic centers.

Each broad response has potential advantages and disadvantages and the critical challenges in effective implementation and management of each response are distinct. In the following section we focus specifically on the potential advantages and disadvantages of the interface approach; identify important issues in planning; and outline potential strategies for avoiding and mitigating common pitfalls. In many instances, however, organizations may elect to focus more on building embedded internal research capacity: additional considerations for this approach can be found in a companion document (Bowen et al. 2021).

Creating a Health System/Academic Interface

There are many potential benefits to healthcare organizations of developing partnerships with academic researchers: universities and other research institutes are centers of research expertise, while healthcare organizations specialize in service delivery. Partnerships allow organizations to have access to a broader range of methodological skills and areas of program expertise than the organization could secure in-house. There may also be increased credibility of findings if research is led from outside the organization. Ideally, partnerships may bring together the best of both the service and academic worlds.

Many organizations begin to strengthen their research role by establishing, or further developing, relationships with individual researchers. While this approach may result in positive experiences with a specific research project, it is not equivalent to developing effective collaborative initiatives at the system level. Potential disadvantages of one-on-one collaborations include risks of staff turnover to research continuity; lack of organizational awareness of, and commitment to, staff time and other resources allocated to support the collaboration; and less likelihood of organization adoption of relevant research findings (Bornstein et al. 2017; Hofmeyer et al. 2012; Wolfenden et al. 2017).

Although there are a number of potential advantages to the organization of creating linkages with academic research centers at the system level, there are also barriers to effective operation of such collaborations: key among them being rigid approaches to definitions of research; lack of researcher flexibility in the complex world of healthcare; dependence on funding from research funding organizations (which may take years to secure); lack of responsiveness to organizational time lines; and, the pressure to fall into a reactive mode based on researcher interests (Bowen et al. 2019; Nyström et al. 2018). Organizations that have developed successful collaborations often report that it takes years of discussion and interaction, skills in negotiation, and academic commitment to learning about healthcare needs and realities for such interfaces to become effective (Gagliardi et al. 2017; Lehmann and Gilson 2015; Wolfenden et al. 2017). In addition, organizations often come to realize that support for key research-related activities (e.g., evaluation and time-sensitive evidence reviews) are not met by this shared structure, and that the just-in-time input they need for decision-making cannot be provided. The often-unresponsive time frames of research funding cycles, and the common lack of priority given by research funding agencies to applied research, may result in organizational needs not being a priority for university researchers, who are evaluated on their ability to obtain research grants and have their research published. Nor do researchers always have the needed preparation to enable them to work effectively in collaborations, or methodological breadth and flexibility to enable them to respond to the variety of research questions of interest to knowledge users.

The organization should consider several questions about the proposed interface, including:

- What are the objectives and scope of the "interface" initiative?
- How will it be funded (if other than investment in time from both parties)?
- How responsive will the initiative be to organizational priorities? How will this be assured?
- At what level of the organization is the initiative developed? Is there support from senior leadership (e.g., CEO; Dean) of both?
- Who from within the organization will take the lead in liaison and coordination roles? Do they have the skills to do this?
- How will organizational staff have input into decisions?
- How will decisions be made about who will partner on the coproduced research (e.g., principal and co-investigators)?
- How will differences and misunderstandings be handled?
- How will the organization address the additional research-related needs (e.g., "just in time" evidence reviews, evaluation) not addressed by the interface?

Recognizing potential challenges and pitfalls can also help achieve the goals of the collaboration, enabling proactive action that may help prevent or mitigate future problems (Table 3.4.3).

TABLE 3.4.3   Potential pitfalls, positioning for success.

Potential Pitfall	Characteristics associated with success
Collaborations limited to research questions for which there are current research funding opportunities rather than organizational priorities	- Appropriate planning dedicated to clarifying goals of the collaboration and organizational expectations, including requirement of academic commitment to addressing organizational priorities - Organizational recognition that the collaborative setting will likely not address all organizational interests and needs - Investment in internal resources to address broader research-related needs - Investment of all partners into development of on-going relationships that will enable proactive response - Clear terms of reference - Clear processes and approval criteria for decisions on joint activity

Potential Pitfall	Characteristics associated with success
Research findings not timely	• Investment in internal resources to address immediate needs • Negotiating access to preliminary findings
Failure to negotiate the different agendas, expectations, and cultures of the academic and health services world	• Initial in-depth orientation for all participants, that includes not only orientation to research and research processes, but also to the organization's structure, decision-making processes and priorities • Clearly identifying areas of expertise of each team member • Clear processes for addressing emerging problems • Ensuring strong negotiation skills on leadership team • Academic commitment to recognizing and rewarding diverse forms of research, dissemination and measurement of impact (Canadian Academy of Health Sciences 2017)
Collaborations developed at a personal, individual (e.g., researcher/manager, CEO/Dean) level rather than institution to institution level	• Negotiated organization-organization agreements • written organization-to-organization memorandums of understanding, and/or specific contracts • Ensuring appropriate organizational policy • Succession plan to address potential loss of organizational leads
Failure to involve appropriate partners with interest, skills in partnership	• Guidelines for partnership that include requirements and expectations of partners • Consideration of identifying organizational "relationship broker" with skills and responsibility to develop partnerships (Bowen et al. 2017) • Proactive identification and recruitment of researchers with partnership experiences and approaches
Inadequate time and resources dedicated to initiative	• Ensuring identified staff have protected time to participate • Clear communication of organization meeting time preferences and availability, as well as preferred communication strategies (e.g., email, phone, in-person. meeting) • Negotiation of compensation for participation where appropriate (e.g., time in proposal development)
Failure to monitor and evaluate development of the interface and participant experience with it.	• Joint development of plan to monitor and assess participation, satisfaction and impact • Regular check-ins at senior leadership levels

Embedding Research Capacity within the Organization

Given the costs of the time needed to develop and maintain an effective collaborative relationship with academic bodies, and the unmet research needs the organization may continue to face, many organizations decide that the best way to have their needs met is to invest in building internal research resources. This response focuses on a different form of partnership than the one of creating an interface, as both "partners" (researchers and organizational leaders and staff) are employed by the same organization. The advantages and disadvantages of developing embedded research, along with guidance for optimizing this approach, are detailed elsewhere (Bowen et al. 2021). As internal research units are unlikely to be able to address all the organization's research-related needs – organizations selecting to develop such units may still benefit from collaboration with academic centers around some research questions.

PLANNING FOR IMPLEMENTATION AND EVALUATION

Careful organizational planning, in and of itself, is insufficient for success. Any research initiative – including initiation and development of research coproduction activities – must be implemented effectively: often, failure of an initiative is not the result of a poorly thought-out idea, but rather the result of failures in implementation (Bauer and Kirchner 2020).

A comprehensive evaluation plan, designed and ready to implement at the time an initiative is launched, is essential. Too often, evaluation is an organizational afterthought, with little or no allocation of resources to support it. Without effective and ongoing evaluation, however, opportunities for early identification (and remediation) of problems may be missed; and opportunities for growth and improvement of the early research initiative may pass unrecognized. Organizations need access to competent evaluation expertise, whether in-house or external. In addition, it is useful to build awareness and appreciation of the range of evaluation purposes and approaches among staff and managers. There are a number of practical resources that can guide an organization through the evaluation process (Bowen 2012). A useful form of evaluation in this context is *developmental evaluation*, intended to support the continued development of an initiative within the organization. Reflecting the principles of complexity theory, developmental evaluation engages organizational members in the evaluation process, supporting an ongoing process of innovation (Patton 2011).

While the focus of an evaluation can be expected to change over time, the first phase of any evaluation should be *implementation* evaluation, designed to assess to what extent the initiative has been implemented as intended. This allows for early intervention and re-direction if needed, optimizing the potential for effective functioning (Bowen 2012).

FUTURE RESEARCH

Future research should ensure that the perspectives of health system personnel are given equal attention to academic perspectives, and that there is broad, multi-dimensional exploration of the impacts of coproduction activities on organizations and programs. Rigorous evaluation research, focusing on the implications for transferability of approaches and principles of specific approaches to coproduction, is also required in order to build a knowledge base that will provide guidance to healthcare organizations in their work of developing effective research responses.

CONCLUSION

The perspectives and experiences of managers and staff of healthcare organizations with research partnerships have received scant attention in the academic literature: few resources are available to support these organizations as they explore any form of research collaboration. Recent research has, however, highlighted the many challenges that healthcare decision-makers may face in engaging in research partnerships.

Not all organizations will be prepared to engage in coproduction of research. We have proposed, based on emerging research of decision-maker experiences, important questions for organizational consideration before decisions are made about whether and how personnel will engage in research partnerships. Organizations are also urged to explore the potential benefits of building embedded organizational capacity to ensure that research activities can be responsive and accountable to organizational needs (Bowen et al. 2021). For research coproduction to be effective, research processes must be ready to respond to the realities of service provision, and researchers who are committed to research coproduction must support decisions that organizations take to ensure that the proposed research benefits, rather than imposes on, their organization.

REFERENCES

1. Barnes, R.O., Holmes, B.J., Lindstrom, R., Trytten, C., and Wale, M.C. (2015). Evidence-informed healthcare through integration of health research. *Healthcare Management Forum / Canadian College of Health Service Executives = Forum gestion des soins de santé / Collège canadien des directeurs de services de santé* 28: 75–78. doi: 10.1177/0840470414562637.

2. Bartunek, J.M. and Rynes, S.L. (2014). Academics and practitioners are alike and unlike: the paradoxes of academic–practitioner relationships. *Journal of Management* 40: 1181–1201. doi: 10.1177/0149206314529160.

3. Bauer, M.S. and Kirchner, J. (2020). Implementation science: what is it and why should I care? *Psychiatry Research* 283: 112376. doi: 10.1016/j. psychres.2019.04.025.

4. Boaz, A., Hanney, S., Borst, R., O'Shea, A., and Kok, M. (2018). How to engage stakeholders in research: design principles to support improvement. *Health Research Policy and Systems / BioMed Central* 16: 60. doi: 10.1186/ s12961-018-0337-6.

5. Boaz, A., Hanney, S., Jones, T., and Soper, B. (2015). Does the engagement of clinicians and organisations in research improve healthcare performance: a three-stage review. *BMJ Open* 5: e009415. doi: 10.1136/bmjopen-2015-009415.

6. Bornstein, S., Baker, R., Navarro, P., Mackey, S., Speed, D., and Sullivan, M. (2017). Putting research in place: an innovative approach to providing contextualized evidence synthesis for decision makers. *Systematic Reviews* 6: 218. doi: 10.1186/s13643-017-0606-4.

7. Bowen, S. (2012). A Guide to Evaluation in Health Research. Ottawa. https://cihr-irsc.gc.ca/e/documents/kt_lm_guide_evhr-en.pdf. Accessed January 11 2022.

8. Bowen, S., Botting, I., Graham, I.D., and Huebner, L.A. (2017). Beyond "two cultures": guidance for establishing effective researcher/health system partnerships. *International Journal of Health Policy and Management* 6: 27–42. doi: 10.15171/ijhpm.2016.71.

9. Bowen, S., Botting, I., Graham, I.D., MacLeod, M., Moissac, D., Harlos, K., Leduc, B., Ulrich, C., and Knox, J. (2019). Experience of health leadership in partnering with university-based researchers in Canada – A call to "re-imagine" research. *International Journal of Health Policy and Management* 8: 684–699. doi: 10.15171/ijhpm.2019.66.

10. Bowen, S., Graham, I.D., and Botting, I. (2021) It's Time to Talk about Our Relationship with Research. [Online]. https://iktrn.ohri.ca/resources/ikt-resources. Accessed August 21 2021.

11. Bowen, S., Martens, P., and Need to Know Team. (2005). Demystifying knowledge translation: learning from the community. *Journal of Health Services Research and Policy* 10: 203–211. doi: 10.1258/135581905774414213.

12. Canadian Academy of Health Sciences. (2017). Academic Recognition of Team Science: How to Optimize the Canadian Academic System. Ottawa: The Expert Panel on Academic Recognition of Team Science in Canada, CAHS. https:// cahs-acss.ca/wp-content/uploads/2017/07/2017-06-22-Team-Science-Report-Eng-FINAL-Web.pdf. Accessed January 11 2022.

13. de Moissac, D., Bowen, S., Botting, I., Graham, I.D., MacLeod, M., Harlos, K., Songok, C.M., and Bohemier, M. (2019). Evidence of commitment to research partnerships? Results of two web reviews. *Health Research Policy and Systems / BioMed Central* 17: 73. doi: 10.1186/s12961-019-0475-5.

14. Ellen, M.E., Lavis, J.N., Horowitz, E., and Berglas, R. (2018). How is the use of research evidence in health policy perceived? A comparison between the

reporting of researchers and policy-makers. *Health Research Policy and Systems / BioMed Central* 16: 64. doi: 10.1186/s12961-018-0345-6.

15. Gagliardi, A.R., Kothari, A., and Graham, I.D. (2017). Research agenda for integrated knowledge translation (IKT) in healthcare: what we know and do not yet know. *Journal of Epidemiology and Community Health* 71: 105–106. doi: 10.1136/jech-2016-207743.

16. Greenhalgh, T., Jackson, C., Shaw, S., and Janamian, T. (2016). Achieving research impact through co-creation in community-based health services: literature review and case study. *The Milbank Quarterly* 94: 392–429. doi: 10.1111/1468-0009.12197.

17. Hoekstra, F., Martin Ginis, K.A., Allan, V., Kothari, A., and Gainforth, H.L. (2018). Evaluating the impact of a network of research partnerships: a longitudinal multiple case study protocol. *Health Research Policy and Systems / BioMed Central* 16: 107. doi: 10.1186/s12961-018-0377-y.

18. Hofmeyer, A., Scott, C., and Lagendyk, L. (2012). Researcher-decision-maker partnerships in health services research: practical challenges, guiding principles. *BMC Health Services Research* 12: 280. doi: 10.1186/1472-6963-12-280.

19. Holmes, B.J. (2020). Re-imagining research: a bold call, but bold enough? Comment on "experience of health leadership in partnering with university-based researchers in Canada: a call to "re-imagine' research." *International Journal of Health Policy and Management* 9: 517–519. doi: 10.15171/ijhpm.2019.139.

20. Jessani, N.S., Siddiqi, S.M., Babcock, C., Davey-Rothwell, M., Ho, S., and Holtgrave, D.R. (2018). Factors affecting engagement between academic faculty and decision-makers: learnings and priorities for a school of public health. *Health Research Policy and Systems / BioMed Central* 16: 65. doi: 10.1186/s12961-018-0342-9.

21. Kothari, A., MacLean, L., Edwards, N., and Hobbs, A. (2011). Indicators at the interface: managing policymaker-researcher collaboration. *Knowledge Management Research & Practice* 9: 203–214. doi: 10.1057/kmrp.2011.16.

22. Lehmann, U. and Gilson, L. (2015). Action learning for health system governance: the reward and challenge of co-production. *Health Policy and Planning* 30: 957–963. doi: 10.1093/heapol/czu097.

23. Marx, J. and Treharne, G.J. (2018). Introduction: researching "down," "up," and "alongside." In: Catriona Ida Macleod, Jacqueline Marx, Phindezwa Mnyaka & Gareth J. Treharne (eds.), *The Palgrave Handbook of Ethics in Critical Research*, 327–338. Accessed January 11 2022.

24. McLean, R.K.D., Graham, I.D., Tetroe, J.M., and Volmink, J.A. (2018). Translating research into action: an international study of the role of research funders. *Health Research Policy and Systems / BioMed Central* 16: 44. doi: 10.1186/s12961-018-0316-y.

25. Nyström, M.E., Karltun, J., Keller, C., and Andersson Gare, B. (2018). Collaborative and partnership research for improvement of health and social

services: researcher's experiences from 20 projects. *Health Research Policy and Systems / BioMed Central* 16: 46. doi: 10.1186/s12961-018-0322-0.

26. Oliver, K., Innvar, S., Lorenc, T., Woodman, J., and Thomas, J. (2014). A systematic review of barriers to and facilitators of the use of evidence by policymakers. *BMC Health Services Research* 14: 2. doi: 10.1186/1472-6963-14-2.

27. Oliver, S., Clarke-Jones, L., Rees, R., Milne, R., Buchanan, P., Gabbay, J., Gyte, G., Oakley, A., and Stein, K. (2004). Involving consumers in research and development agenda setting for the NHS: developing an evidence-based approach. *Health Technology Assessment* 8: 1–148, III–IV. doi: 10.3310/hta8150.

28. Patton, M. (2011). *Developmental Evaluation: Applying Complexity Concepts to Enhance Innovation and Use.* New York: The Guilford Press.

29. Rycroft-Malone, J., Burton, C.R., Wilkinson, J., Harvey, G., McCormack, B., Baker, R., Dopson, S., Graham, I.D., Staniszewska, S., Thompson, C., Ariss, S., Melville-Richards, L., and Williams, L. (2016). Collective action for implementation: a realist evaluation of organisational collaboration in healthcare. *Implementation Science: IS* 11: 17. doi: 10.1186/s13012-016-0380-z.

30. Wehrens, R., Bekker, M., and Bal, R. (2010). The construction of evidence-based local health policy through partnerships: research infrastructure, process, and context in the Rotterdam "Healthy in the City' programme. *Journal of Public Health Policy* 31: 447–460. doi: 10.1057/jphp.2010.33.

31. Wolfenden, L., Yoong, S.L., Williams, C.M., Grimshaw, J., Durrheim, D.N., Gillham, K., and Wiggers, J. (2017). Embedding researchers in health service organizations improves research translation and health service performance: the Australian Hunter New England Population Health example. *Journal of Clinical Epidemiology* 85: 3–11. doi: 10.1016/j.jclinepi.2017.03.007.

3.5 Managing Academic-Health Service Partnerships

Alison M. Hutchinson, Cheyne Chalmers, Katrina Nankervis, and Nicole (Nikki) Phillips

Key Learning Points

- Partnerships are key to coproduction. Academic-health service partnerships help advance common research, education, and practice interests for mutual benefit.
- Coproduction of knowledge through such partnerships is more likely to be meaningful and have impact.
- Sustaining academic-health service partnerships requires deliberate and concerted effort.
- Principles guiding the management and sustainment of partnerships highlight the importance of mutual respect, trust, transparency, flexibility, open communication, shared knowledge, and commitment.
- A shared mission and vision, and mutually agreed objectives are required. The partnership strategic plan should evolve as the strategic plans for the respective organizations evolve.

Research Coproduction in Healthcare, First Edition. Edited by
Ian D. Graham, Jo Rycroft-Malone, Anita Kothari, and Chris McCutcheon.
© 2022 John Wiley & Sons Ltd. Published 2022 by John Wiley & Sons Ltd.

- A formal governance structure is essential to ensure the values of the partners remain aligned, and priorities and future research directions are mutually agreed.
- Clear lines and agreed processes for communication are necessary.
- Researchers within the partnership require a clear understanding of their roles and expectations to ensure they address the imperatives of each organization. A formal agreement between the partners is necessary to ensure the partnership meets the expectations and needs of both organizations and to agree on and confirm the commitment of infrastructure and resources to support the partnership.
- Evaluation of the partnership should occur at mutually agreed times; likewise, the formal agreement should be reviewed and re-negotiated at predetermined time points.
- Research conducted within the partnership needs to be relevant and meaningful, and to address a health service priority. Partnership researchers need to respond nimbly to requests for research and evidence reviews, and to be flexible in the conduct of research in environments that are constantly adapting to change.

INTRODUCTION

Partnerships are central to research coproduction. This chapter will focus on how to manage academic-health service partnerships during the research process, how to sustain such partnerships and how to assess their sustainability. Academic-health service partnerships provide a platform for the nexus between research, education, and practice to be realized and to flourish, benefiting all three domains: the respective partner organizations, their employees, and most importantly the recipients of their services and education (Bakewell-Sachs 2016). Such partnerships have been defined as strategic arrangements, formal or informal, between universities and health services that are established to advance common research, education and practice interests (American Association of Colleges of Nursing 1990). Academic-health service partnerships can leverage the combined strengths and resources of the partners to generate and translate knowledge for mutual advantage and to an extent that would not have been achieved in isolation, resulting in the whole being greater than the sum of its parts. Coproduction of knowledge through established academic-health service partnerships is more likely to have substantial, meaningful, and lasting impact (Beckett et al. 2018); ultimately leading to better outcomes for patients (Granger et al. 2012) by addressing clinically relevant issues using rigorous research approaches. Additionally, such partnerships can contribute to research capability development among clinicians, promote development of a research culture in health services, and strengthen the network and depth of researcher-clinician collaborations (Bakewell-Sachs 2016).

Sustaining academic-health service partnerships, however, can be challenging and requires concerted efforts from the partners (Nabavi et al. 2012). The different sectors (university and health service) have fundamentally different purposes, priorities, performance measures, cultures, and funding models (De Geest et al. 2010). Hence, finding common values and goal alignment is necessary for sustained partnership. The stresses (for example financial pressures and service demand) on the different sectors vary in timing and nature and each partner needs to be sensitive to and accommodate the other's needs.

BACKGROUND

In this chapter, we draw on our experience in a formal, long-standing academic-health service partnership. Established in 2006, our research center represents a sustained partnership between the disciplines of nursing and midwifery at Monash Health (one health authority in the state of Victoria, Australia) and the School of Nursing and Midwifery at Deakin University. In the previous decade, the School had established formal partnerships with a number of other health services. Hence, our Monash Health-Deakin University partnership was part of a wider network of academic-health services partnerships with the School. In essence, the partnerships were established for mutual benefit in the conduct of relevant and meaningful research, development of research capability in nurse clinicians, and ensuring the nursing education undergraduate and postgraduate curricula is contemporaneously informed by developments in the health services.

The center is led by the Chair in Nursing at Monash Health, who is also a Professor of Nursing at the University. The Chair in Nursing reports to the Chief Nursing and Midwifery Officer at Monash Health and the Head of the School of Nursing and Midwifery at Deakin University. The Chair in Nursing's links with the school and the health service provide a conduit for rapid sharing of information and escalation of issues between the organizations, enabling fast problem resolution and decision-making for mutual benefit. The center also includes a jointly appointed Associate Professor and Research Fellow. In addition, a Research Assistant and administrative officer are employed by the health service to work with the jointly appointed researchers. These appointments involve a significant financial commitment from both partners. The health service provides office space and computers for the researchers. This also includes space for research assistants who are employed on casual or short-term contracts and research-focused students of the center. Co-location of the researchers with the health service nursing and midwifery education and strategy team facilitates collaboration, communication, and sharing of information between the researchers and key nursing personnel.

Under the auspices of the partnership, researchers, in collaboration with health service personnel, undertake multiple studies and programs of research. The work of the researchers within the center spans three broad domains: knowledge generation, knowledge translation and brokerage, and capability-building. Knowledge generation occurs through the conduct of primary and secondary research. Knowledge translation is facilitated through research designed to implement the best available evidence in policy and practice. Knowledge brokerage occurs through the researchers' responding to requests for current evidence and the researchers' active involvement in a range of committees, advisory and working groups across the health service. In terms of capability building, the center's researchers supervise a number of research students (e.g., master and doctoral level) working within the health service as well as external students undertaking research at Monash Health. Additionally, the researchers support staff who are undertaking clinician-initiated research and link them with other university researchers who have relevant expertise. The Chief Nursing and Midwifery Officer at Monash Health holds an Adjunct Professor role with Deakin University, and contributes to key clinical education governance activities in Deakin's School of Nursing and Midwifery, such as curriculum development and chairing the School's Advisory Board. This hard-wired mechanism enables the Chief Nursing and Midwifery Officer to be a visible champion for the university and the agreed objectives of the partnership.

Our partnership is part of a wider network of partners. The Deakin University School of Nursing and Midwifery has similar partnerships with five other health services in the state of Victoria. Collectively, we refer to all the partnerships as *Deakin Partners in Nursing and Midwifery*. This hub and spoke model enables research to be undertaken in multiple health services across the network, to address issues or problems that are common to the health service partners. Workshops and meetings of senior leaders are held to facilitate discussion, conceptualization, prioritization, and decision-making about research across Deakin Partners in Nursing and Midwifery. In the following sections we address the evidence and our experience in relation to the management and sustainment of an academic-health service partnership.

HOW TO MANAGE PARTNERSHIPS DURING THE RESEARCH PROCESS

In 2012, the American Association of Colleges of Nursing and the American Organization of Nurse Executives Taskforce produced a set of guiding principles for academic-practice partnerships (Table 3.5.1). While these principles were specifically established for the discipline of nursing, they could be readily applied to other disciplines. Adherence to principles by both partners is necessary in the ongoing management of partnerships.

TABLE 3.5.1 Guiding principles for academic-practice partnerships.

1. Collaborative relationships between academia and practice are established and sustained.
2. Mutual respect and trust are the cornerstones of the practice/academia relationship.
3. Knowledge is shared among partners.
4. A commitment is shared by partners to maximize the potential of each registered nurse to reach the highest level within his/her individual scope of practice.
5. A commitment is shared by partners to work together to determine an evidence-based transition program for students and new graduates that is both sustainable and cost effective.
6. A commitment is shared by partners to develop, implement, and evaluate organizational processes and structures that support and recognize academic or educational achievements.
7. A commitment is shared by partners to support opportunities for nurses to lead and develop collaborative models that redesign practice environments to improve health outcomes.
8. A commitment is shared by partners to establish infrastructures to collect and analyze data on the current and future needs of the RN workforce.

(American Association of Colleges of Nursing and American Organization of Nurse Executives Taskforce 2012).

More recently, Hoekstra and colleagues reviewed 86 published reviews of research partnership literature (Hoekstra et al. 2018, 2020), identifying 17 over-arching principles, grouped into the following six sub-categories: relationship between researchers and stakeholders; coproduction of knowledge; meaningful stakeholder engagement; capacity-building, support, and resources; communication between researchers and stakeholders; and ethical issues of collaborative research activities. The most frequently reported principles identified in the included studies related to: the development and maintenance of relationships "based on trust, credibility, respect, dignity and transparency" (Hoekstra et al. 2020, p. 12); the coproduction of knowledge through engagement of partners throughout the research process; being "flexible and creative in collaborative research activities;" and adopting a tailored approach (Hoekstra et al. 2020, p. 12).

Specifically, in the field of spinal injury research, Gainforth and colleagues (2021) co-developed, with an expert panel, researchers, knowledge users, and funders, a set of eight guiding principles for the conduct and dissemination of research in partnership with knowledge users (Table 3.5.2) (Gainforth et al. 2021).

Not surprisingly, there are commonalities across these sets of principles and they also closely align with our first-hand experience of partnering between a university and health service. In their review of reviews, Hoekstra et al. (2020) also identified a set of 11 overarching strategies used to conduct research through partnerships; the strategies were grouped into six sub-categories: relationship between researchers and stakeholders; capacity-building, support and resources;

TABLE 3.5.2   Guiding principles to engage in research

1. Partners develop and maintain relationships based on trust, respect, dignity and transparency.
2. Partners share in decision-making.
3. Partners foster open, honest, and responsive communication.
4. Partners recognize, value, and share their diverse expertise and knowledge.
5. Partners are flexible and receptive in tailoring the research approach to match the aims and context of the project.
6. Partners can meaningfully benefit by participating in the partnership.
7. Partners address ethical considerations.
8. Partners respect the practical considerations and financial constraints of all partners.

(Gainforth et al. 2021)

communication between researchers and stakeholders; stakeholder engagement in the planning of the research; stakeholder engagement in conducting the research; and stakeholder engagement in dissemination and application of the research. These strategies resonate closely with the approaches that are integral to our partnership and are illustrated in the following sections.

Experiential Knowledge of Managing a Partnership

Taking a strategic approach to the academic-health service partnership is critical (De Geest et al. 2013). This requires a shared mission and vision, and mutually agreed objectives for the partnership. Alignment of these with the values and strategic direction, particularly for research and education, of the health service as well as the university, is fundamental (Beal 2012). As the strategic plans and directions for the respective organizations evolve, the strategic plan for the partnership should evolve in unison. For the ongoing management of the partnership, a clear and joint governance structure is important to the day-to-day management of the center and the strategic planning (Sebastian et al. 2018).

Formal governance meetings are essential to ensuring the values of the partners remain aligned and are reflected in the work of the partnership, to discuss and reach mutual agreement on priorities, to reflect on outputs and achievements (such as research completion, relevance of the research to organizational policy and practice, students undertaking research through the center, publications, presentations) and to determine future research directions. We hold biannual governance meetings that include: from the health service, the Chief Executive Officer and the Chief Nursing and Midwifery Officer; from the University, the Executive Dean, Faculty of Health, and the Head of the School of Nursing and Midwifery; and from the partnership center, the Chair in Nursing and the Associate Professor, who each hold joint appointments between the university and the health service.

The personnel with joint appointments need to have clear lines and agreed processes for communication to promptly address issues such as endorsement and formal approval for research and resourcing. Similarly, clear roles and expectations are required to ensure the researchers are addressing the imperatives of each organization. Periodic evaluation and re-negotiation of a formal agreement between the University and Health Service is important to ensure the partnership still meets the expectations and needs of both organizations and to confirm the commitment of infrastructure and resources to support the partnership (De Geest et al. 2013). Set and forget is not an option for research partnership agreements. Typically, the health service and university re-negotiate agreements on three- to five-year cycles.

A title for the partnership is important; it provides credibility and legitimizes the work of the partnership. From establishment, the health service and university agreed to the term Center. However, the name of the center has changed and evolved over the years. Because our center is part of a wider network of similar partnerships, between the School of Nursing and Midwifery and other health services, in recent years it was mutually agreed by the chief nurses of all the partner health services and the Head of the School of Nursing and Midwifery that the title of each academic-health service partnership would include the title of the research center (the Center for Quality and Patient Safety Research) located within the School and the name of the respective health service. Hence, our center is titled, the Center for Quality and Patient Safety Research – Monash Health Partnership.

One of the keys to ongoing management of a partnership is the relationships between the health service and university personnel. Trust and mutually respectful and transparent communication are imperative (Gaskill et al. 2003). It is essential that the key representatives from each partner make a concerted effort to understand the purposes, priorities, performance measures, cultures, and funding models which, as noted previously, are different for different sectors. An understanding of these elements enables each partner to be aware of and sensitive to the pressure points for each. Additionally, it is important for the researchers to network across the health service to build professional relationships and to gain knowledge of who they need to consult or collaborate with to ensure research is supported at operational and clinical levels.

In our partnership, identification of research questions for knowledge generation occurs in one of three ways: health service personnel initiated, researcher initiated, or coproduced by health service personnel and researchers. Health service personnel propose research ideas to the researchers based on their operational and/or practice experience; the ideas are then framed as researchable questions in collaboration with the researchers. Health service nursing and midwifery leaders may also ask the researchers to undertake specific research, such as a review of the evidence to address a key question in relation to a clinical or operational issue, or an evaluation of a health service initiative or quality data.

Examples of the latter include an evaluation of the impact of electronic medical record implementation on nurses and midwives and an analysis of complaints and compliments data relating to nurses and midwives. These inform initiatives to prevent circumstances that lead to complaints and to optimize processes and practices that elicit compliments.

The center-based researchers also proactively propose research ideas and researchable questions based on their knowledge and observations of challenges and activities within the health service and their knowledge of available funding opportunities and priorities. Finally, health service personnel and researchers collaboratively generate research ideas and frame them as researchable questions. These coproduced research ideas emerge from discussions and brainstorming about current issues, typically occurring at nursing leadership meetings or interdisciplinary forums addressing quality and standards. The biannual meetings are also an opportunity to discuss and co-create research ideas and opportunities in relation to forthcoming initiatives within the health service. Integral to all research ideas and questions is that they address a relevant quality and safety issue for the health service and align with the health service priorities and strategic research plan. Operational approval to pursue research related to the health service is obtained from the Chief Nursing and Midwifery Officer and other relevant managers. Their endorsement and support are critical, not only from a governance perspective but also in demonstrating the relevance and importance of the research to the health service.

Also key to the success of an academic-health service partnership is ensuring, not only that research is relevant and addresses an important health service issue, but also that the researchers are able to respond nimbly to requests for research and evidence reviews, and to be flexible in the conduct of research in environments that are constantly adapting to change (Bowen et al. 2019, 2021). On a day-to-day basis, changes within a clinical setting can be rapid and unpredictable. This is not to say that the rigor of the research should be compromised, but rather it is about being flexible and agilely adapting data collection processes and timing in conjunction with the demands and dynamics of the health service settings (Holly et al. 2014). It is vitally important to be respectful of, and sensitive to, the primary activities of health service personnel, and to manage research so as not to compromise their work or unduly burden them.

Being truly embedded in the health service by having a physical presence, as well as being actively engaged in committees and advisory groups, is critical to building strong connections between researchers and health service personnel. The researchers' presence in the health service and their attendance at key operational and governance meetings is important for a range of reasons. This enables them to build professional relationships with health service personnel, so that both parties know with whom and how to make contact, when required, and learn about one another's capabilities. Being present enables the researchers to maintain a contemporaneous knowledge and understanding of the key issues facing the health service; issues that reveal research gaps or opportunities for translation, as well as issues the researchers need to take into account when planning research. Finally, having a presence enables the researchers to respond quickly to identified knowledge gaps, whether that be through synthesizing existing knowledge or embarking on research to address a knowledge gap. For the researchers, an understanding of the quality and safety issues within the health service enables them to respond swiftly and opportunistically when relevant funding opportunities are released.

With an established partnership and infrastructure, acquisition of institutional support can be achieved rapidly, relevant personnel can be coalesced and an application generated quickly; letters of support can be obtained in a timely manner (Gaskill et al. 2003). Cash and in-kind contributions can also be agreed on promptly. Additionally, being able to demonstrate in the application a sustained and strong partnership is highly advantageous. The ability to respond to such opportunities nimbly and promptly offers a substantial advantage over others in the competition who need to address these requirements in the absence of an established and mature partnership foundation.

HOW TO SUSTAIN PARTNERSHIPS

Sustainment of academic-health service partnerships requires commitment from each partner to the partnership goals and flexibility to adjust the terms of agreement as priorities change (Davis et al. 2019). Acknowledging that challenges to maintaining a strong partnership will arise, regular reflection and communication to address challenges are important. In undertaking research in partnerships, it is important to keep sight of the availability of resources, such as staff, and be prepared to adapt and adjust processes, such as data collection, in response to changes in the setting. The nature of the research process, which is slow and often complex in a dynamic environment, requires patience and an understanding of the importance of rigor among the partners.

Experiential Knowledge of Sustaining a Partnership

While governance is key to managing a partnership, as discussed above, it is also fundamental to sustaining partnerships. A rigorous governance mechanism includes contracts with agreed key performance indicators and a reporting and meeting structure to ensure expectations are being met. Governance meetings are used to share and understand changing priorities and emerging issues and trends. These meetings are also an opportunity for partners to discuss intellectual and operational challenges and enable discourse to create mutually agreed strategic priorities and future directions for the center and research.

To support the partnership, having an established organizational structure, career development opportunities for center researchers, and a succession plan are important for partnership success and sustainability. The partnership needs to be an integral part of the organization, and the partnership goals need to be deeply aligned with the health service's values and priorities, so the partnership can withstand changes in staff, threats to funding, and external threats. The COVID-19 pandemic has been a good example of an external threat, with the health service thrust into a full-scale pandemic response which required the cessation of health services research and the university seriously impacted by financial loss and major challenges in securing health service placements for nursing and midwifery students.

Development of, and revision to, the strategic directions of the partnership involve mutual investment over time, with wins scored for both partners. As such, the strategy needs to align with the organizational and research strategies of each partner. As the partnership matures the researchers become more embedded in the health service and they develop strong professional relationships with knowledge users. With this, the strategy alignment becomes inherent in all research planning.

With maturity of the partnership comes greater engagement in group think between researchers and knowledge users. Providing the opportunity for each other's perspectives to be shared, deeply considered and challenged is important. Researchers and knowledge users bring different lenses to a problem and robust discussions can result in creative solutions for exploration and testing. The chemistry between researchers and knowledge users is key to the success of such engagement. This is predicated on the mindsets of individuals in the partnership, being open to exploring new directions, which at first may not appear to align with the strategic plan, but may ultimately advance the partnership towards the overall goal.

Team-building and getting to know members of the academic-health service partnership on a personal level helps contribute to the success and sustainability of the partnership by increasing approachability and ease of communication among partners. Having good interpersonal relationships is also critical to constructive and transparent communication. Part of the success of the partnership relates to the people involved and their fit with each other and the respective organizations (how they get along and work together). Thus, investing in getting to know each other as individuals becomes important to the overall success of an academic-health service partnership and can bring about momentum that can be transformative. Fundamental to strong interpersonal relationships is the ongoing governance and supporting structures that provide an environment that is conducive to relationship building, enabling the partnership to flourish.

Sustainability of the academic-health service partnership also requires recognition by partners that failure is acceptable. For partners, the power of a strong partnership helps to weather periods when grant funding is limited and funding applications are unsuccessful. In solid academic-health service partnerships, partners can buoy one another to maintain motivation and energy for future funding rounds. Sustainment of the partnership, in part, also hinges on strong institutional reputations of each partner organization for the quality of their services and outcomes, which adds to the credibility of the research. While the reputations of partner organizations are important when initiating partnerships, such reputations need to be sustained or strengthened for ongoing partnership to be attractive.

HOW TO ASSESS THE SUSTAINABILITY OF PARTNERSHIPS

Collaborations for Leadership in Applied Health Research and Care (CLAHRCs) were established in England as partnerships between health services and universities to promote translation of research by bringing together researchers and knowledge users. In evaluating CLAHRCs, Rycroft-Malone and colleagues concluded that sustaining the partnership may be "a function of how successfully they worked with different agendas, drivers and motivations while realising planned goals in parallel to being responsive to issues that arose through continued interaction" (Rycroft-Malone et al. 2015, p. vi). This resonates with our experience, whereby researchers within the partnership are required to recognize and work within the agendas of the health service and university while undertaking research that is responsive to the needs and priorities of both organizations. This can require some lateral and creative thinking in creating outputs and ensuring outcomes are achieved that benefit both communities.

In terms of sustaining academic-health service partnerships, evidence of impact is necessary. Focussing on academic-health service partnerships in the nursing profession, Beal (2012) reports an integrative review of the literature, based on which, a range of outcome measures are proposed at individual partner and regional levels. The quantification measures relate mostly to outcomes associated with students (for example, clinical placements, student enrolment, student retention, and student satisfaction) and nurses (for example, the proportion of nurses who become leaders and the proportion of nurses who return to university to undertake advanced degrees). In terms of research and the quality of patient outcomes two indicators are proposed: increased research productivity and improved patient safety and quality indicators (Beal 2012).

Beckett and colleagues (2018) highlight the emphasis typically placed on more tangible, quantifiable (for example, publications and conference presentations), and economic impacts (for example, grant funding success) of such partnerships, and the failure to capture the social impacts. As such, they recommend capturing both the process and outcomes of coproduced research. Recognizing the potential for impact at multiple levels (individual, groups or teams, organizational, and societal), Beckett et al. developed a Social Impact Framework to guide measurement of the impact of coproduced research. The framework is designed to elicit the research process (Who, When, Why and How the levels were involved), impacts (including outputs, uses, and outcomes of the research as they apply at the different levels), and the mechanisms at the different levels that enabled the research to be undertaken (Beckett et al. 2018).

Assessing the Sustainability of Our Partnership

To assess the sustainability of our partnership, six-monthly reporting on activity is used to ensure the research aligns with the values of the health service and university and the outputs and outcomes are acceptable to both partners. Governance meetings provide an opportunity for the key leaders from both partners to connect and discuss the achievements, opportunities, challenges and future directions. Adjustments in direction based on mutually agreed priorities are made collaboratively.

Agreed key performance indicators (health service and academic) are used in reporting, which addresses research that has been completed since the previous review, research in-progress, and commencing or planned research, according to each of the center's three pillars of research: patient experience, patient safety, and health workforce. Additionally, we report on the commencement, progress and completion of research students (master's and doctoral) under the supervision of the partnership researchers, including details about the students' study topics. We report on scholarly activities by clinicians that we have advised (publications, conferences, funding applications) on or to which we have contributed. All publications and presentations authored by researchers within the center include both organizations as affiliations. We report on funding application outcomes, as well as applications under review and in preparation. We also report on awards and honors, publications, presentations, and media activity since the previous review. In terms of translation activities, we report on the contributions of the researchers to health service committees and advisory groups, activities such as providing evidence summaries or rapid reviews to inform practice, and influences of our research on health service practice or policy. The outcomes are included in both the health service's and the university's annual reports.

Agreeing on key performance indicators enables the university and health service leaders to recognize and understand the priorities of each organization. For university leaders, gaining an understanding of, and valuing, the health service priorities relating to research impact on service delivery (non-academic outputs) is important. As funding bodies are increasingly focussing on translation and impact, evidence of impact is becoming increasingly important to the academic community. Conversely, in establishing key performance indicators, health service leaders gain an understanding of, and appreciation for, the traditional outputs valued by the university. Even if such outputs are of less relevance to the health service, they do provide a means for showcasing the research undertaken in the health service and contribute to the reputation of the health service. Overall, expanding understanding of what is valued and incentivized across the partners is important to a strong partnership.

BARRIERS/FACILITATORS AND STRATEGIES TO OVERCOME THEM

Interviews with Canadian health service leaders about their experiences of partnerships between health services and universities identified the value of the partnership to coproduction of university curricula, which was considered important in ensuring the health service was not simply a passive recipient of university curricula (DeBoer et al. 2019). The leaders also perceived that support from university personnel to help clinical staff advance their education was beneficial. While some interview participants argued that universities received more tangible benefits from the partnership than did health services, the health services were reported to value their association with the university because of the reputational benefits of status and prestige. Academic-health service partnerships were also described as demonstrating, in part, the health service's commitment to strategic values relating to education and research. Mutual benefits to the health service and university reported by Canadian health service leaders included access to research opportunities and resources, including human resources, to undertake research. Health services were also perceived to benefit from clinicians being kept up-to-date with the best available evidence, being prompted to question practices, and the quality outcomes and knowledge translation that resulted from exposure to research (DeBoer et al. 2019). According to the health service leaders, the extent of collaboration between the health service and university varied from highly collaborative to less than desired, and explicit and ongoing communication was identified as necessary for strengthening the collaboration. Face-to-face communication with university partners was also identified by the health service leaders as important to collaboration (DeBoer et al. 2019).

A range of barriers to and facilitators of successful partnerships exist. To manage and overcome barriers and challenges, both partners need to work in unison. Contributions in terms of funding and infrastructure need to be balanced, with no one partner feeling they are contributing more than the other. Or, if one partner is contributing the greater portion, they must feel satisfied they are receiving a proportionally equivalent return on their investment. Discussions about contributions and returns need to be open and transparent.

One challenge that can be experienced by researchers employed through an academic partner, is the feeling that they are viewed as guests within the health service (Bakewell-Sachs 2016). This can be experienced by researchers through lack of access rights to certain electronic systems and processes normally enjoyed by health service employees. It is important to ensure that researchers are given a health service identification number, email address, and access rights to health service systems. This enables them to not only feel part of the organization and gain credibility, but also to facilitate their ability to undertake research within the health service. Having a formally recognized honorary system, which includes provision of a health service name badge, for example, also promotes the researchers' visibility and legitimizes their presence in the health service.

Researchers need to balance different and shifting institutional cultures, demands, and priorities, which requires a sophisticated insight into how both health services and universities function and how to skilfully reconcile the two. Having two reporting lines can also present challenges for researchers who need to ensure they manage and meet the expectations of two organizations. Workload can easily become unmanageable if strategies are not adopted to ensure the requirements of both organizations are met in a mutually acceptable manner. Having a clear understanding of expectations and performance measures helps the researchers navigate a path to satisfying these.

Budget constraints are possibly the biggest challenge encountered in academic-health service partnerships, with both organizations having to commit funds to support the partnership. This may be the biggest threat to partnership sustainability. Forward planning is necessary to ensure budgets are feasible and can be adhered to. A cost-benefit analysis is also important in justifying ongoing financial commitments.

Despite a number of barriers to maintaining and sustaining partnerships, these are counterbalanced by a range of facilitators. The commitment to the partnership from both organizations is critical (see Davis et al. 2019). Additionally, it is important that both partners are willing and flexible when negotiating the terms of agreements as circumstances change. As discussed above, a shared and evolving vision and mission, value alignment, joint governance, and establishment of a formal agreement are all key to maintaining and sustaining partnerships.

In our example, some key factors to consider are the measure of performance used by health services and universities, how members of the partnership are held accountable by the partner organizations' governance mechanisms, and the tension that this can create in a partnership. The health service in this example, a publicly funded and managed organization, is overseen by government and has key metrics against which it is held accountable, such as waiting times in emergency departments, waiting lists for elective surgery, overall access to care by the community, financial targets, budget requirements, and staff satisfaction. University researchers are traditionally measured according to funding income, publications, and presentations. The key is to find some common ground, a thread that traverses both organizations, aligning goals and priorities. Fruitful opportunities may include research relating to the skills and capabilities of the workforce, implementation and testing of different service delivery models, and measurement of the efficiency of care delivery and the extent to which it aligns with best available evidence for practice.

IMPLICATIONS FOR THE PRACTICE OF RESEARCH COPRODUCTION

A sustained partnership, built on trust, respect, transparent communication, and close interprofessional relationships, positions researchers and knowledge users to meaningfully coproduce research that is relevant to health service issues and priorities. Such research is therefore more likely to be impactful, through local policy and practice change as well as development of research capability among knowledge users. Involvement of knowledge users (including health professionals and consumer representatives) in the process of coproduction not only ensures that the research addresses issues of importance, it also promotes feasibility of the research methods and processes, innovations and solutions.

FUTURE RESEARCH

Evaluation is key to understanding what types and how academic-health service partnerships work and under what circumstances they function best to promote generation of new knowledge, innovation, and translation of evidence into practice (Bowen et al. 2021). Greater attention needs to be paid to the adoption of evaluation approaches to further knowledge about how to optimize partnerships in order to achieve positive outcomes and impact regarding quality and safety of patient care. Use of innovative approaches to the assessment of research quality would further knowledge on the impact of academic-health service partnerships on the quality of science and impact. Such approaches could also enable appropriate recognition for the achievements of researchers that straddle the academic and practice environments. Research to measure the impact of academic-health service partnerships on nurse and others' capability building and career progression is also warranted. Additionally, further research is needed to understand the requirements (resources, processes, and mechanisms) for sustainable partnerships and how they may differ based on characteristics such as the partners' mission, size, complexity, and location (geographic region).

CONCLUSION

Effectively managing academic-health service partnerships is crucial to research coproduction and sustainability of the partnership and, importantly, to patient outcomes. While there are challenges to managing and sustaining academic-health service partnerships, as outlined in this chapter, if the partners recognize the challenges and are proactive in their efforts to collaboratively pursue the purpose of the partnership for mutual benefit, such partnerships can lead to transformative and impactful outcomes. One academic-health service partnership, that is part of the broader Deakin Partners in Nursing and Midwifery network, has been described in this chapter as capturing the essence of an effective and highly functioning, transformative partnership that impacts the workforce of the health service, the curricula of the nursing and midwifery courses offered at the university, and, most importantly, the quality and safety of patient care.

REFERENCES

1. American Association of Colleges of Nursing. (1990). *Resolution: Need for Collaborative Relationships between Nursing Education and Practice.* Washington, DC: AACN.

2. American Association of Colleges of Nursing and American Organization of Nurse Executives Taskforce. (2012). *Guiding Principles to Academic-Practice Partnerships.* https://www.aacnnursing.org/Academic-Practice-Partnerships/The-Guiding-Principles (accessed 11 January 2022).

3. Bakewell-Sachs, S. (2016). Academic-practice partnerships: driving and supporting educational changes. *The Journal of Perinatal & Neonatal Nursing* 30: 184–186. doi: 10.1097/JPN.0000000000000196.

4. Beal, J.A. (2012). Academic-service partnerships in nursing: an integrative review. *Nursing Research and Practice* 2012: 501564. doi: 10.1155/2012/501564.

5. Beckett, K., Farr, M., Kothari, A., Wye, L., and le May, A. (2018). Embracing complexity and uncertainty to create impact: exploring the processes and transformative potential of co-produced research through development of a social impact model. *Health Research Policy and Systems/BioMed Central* 16: 118. doi: 10.1186/s12961-018-0375-0.

6. Bowen, S., Botting, I., and Graham, I.D., and The Building And Managing Effective Partnerships In Canadian Health Research Research/Advisory Team. (2021). Re-imagining health research partnership in a post-COVID world: a response to recent commentaries. *International Journal of Health Policy and Management* 10: 39–41. doi: 10.34172/ijhpm.2020.69.

7. Bowen, S., Botting, I., Graham, I.D., MacLeod, M., Moissac, D., Harlos, K., Leduc, B., Ulrich, C., and Knox, J. (2019). Experience of health leadership in

partnering with University-based researchers in Canada – A call to "Re-imagine" research. *International Journal of Health Policy and Management* 8: 684–699. doi: 10.15171/ijhpm.2019.66.

8. Davis, K.F., Harris, M.M., and Boland, M.G. (2019). Ten years and counting: a successful academic-practice partnership to develop nursing research capacity. *Journal of Professional Nursing: Official Journal of the American Association of Colleges of Nursing* 35: 473–479. doi: 10.1016/j.profnurs.2019.04.013.

9. De Geest, S., Dobbels, F., Schönfeld, S., Duerinckx, N., Sveinbjarnardottir, E.K., and Denhaerynck, K. (2013). Academic Service Partnerships: what do we learn from around the globe? A systematic literature review. *Nursing Outlook* 61: 447–457. doi: 10.1016/j.outlook.2013.02.001.

10. De Geest, S., Sullivan Marx, E.M., Rich, V., Spichiger, E., Schwendimann, R., Spirig, R., and Van Malderen, G. (2010). Developing a financial framework for academic service partnerships: models of the United States and Europe. *Journal of Nursing Scholarship: An Official Publication of Sigma Theta Tau International Honor Society of Nursing/Sigma Theta Tau* 42: 295–304. doi: 10.1111/j.1547-5069.2010.01355.x.

11. DeBoer, S., Dockx, J., Lam, C., Shah, S., Young, G., Quesnel, M., Ng, S., and Mori, B. (2019). Building successful and sustainable academic health science partnerships: exploring perspectives of hospital leaders. *Canadian Medical Education Journal* 10: e56–e67. https://www.ncbi.nlm.nih.gov/pubmed/30949261.

12. Gainforth, H.L., Hoekstra, F., McKay, R., McBride, C.B., Sweet, S.N., Martin Ginis, K.A., Anderson, K., Chernesky, J., Clarke, T., Forwell, S., Maffin, J., McPhail, L.T., Mortenson, W.B., Scarrow, G., Schaefer, L., Sibley, K.M., Athanasopoulos, P., and Willms, R. (2021). Integrated knowledge translation guiding principles for conducting and disseminating spinal cord injury research in partnership. *Archives of Physical Medicine and Rehabilitation* 102: 656–663. doi: 10.1016/j.apmr.2020.09.393.

13. Gaskill, D., Morrison, P., Sanders, F., Forster, E., Edwards, H., Fleming, R., and McClure, S. (2003). University and industry partnerships: lessons from collaborative research. *International Journal of Nursing Practice* 9: 347–355. doi: 10.1046/j.1440-172x.2003.00448.x.

14. Granger, B.B., Prvu-Bettger, J., Aucoin, J., Fuchs, M.A., Mitchell, P.H., Holditch-Davis, D., Roth, D., Califf, R.M., and Gilliss, C.L. (2012). An academic-health service partnership in nursing: lessons from the field. *Journal of Nursing Scholarship: An Official Publication of Sigma Theta Tau International Honor Society of Nursing/Sigma Theta Tau* 44: 71–79. doi: 10.1111/j.1547-5069.2011.01432.x.

15. Hoekstra, F., Mrklas, K.J., Khan, M., McKay, R.C., Vis-Dunbar, M., Sibley, K.M., Nguyen, T., Graham, I.D., SCI Guiding Principles Consensus Panel, and Gainforth, H.L. (2020). A review of reviews on principles, strategies, outcomes and impacts of research partnerships approaches: a first step in synthesising the

research partnership literature. *Health Research Policy and Systems / BioMed Central* 18: 51. doi: 10.1186/s12961-020-0544-9.

16. Hoekstra, F., Mrklas, K.J., Sibley, K.M., Nguyen, T., Vis-Dunbar, M., Neilson, C.J., Crockett, L.K., Gainforth, H.L., and Graham, I.D. (2018). A review protocol on research partnerships: a Coordinated Multicenter Team approach. *Systematic Reviews* 7: 217. doi: 10.1186/s13643-018-0879-2.

17. Holly, C., Percy, M., Caldwell, B., Echevarria, M., Bugel, M.J., and Salmond, S. (2014). Moving evidence to practice: reflections on a multisite academic-practice partnership. *International Journal of Evidence-based Healthcare* 12: 31–38. doi: 10.1097/XEB.0000000000000001.

18. Nabavi, F.H., Vanaki, Z., and Mohammadi, E. (2012). Systematic review: process of forming academic service partnerships to reform clinical education. *Western Journal of Nursing Research* 34: 118–141. doi: 10.1177/0193945910394380.

19. Rycroft-Malone, J., Burton, C., Wilkinson, J., Harvey, G., McCormack, B., Baker, R., Dopson, S., Graham, I., Staniszewska, S., Thompson, C., Ariss, S., Melville-Richards, L., and Williams, L. (2015). Collective action for knowledge mobilisation: a realist evaluation of the Collaborations for Leadership in Applied Health Research and Care. *Health Services and Delivery Research* 3. doi: 10.3310/hsdr03440.

20. Sebastian, J.G., Breslin, E.T., Trautman, D.E., Cary, A.H., Rosseter, R.J., and Vlahov, D. (2018). Leadership by collaboration: nursing's bold new vision for academic-practice partnerships. *Journal of Professional Nursing: Official Journal of the American Association of Colleges of Nursing* 34: 110–116. doi: 10.1016/j.profnurs.2017.11.006.

Grant-Writing, Dissemination, and Evaluation

4.1 Writing a Research Coproduction Grant Proposal

Ian D. Graham, Chris McCutcheon, Jo Rycroft-Malone and Anita Kothari

Key Learnings Points

- Collectively, the team (researchers and knowledge users) should come to agreement at the outset on how they want to work together (i.e., principles of coproduction/partnership, roles, governance, involvement during the lifecycle of the project).
- Start researcher–knowledge user discussions as early as possible, and allow a lot of time to coproduce the grant proposal.
- Read all instructions related to the call for grant proposals carefully, paying particular attention to the funder's evaluation or adjudication criteria.
- Describe clearly how the proposal writing followed a coproduction approach and how the research is coproduction (i.e., how knowledge users were and will be involved, their roles and how they will be involved in the governance and conduct of the study throughout the life of the project).

Research Coproduction in Healthcare, First Edition. Edited by
Ian D Graham, Jo Rycroft-Malone, Anita Kothari and Chris McCutcheon.
© 2022 John Wiley & Sons Ltd. Published 2022 by John Wiley & Sons Ltd.

- Demonstrate the authenticity of the researcher–knowledge user relationship in the grant proposal and in supporting documents (e.g., authentic letters of support)
- Budget for knowledge user costs related to participating on the team and the research endeavor.
- Submit the proposal to an internal review by knowledge users and researchers before submitting it to the funder. Revise accordingly.

BACKGROUND

Around the world, public and private research funders are increasingly funding coproduction research (McLean et al. 2018 and see Chapter 5.3). As has been noted in previous chapters, funder interest in coproduction has often been generated by the strong desire to reduce the delay in translating research findings into practice and policy and accelerating the return on their investment in research funding (i.e., optimizing research impact). Funders have also been influenced by the growing societal movements demanding greater involvement of patients' and citizens' in determining the research and services they need and want and how services should be delivered in ways that best meet their needs. Funder interest has also been supported by the movements advancing the democratization of science. There is a shift from the researcher/scientist as all-knowing and "non-researchers" as simply "research subjects" to researchers and knowledge users working together to create synergies by bringing their unique expertise together to strengthen research projects and improve study outputs and impacts. A critical step in embarking on research coproduction, once it has been decided the team wants to work together and address an issue of concern for the knowledge users, is obtaining funding for the research. This chapter focuses on the strategies to increase the likelihood of successfully obtaining research funding for coproduction projects.

To provide some context, three of the authors (IDG, CM, JRM) have had responsibility for overseeing research coproduction funding opportunities at the Canadian Institutes of Health Research (CIHR), the Canadian Health Services Research Foundation, and the UK National Institute of Health Research. We have extensive experience writing research coproduction grant calls for proposals. All authors have also chaired and been members of research coproduction grant funder review panels. We all also have considerable experience writing research coproduction grant proposals, some being successful! In this chapter, we will provide general advice on grant writing but specifically focus on the art of research coproduction grant proposal writing. We incorporate advice from published sources when available and from colleagues along with our experiential knowledge of coproduction grant writing. While there may be some general promising practices to consider when grant writing, for the most part, grant writing is a creative endeavor and often more art than science. With two exceptions, there are no right or wrong ways to write coproduction proposals, the exceptions being: 1) failing to address the objective of the call for proposals or its evaluation/adjudication criteria, and 2) not demonstrating authentic and meaningful partnership between the researchers and the knowledge users on the team. Always keep in mind that, with these types of proposals it is all about demonstrating how the proposal was truly coproduced and how the research project, if funded, will be coproduced.

In addition to empirically demonstrating many of the benefits of research coproduction grants (integrated knowledge translation (IKT) using CIHR terminology), the evaluation of CIHR's Knowledge Translation Funding Program (McLean and Tucker 2013) also identified several key elements for success of IKT funding opportunities: engaging knowledge users in and throughout the research process; assuring commitment and buy-in from partners (not necessarily financial); tailoring and timing the dissemination of results to the audience(s); and, engaging both researchers and knowledge users in the review of the IKT funding application. The challenges to conducting research using an IKT approach included: the substantial effort required to do IKT research (i.e., engaging knowledge users in a meaningful way); timing the research with knowledge user needs; submitting a knowledge user's non-academic curriculum vitae to CIHR; and describing the parameters of a research partnership in a grant application. In our experience, these observations have relevance to writing all research coproduction grant proposals.

SO WHAT DOES IT TAKE TO WRITE A SUCCESSFUL COPRODUCTION RESEARCH GRANT PROPOSAL?

General Advice on Writing a Grant Proposal

In many ways, writing a coproduction research grant proposal is very similar to writing a researcher-driven grant proposal. A recent synthesis of recommendations for promoting faculty grant proposal success in academic medical settings examined articles published on the topic between 2012 and 2020 (Wisdom et al. 2015). From 53 articles, they identified 10 recommendations for writing successful grants. These recommendations apply equally to research coproduction grants and provide solid advice for writing any grant proposal. The recommendations are:

1. Research and identify appropriate funding opportunities. Align the proposal with the funder's priorities, mission, and language.
2. Use key proposal components to persuade reviewers of project significance and feasibility.

3. Describe the proposed activities and their significance persuasively, clearly, and concisely.

4. Seek advice from colleagues to help develop, clarify, and review the proposal.

5. Keep study design simple, logical, feasible, and appropriate for the research questions.

6. Develop a timeline that includes time for possible resubmission to guide the grant proposal process.

7. Choose a novel, high-impact project with long-term potential.

8. Conduct an exhaustive literature review to clarify the present state of knowledge about the topic.

9. Ensure the budget requests only essential items and is an honest portrayal of the funding that the team needs to successfully carry out the work.

10. Consider interdisciplinary collaborations.

Additional generic advice worth considering comes from a CIHR guide to grant writing (McInnes et al. 2005). McInnes and colleagues identify the top eight things to do when writing a grant proposal as:

1. Organize an internal review of your proposal by individuals familiar with the competition and its requirements. Identify and address weakness in the proposal before submitting it.

2. Start writing early. Start preparing three months before the due date.

3. Write daily. Spending as little as 30 minutes per day will improve the quality of the ideas and writing.

4. Finish the "junk" in month one. This refers to things such as CV modules, letters of collaboration, collaborative details, references, cost quotes, etc.

5. Consider tips on good grant writing (they suggest getting the grant style. Get copies of highly rated grants from other researchers; get it down and don't be a sentence "caresser"; tailor the proposal to the audience; give the big picture, don't drown the reviewer in details, and state rationales; use illustrations; use the first or third person).

6. Write the application. Follow the structure of the grant application.

7. Carefully consider the number of proposals you will submit and external reviewers you suggest. Do not overextend yourself by submitting multiple proposals at the same time. Choose potential reviewers known to be fair and respected if submitting names of potential reviewers is required.

8. Apply for an appropriate budget and term.

Sources of information on general grant writing are plentiful. Start with the funding agency to which you are applying and check whether it has advice on grant writing in general or for the specific funding opportunity; for example, tips for writing PHSI grants (Canadian Institutes of Health Research 2014); tips for writing knowledge synthesis grants (Canadian Institutes of Health Research 2013). A quick google search will identify articles (Zlowodzki et al. 2007), books (Rothstein 2019), and book chapters (Hickman and Ferguson 2020) that may be helpful in guiding grant writing. Speak with successfully funded colleagues about their approaches to grant writing. To gain general knowledge about grant writing, it can also be fruitful to ask colleagues to share examples of their successful proposals to get a sense of how they frame winning proposals (especially if you are applying to the same competition or to the same panel). Try to speak to someone who was on the adjudication panel the previous year to understand the culture and expectations of the panel. Taking advantage of funder opportunities to observe adjudication panels is a great way to get a sense of what reviewers are looking for, as is becoming a peer reviewer. Attend an information session about the grant opportunity, if one is available.

Turning to research coproduction grant writing, we have only been able to find a few resources devoted specifically to providing advice on writing these sorts of proposals. We next review these resources before offering our own suggestions as to what makes a strong and compelling coproduction proposal.

Coproduction Grant Proposal Writing Advice

When considering how to start coproducing a grant proposal, the UK National Institute for Health Research's document, *Guidance on Coproducing a Research Project* is a good starting point. Keep in mind that this document is specifically focused on working with patients and the public (Hickey et al. 2021). It describes coproducing a research project as "An approach in which researchers, practitioners and members of the public work together, sharing power and responsibility from the start to the end of the project, including the generation of knowledge. The assumption is that those affected by research are best placed to design and deliver it and have skills and knowledge of equal importance" (p. 3). This document lays out many of the principles and features of coproducing research that teams should adopt to ensure they are actually using a coproduction approach (see Table 4.1.1). It also provides advice on how to achieve the key features. (Much of this advice is similar to what is presented in Chapters 2.2, 3.1, 3.2, 3.3, and 3.5. We encourage you to read those chapters for this foundational knowledge, if you have not already done so.) These key principles and features contribute to "the necessary preconditions" for a quality coproduction grant proposal and eventual project (University of British Columbia 2021).

TABLE 4.1.1　Principles and features described in the UK NIHR document, Guidance on Coproducing a Research Project.

Key principles	Key features
• Power sharing (the research is jointly owned) • Including all perspectives and skills • Respecting and valuing the knowledge of all those working together on the research (everyone is of equal importance) • Reciprocity (everyone benefits)	• establishing ground rules • continuing dialogue • joint ownership of key decisions • a commitment to relationship building • opportunities for personal growth and development • flexibility • continuous reflection

Our experience is that it takes several meetings between researchers and knowledge users to figure out what is at stake and whether there is enough in common to want to work together, to reach consensus on what needs to be studied and why, and to decide how to work together; for example, how the team will operationalize the NIHR or others' key coproduction principles and features in the budding partnership. Although absent from the lists above, we would add ethical partnership behavior as another key principle.

Researcher–knowledge user partnerships can begin in one of three ways: 1) researchers approach knowledge users with an idea for a project, 2) knowledge users seek out researchers with an issue or problem they would like to solve through research, and 3) researchers and knowledge users come together and co-create research projects around particular challenges or funding calls (see Chapters 3.1 and 3.3). Each approach can work as research coproduction. What is critical with each approach is that there is genuine respect and engagement of all parties. This is particularly important for researcher-initiated (#1) and knowledge user-initiated (#2) partnerships. There must be an openness to negotiate and compromise, and move forward with building together what is to be achieved and what the project will look like (i.e., the enactment of the principles and features above).

The time and effort that is needed to initiate and develop this working relationship should not be underestimated. Like all relationships, it takes time to learn about each other and to develop trust. Researchers often become aware of a special grant call with tight timelines and want to quickly pull a team together so that they can apply. They may approach knowledge users at the last moment or next-to-last moment (researcher-initiated approach). This sort of time pressure is seldom conducive to creating meaningful relationships and solid coproduction proposals between new research partners. It could also put prospective knowledge users off by suggesting to them that the researcher is not really committed to the concept of coproduction. Having said that, we have seen this scenario create the impetus for researchers and knowledge users to start to talk with each other, even if they subsequently realized there was insufficient time to create the conditions for coproduction before the proposal submission due date.

Once the conversations have started, the researchers and knowledge users are more ready to apply to the next funder call when it is launched because they have already initiated many of the necessary partnership preconditions.

While the temptation is for researchers to apply to any and all funding opportunities, with research coproduction a more judicious approach, that better reflects the joint venture of coproduction, will lead to a more credible proposal. On the other hand, if researchers and knowledge users have a pre-existing relationship, they may be well positioned to take advantage of applying to calls with short timelines. This situation of coproduction research not being amenable to short funder application timelines could be remedied if funders acknowledged the unique aspects of coproduction and tailored funding opportunities to better support research partnership building and the time needed to coproduce grant proposals.

In general, one way to start discussions and partnership building is by seeking out small funding opportunities to provide the resources to host meetings to bring researchers and knowledge users together. While early face-to-face meetings during the research relationship building phase have worked best for us, in the pandemic and post-pandemic era, virtual meetings will likely continue as the next best partnership building approach (and typically does not require funding to bring people together) (Hickey et al. 2021 and also Chapter 3.3).

The UK NIHR has another guidance document, *Public Co-Applicants in Research: Guidance on Roles and Responsibilities* (Elliott et al. 2019), written specifically for researchers who want to include public co-applicants and public contributors wanting to become a co-applicant. The term public refers to "patients, potential patients, carers and family members, people who use health and social care services, as well as people from organisations that represent people who use services" (p. 2). Keep in mind that this concept of "public" may not be equivalent to the term knowledge user as it is being used in this book, as public co-applicants may not always be the ones who use the research findings or make decisions based on the research findings. Also, the term public does not cover other types of knowledge user co-applicants, such as clinicians, managers, and policy makers, although much of what is covered in the document does apply to all types of knowledge users. The document discusses important issues, such as the need for role clarity of public co-applicants, what should be included in their CVs, budgeting considerations for, and contracts with public co-applicants, and the legal responsibilities of the researchers and public co-applicants. It also points to a number of useful resources, such as the INVOLVE Cost Calculator. While the advice is directed at those conducting research in the UK, much of it applies to all researcher–knowledge user partnerships in any country.

Turning now to the components of a strong coproduction research proposal, the *Guide to Knowledge Translation Planning at CIHR: Integrated and End-of-Grant Approaches* (Canadian Institutes of Health Research 2012) identifies four key factors CIHR IKT grant proposals should address: the research question, the research approach, feasibility, and outcomes. Table 4.1.2 presents the factors, their description, and how to address them in a proposal. The questions the

Table 4.1.2 CIHR's Integrated knowledge translation (iKT) project proposal worksheet

Factor	What is it?	Key Questions	What does this really mean?
Research Question	An explanation of what the research project is aiming to achieve and a justification for the need to conduct the research (i.e., how/why was this topic chosen? What gap will it fill?)	• To what extent does the project respond to the objectives of the funding opportunity? • To what extent does the research question respond to an important need identified by the knowledge users on the research team?	• Clearly articulate the research question • Be clear about the origin of the research question. Why is it interesting? Who is interested in it? How do the knowledge user partners view it? What potential benefit does it bring to the knowledge users?
Research Approach	A detailed description of the research approach and a justification for the proposed methods/ strategies	• To what extent is it likely that the proposed methods will address the research question? • To what extent is the study design appropriate and rigorous? • To what extent are the knowledge users meaningfully engaged in informing the research plan? • To what extent does the research team have the appropriate expertise to utilize the best methodologies?	• Be clear and specific about the proposed methods – it should be evident that the project team knows what it wants to do/study • Demonstrate the participation of and commitment to the project by the knowledge users – this can be written into the text or shown through letters of support. These letters are important; they need to show true IKT-style collaboration, describe the feasibility of the project and speak to methods of study design. These letters should not be "cookie cutter"; ensure that they are unique and specific about the knowledge users' expectations

Factor	What is it?	Key Questions	What does this really mean?
Feasibility	A clear demonstration that the researcher/ knowledge user team has the requisite skills, experience and resources to complete the project in the proposed time frame	• To what extent are the knowledge users committed to considering application of the findings when they become available and is this application achievable in the particular practice, program and/or policy context? • To what extent does the researcher/ knowledge user team have the necessary expertise and track record to deliver on the project's objectives, including the objectives of the end-of-grant KT plan? • To what extent is the project accomplishable in the given time frame with the resources available/described?	• Document the expertise of all team members and their role in the proposed study • Demonstrate that this is a doable study from both a scientific and a practical perspective • Demonstrate an interest by the knowledge user partners in the results of the study and the willingness and ability to use the results and move them into action (when appropriate) • Demonstrate that the budget is appropriate for the IKT plan, including the engagement activities/ communication needed.
Outcomes	A description of the potential results expected from the successful completion of the project	• To what extent will the project have relevant findings that may ultimately have a substantive and sustainable impact on health outcomes, practice, programs and/ or policies? • To what extent will the project's findings be transferable to other practice, programs and/ or policy contexts?	• Consider the potential impact of the study and its transferability. If it is not transferable, acknowledge and justify this • Include a detailed plan for end-of-grant KT • Develop a reasonable evaluation plan to be able to measure the outcomes and impacts of the study

(Continued)

TABLE 2.3.3   (Continued)

Factor	What is it?	Key Questions	What does this really mean?
		• To what extent will knowledge users be involved in interpreting results and informing KT plans/activities? • To what extent does the end-of-grant KT plan detail strategies appropriate for its goals and target audiences? • To what extent does the evaluation plan demonstrate that it will enable researchers to assess the project's impact?	

(Table 4.1.2 reprinted with permission from CIHR – https://cihr-irsc.gc.ca/e/45321.html)

research team should answer in their proposal are specific to CIHR proposals, but we believe these questions relate to all coproduction proposals and answering them will strengthen any proposal. The document also includes examples from actual proposals to illustrate how the factors have been addressed in successful proposals. While the column titled "What is it?" can apply to any grant proposal, the columns titled "Key Questions" and "What does this really mean?" flesh out many of the coproduction issues that are important to describe in the proposal; pay particular attention to these columns.

When preparing a coproduction grant proposal, keep in mind that coproduction is an approach and framing rather than a method per se: it can be applied to any study design and any research method. We have found that it works well to declare early on in the proposal that a coproduction approach is being taken and the coproduction principles and strategies that are guiding the partnership. Then, in the methods and other sections of the proposal interweave, as appropriate: who the knowledge users are, why they are particularly interested in this project, what their roles are during the conduct of the project, their commitment to the project, and how specifically they will be involved.

Given coproducing research is about engagement, consider using or referring to a research engagement framework to guide the coproduction process. Jull and her colleagues (Jull et al. 2019) have synthesized 54 articles about frameworks for knowledge user engagement in health research and identified

15 common concepts of engagement related to preparing (a precursor to the study), planning the design of the study, conducting the study and applying the study's findings. These concepts are: prepare and support researchers for coproduction, prepare and support knowledge users for coproduction (including training), relational processes (relationship-building and sustaining), the research agenda, ethics principles/values specific to coproduction, research questions, resources, ethics policy/rules related to conducting the research, methodology, methods, data collection, analysis, dissemination, evaluation of study processes, and sustainability of the study benefits. Twenty-eight of the articles reported on engagement that had occurred during studies while the remaining 26 articles reported on what should be done when engaging knowledge users. If other frameworks or theories are being used to guide the proposed study, when possible describe how they have been adapted to incorporate a coproduction lens or approach.

A common challenge reported by teams writing coproduction research proposals is that they are not able to provide all the methodological details that would usually be expected in a researcher-driven grant proposal. This is because decisions about methods may evolve during the course of the project because of the nature of coproduction. This is a dilemma facing all grant proposals which use participatory research approaches or some researcher-driven qualitative methodologies. While the exact methodological decisions may be unknown at the time the proposal is being written, grant applicants can be very clear about the participatory process being used, the decisions that will be made during the project, and the process(es) that will be used to make the relevant decisions. When appropriate, discuss stop/go criteria which will determine whether or not to proceed to the next phase of the project. Applicants can also clearly describe how the knowledge users are involved in the lifecycle of the research. Our advice is to be as detailed and explicit as possible about the coproduction process and identify what methodological decisions will need to be made during the course of the project and the process(es) that will ensure rigor in these decisions.

Tips on Writing Coproduction Research Grant Proposals

In preparation for writing this chapter, we tweeted out a request for experiential knowledge on writing and reviewing coproduction research proposals. We were specifically seeking critical factors that should be included in proposals to optimize funding success. Nineteen researchers and patient partners responded, some with experience as researchers and others as knowledge user grant reviewers. What follows is a synthesis of factors offered by our Twitter colleagues, as well as factors we believe are critical (or desirable) for grant success. When drafting the proposal, do not lose sight of the goal, which is convincing the grant reviewers that the proposed project is important and that the proposed coproduction and research processes are reasonable, appropriate, feasible, and can be trusted to generate the expected outcomes.

PRECONDITIONS THAT LEAD TO SUCCESSFUL PROPOSAL DEVELOPMENT – THE RELATIONSHIP AND PREPARATORY WORK

- Invest in research coproduction partnerships early, ideally before knowing of a relevant funding opportunity and certainly well in advance of a grant deadline. If approaching knowledge users, start at the idea stage, at the very beginning, not after the proposal has been written. Create space to jointly generate ideas.
- Work with an experienced knowledge or relationship broker (Bowen et al. 2019; Kislov et al. 2016) if possible – someone who understands the knowledge users' world, can translate for the researcher, and help the researcher navigate knowledge user organizations. They can also assist the knowledge user in managing the research relationship.
- To avoid tokenism, the partnership needs to involve meaningful engagement of knowledge users and the building of trusting relationships. Reviewers can spot tokenistic behavior towards knowledge users very quickly in a proposal.
- Jointly define what research coproduction means for the team and project. Consider using a research engagement or coproduction framework or theory to guide discussions and the project.
- Agree on coproduction principles to work by.
- Negotiate the overarching goal(s) of the partnership.
- Agree on the research question and the key elements of the project.
- Decide on processes and structures to enable equity and meaningful engagement of all knowledge users and stakeholders (see Chapters 3.1 and 3.3).
- Consider whether there might be benefit in training/learning opportunities for the researchers and knowledge users on how to work together, how their roles complement each other, and what might be needed to ensure the most productive research partnership. These activities can be built into the research proposal.
- Remember that equality in partnerships does not mean all members give and receive equally, but rather all parties play a role in negotiating roles and expectations (McLean and Tucker 2013).
- Come to agreement about what a meaningful partnership looks like for this particular partnership and consider such things as: mutual learning,

mutual respect, mutually agreed-upon roles and responsibilities, mutual recognition of efforts, mutual exchange of information, and mutual benefits (McLean and Tucker 2013).

- Decide on a governance model that reflects coproduction. Include decision-making processes that support consensus-based decisions about priorities, research questions, study design, etc.

Proposal Elements

- Understand the aim of the funding call and its evaluation/adjudication criteria and be sure to address these in the proposal. Make it really easy for reviewers to see how the proposal is addressing the funding aim and the adjudication criteria.
- In the proposal provide a definition of research coproduction and what frameworks, models, or theories guide your approach to it. It is better for the team to define what it is and how it will do it than assume reviewers will see it the same way.
- Demonstrate how the partnership and research question are responding to the needs of the knowledge user partners.
- Articulate both how the grant proposal is a result of coproduction and how the proposed research will be coproduced.
- Articulate how the partners have been involved in coproducing the proposal and how they will benefit from the work.
- Be explicit about when and how knowledge users will be engaged in the research process. Think in terms of the life cycle or stages of the research; for example, their role in deciding on study design, study methods, study outcomes, ethics application, data collection, analysis and interpretation of the data, dissemination of findings and co-authoring publications/presentations, using the findings, etc. In other words, demonstrate all of the ways the research will be coproduced (i.e., contributions by knowledge users). It is often desirable to also explain how during the project there will be sharing and ongoing learning from each other.
- Describe how knowledge users have been integrated into the project's governance. Explain how decision-making is being shared with knowledge users and the strategies for managing team conflicts.
- Notwithstanding the uncertainties about aspects of the study methods resulting from the coproduction approach (i.e., methodological decisions that can only be made once the study is underway), are the research methods adequately described? Reviewers will understand that coproduction means not being able to a priori determine all of the aspects of the

methods as is expected with researcher-driven studies, but they will still want to be convinced that in general, the study methods as presented are appropriate, reasonable and feasible.

- Articulate knowledge user commitment to the project including plans to potentially implement the findings. Commitment can be demonstrated in words but also in cash and in-kind contributions (i.e., describe how the partners have "skin in the game"). Dedicating staff (knowledge user) time to work on the project can be a strong signal that a knowledge user organization values the project, has confidence in the research team, and is anticipating the findings will be useful to them. Describe knowledge user willingness and ability to implement the study findings, when appropriate.

- If permitted, use letters from knowledge users to further illustrate their support for the project by highlighting their involvement and commitment (including in-kind and cash contributions) and intentions to act on the findings, when appropriate. The letter should be tailored to the grant proposal. The knowledge users' own words can be very persuasive. Letters written by the researchers and simply signed by knowledge users should be avoided as once reviewers suspect this is the case, they lose confidence that a true coproduction approach is at play. See the advice by CIHR on letter writing in Appendix 4.1.A of this chapter.

- Describe the contributions of all the team members and how the knowledge users' participation strengthens the team and adds value. When possible, highlight the team's experience with research coproduction as well as their track record of working together (and ideally demonstrating a sustained and strong partnership within the team). When possible, demonstrate the ongoing relationships between the knowledge users and researchers. All of these things contribute to reviewers' trust in the team and what is being proposed, which can be highly advantageous.

- Describe the overall feasibility of coproducing the research.

- Anticipate challenges to the coproduction process and offer mitigating strategies. For example, what is the plan if one of the primary knowledge users is promoted within the organization and can no longer participate in the project? How will the team deal with the situation where a knowledge user is no longer able to provide the promised cash contribution to the project because of changes in their situation (for example, the impact of COVID-19 on their organization)?

- Describe the transferability of the study results to other contexts; if they are not transferable, justify why not.

- Provide an appropriate dissemination plan for the study findings and describe how it will be coproduced. The plan should consider what products/findings will be ready for dissemination and distinguish between how the findings will be shared with the knowledge user partners and external audiences (see Chapter 4.2).

- Budget for knowledge user expenses, including for reimbursement for time if appropriate. Budget for partnership activities (e.g., funding for knowledge users to attend conferences to copresent the findings). Use the budget justification to underscore the commitment to authentic partnering and to recognize that there may be costs to the partners when they participate on research teams that should be covered by the grant. The budget justification can also be used to highlight knowledge users' commitments via cash and in-kind contributions.
- If knowledge users are included in the grant review process, write the proposal with this in mind, realizing that they will likely be focusing on the project's relevance and potential for impact in addition to its scientific merit.
- Consider including in the proposal an evaluation of the functioning of the partnership during and/or after the research is completed. This is seldom required in grant calls but assessing team functioning during coproduction research can identify any partnership issues early so they can be addressed before becoming too problematic. This sort of process or developmental evaluation data can also contribute to advancing the practice of coproduction.
- After the proposal is written, check one last time that the call adjudication criteria have been met in a comprehensive way.
- Organizing an internal review of the proposal by sharing it with some knowledge users and researchers who have not been part of developing it can be very helpful in revealing gaps in logic or flow and identifying text that might be improved to strengthen the proposal.

To sum up, throughout the proposal, continuously demonstrate (by providing evidence of) authentic, meaningful, and respectful partnerships. Describe all of the decisions and aspects of the relational work listed under the preconditions section above. Similarly, reveal how the team has and intends to work together and the impact potential of the proposed grant.

Tips for Researchers on Working with Knowledge Users During and After Proposal Writing

- Consider including knowledge user partners as co-applicants and co-principal applicants, when appropriate. Some knowledge users prefer to remain collaborators to avoid the administrative burden of submitting CVs or meeting other funder requirements. It is always best to ask knowledge users their preferred "official" role on the grant proposal, which may be different from their actual role on the project.
- Include more than one knowledge user on the team. This is in part about the value of having greater diversity on the team. It also relates to acknowledging and addressing power and status imbalances between the

researchers and knowledge users. Consider how the knowledge users may feel when they are greatly outnumbered by researcher team members who are "experts." This is a particularly important consideration when it comes to patients and caregivers, where the perceived power and status differential between themselves and the researchers may be large. Patients report higher comfort levels when they are not the lone patient at the table.

- Offer to coach knowledge users on the finer points of the study design and research methods.

- Listen to the knowledge users, ask them for their views and opinions, value their knowledge and experience and accord it the same respect as research expertise. Do not rush them.

- Ensure partners have an opportunity to talk through the proposal with the researchers, and within their organization, before they are asked to provide formal feedback. This may facilitate the knowledge users providing better feedback on the proposal.

- Knowledge users want to be kept up-to-date throughout the proposal development process and the conduct of the research. Consider the use of multiple communication channels (e.g., emails, newsletters, meetings) and use them frequently. These processes can also be described in the proposal to illustrate the importance the team places on the knowledge users and the intent to work with them in respectful ways.

- While jointly generating the proposal from the very beginning is ideal, if the research relationship is researcher initiated, one strategy to get it on a coproduction track is to approach potential partners before writing any of the proposal. Use two to three PowerPoint slides to present some ideas to the knowledge users to start the discussion.

- Celebrate the submission of the proposal. This is a milestone for the research partnership that should acknowledge the knowledge users' contributions to date.

- Continue to keep knowledge users informed during the (possibly long) period that the grant is under review by the funder. Knowledge users may not realize how long it can take to hear if a proposal has been funded and assume the researchers have abandoned the project when they do not continue to hear from them. Keep the lines of communication open while the team is waiting to hear the competition results. In the event the proposal is not funded, the team and in particular the knowledge users, may need to be prepared for the disappointment and what might be the next steps. This may mean preparing a resubmission or abandoning the proposal because the knowledge user context has changed significantly since the proposal submission such that the initial research question has been supplanted by more pressing issues.

- Offer knowledge users co-authorship on publications and explain what would be required to meet authorship criteria (Ellis et al. 2021; Richards et al. 2020).

Tips for Knowledge Users Working with Researchers During and After Proposal Writing

- Reach out to researchers if you have ideas for projects. Knowledge users can and should initiate research discussions.
- When researchers approach knowledge users (researcher initiated projects), carefully determine whether the proposed project addresses a priority issue. If not, explain what would make the proposed project work for you or decline to partner.
- Ask the researcher to discuss their conceptualization of research coproduction and how they see the research partnership unrolling. Express your views on what coproduction means to you. Is there a match? Is alignment of views possible? If not, it is okay to say "No thank you."
- Discuss how to move forward together with the proposal (consider the relational preconditions described above).
- Express the role you would like to have in proposal writing and in the conduct of the grant should it be funded.
- Offer your views to the researchers and team during co-development of the proposal. Your knowledge and experience are why you are on the team.
- Ask for clarification if you do not understand something or when team members use acronyms or scientific jargon you do not know.
- Some knowledge users have had unfortunate experiences with researchers in the past (e.g., researchers saying the study would be coproduced when it wasn't, researchers conducting the research and then not sharing the findings, the plan was for grant funding to help offset the organizational costs related in participating in the study and then when the grant was awarded no funding was transferred, etc.). Don't assume all researchers partner in bad faith. Keep an open mind about your researcher partner and raise any issues of concern as soon as possible so they may be addressed.
- Be clear to the team about your commitment to the project, the team, how you intend to act on the findings and how your commitment will be operationalized in the proposal and during the project.

- Be clear about what you see as the benefits for the organization from being a knowledge user partner on the project and continuously check that the project is positioned to deliver on those benefits.
- Consider succession planning should knowledge users on the team change jobs or can no longer continue being part of the team.
- Discuss opportunities to be co-authors on papers generated from the project, if that is of interest (Richards et al. 2020).

Appendix 4.1.B provides an applicant and reviewer coproduction research proposal checklist.

FUTURE RESEARCH

There is currently a paucity of research on how best to design and undertake research coproduction. There is also a need for studies and evaluations on the effectiveness of funder coproduction granting programs and to find how best to encourage and support research teams to embrace and undertake coproduction. Research on how best to train researchers and knowledge users to undertake research coproduction is warranted. Reporting guidelines for coproduced research should be developed.

CONCLUSION

Coproducing a proposal for conducting coproduced research involves not only describing the science but describing all the relational aspects of the research partnership. Strong proposals discuss the coproduction of the proposal, the pre-conditions that have led to it, and why the research question is of particular relevance to the knowledge users on the team. Strong proposals also describe how the coproduction team intends to continue to work together during the research, how they are involved in project governance and decision-making, and how the findings will be relevant to them and other knowledge users. A strong proposal will describe how coproduction has, and will continue to, influence stages of the life cycle of the project. The key is to demonstrate to the reviewers of the grant proposal that having adopted a coproduction approach is appropriate, has been carefully negotiated, and the research partnership is genuine.

As with all relationships, to make them work, research coproduction partnerships take time to develop, require much good will, effort, flexibility, and concern for the other. Enjoy getting to know each other and learning from each other. If the relationship survives the grant writing and peer review process, you are well on your way.

REFERENCES

1. Bowen, S., Botting, I., Graham, I.D., MacLeod, M., Moissac, D., Harlos, K., Leduc, B., Ulrich, C., and Knox, J. (2019). Experience of health leadership in partnering with University-based researchers in Canada – A call to "Re-imagine" research. *International Journal of Health Policy and Management* 8: 684–699. doi: 10.15171/ijhpm.2019.66.

2. Canadian Institutes of Health Research. (2012). *Guide to Knowledge Translation Planning at CIHR: Integrated and End-of-Grant Approaches.* Ottawa: Canadian Institutes of Health Research. https://cihr-irsc.gc.ca/e/documents/kt_lm_ktplan-en.pdf.

3. Canadian Institutes of Health Research. (2013). *Knowledge Synthesis – Tips for Success.* [Online]. https://cihr-irsc.gc.ca/e/46891.html (accessed 31 August 2021).

4. Canadian Institutes of Health Research. (2014). *Tips for PHSI Success.* [Online]. https://cihr-irsc.gc.ca/e/38778.html (accessed 31 August 2021).

5. Elliott, J., Lodemore, M., Minogue, V., and Wellings, A. (2019). *Public Co-Applicants in Research – Guidance on Roles and Responsibilities.* Southampton: INVOLVE. http://www.donorhealth-btru.nihr.ac.uk/wp-content/uploads/2019/02/NIHR-Guidance-on-Public-Co-applicants-2019.pdf.

6. Ellis, U., Kitchin, V., and Vis-Dunbar, M. (2021). Identification and reporting of patient and public partner authorship on knowledge syntheses: rapid review. *Journal of Participatory Medicine* 13: e27141. doi: 10.2196/27141.

7. Hickey, G., Brearly, S., Coldham, T., Denegri, S., Green, G., Staniszewska, S., Tembo, D., Torok, K., and Turner, K. (2021). *Guidance on Co-producing a Research Project.* Southampton: INVOLVE. https://www.learningforinvolvement.org.uk/wp-content/uploads/2021/04/NIHR-Guidance-on-co-producing-a-research-project-April-2021.pdf.

8. Hickman, L. and Ferguson, C. (2020). Writing research proposals and grant applications. In: *Nursing and Midwifery Research* (ed. D. Whitehead and C. Ferguson), 329–345. Chatswood, NSW: Elsevier.

9. Jull, J.E., Davidson, L., Dungan, R., Nguyen, T., Woodward, K.P., and Graham, I.D. (2019). A review and synthesis of frameworks for engagement in health research to identify concepts of knowledge user engagement. *BMC Medical Research Methodology* 19: 211. doi: 10.1186/s12874-019-0838-1.

10. Kislov, R., Hodgson, D., and Boaden, R. (2016). Professionals as knowledge brokers: the limits of authority in healthcare collaboration. *Public Administration* 94: 472–489. doi: 10.1111/padm.12227.

11. McInnes, R., Andrews, B., and Rachubinski, R. (2005). *Guidebook For New Principal Investigators.* Ottawa, ON: Canadian Institutes of Health Research. https://publications.gc.ca/collections/collection_2012/irsc-cihr/MR21-61-2005-eng.pdf.

12. McLean, R.K.D., Graham, I.D., Tetroe, J.M., and Volmink, J.A. (2018). Translating research into action: an international study of the role of research funders. *Health Research Policy and Systems/BioMed Central* 16: 44. doi: 10.1186/s12961-018-0316-y.

13. McLean, R.K.D. and Tucker, J. (2013). *Evaluation of CIHR's Knowledge Translation Funding Program*. Canadian Institutes of Health Research. https://cihr-irsc.gc.ca/e/documents/kt_evaluation_report-en.pdf.

14. Richards, D.P., Birnie, K.A., Eubanks, K., Lane, T., Linkiewich, D., Singer, L., Stinson, J.N., and Begley, K.N. (2020). Guidance on authorship with and acknowledgement of patient partners in patient-oriented research. *Research Involvement and Engagement* 6: 38. doi: 10.1186/s40900-020-00213-6.

15. Rothstein, A.L. (2019). *Creating Winning Grant Proposals: A Step-by-Step Guide*, 1e. New York: Guilford Press.

16. University of British Columbia. (2021). *IKT Guiding Principles*. [Online]. https://ikt.ok.ubc.ca (accessed 31 August 2021).

17. Wisdom, J.P., Riley, H., and Myers, N. (2015). Recommendations for writing successful grant proposals: an information synthesis. *Academic Medicine: Journal of the Association of American Medical Colleges* 90: 1720–1725. doi: 10.1097/ACM.0000000000000811.

18. Zlowodzki, M., Jonsson, A., Kregor, P.J., and Bhandari, M. (2007). How to write a grant proposal. *Indian Journal of Orthopaedics* 41: 23–26. doi: 10.4103/0019-5413.30521.

APPENDIX 4.1.A   CIHR advice on knowledge user letters of support – a quick reference https://cihr-irsc.gc.ca/e/45246.html

Criteria	Key questions	Options
Style	Is the letter original (as opposed to using a template)?	Style could include: • Intent of letter stated up front • Well organized and clear • Personalized to applicant
Background information	Is the relationship of the letter writer/ organization to the research project clearly outlined? Is the relationship of the letter writer/ organization to the applicant clearly delineated?	Background could include: • Credentials of letter writer • Letter writer's role in organization • How organization is linked to project • Background information of organization – demonstrates link to project • Previous involvement in topically similar research • Previous support of valuable research • Role letter writer will play in project • Letter writer's familiarity with credentials, work and goals of applicant • History of prior work with, collaboration with or support of applicant's research • Status of partnership
Relevance	Is the timeliness of the research project articulated? Is the applicability of the research project to the letter writer and/or the organization (goals, vision, mandate) outlined?	Relevance could include: • How/why this project addresses a research need or gap • How/why this project improves/ develops previous research • How/why this project can serve as foundation for future work • How this project addresses/fulfills the goals, vision, and/or mandate of the organization • How the letter writer and/or organization will move the results into practice (this point bridges both relevance and impact)
Impact	Are the potential outcomes and impact of the research project and findings described with some detail?	Impact could include: • How the letter writer and/or organization will move the results into practice (this point bridges both relevance and impact) • What the project results will contribute to the proposed health research topic/ area

(Continued)

TABLE 4.1.A   (Continued)

Criteria	Key questions	Options
Support	Is the extent and level of support that the letter writer and/or organization will provide specified?	• Support could include:Dollar amount and duration of support • Time allotted to, and type of in-kind contributions (e.g., time volunteered, staff or student assistance, help/mechanisms in place to facilitate dissemination etc.) • Specific tasks that in-kind support will consist of • Names, expertise and titles of people willing to contribute support • Contributions that the letter writer and/or organization have made to date

APPENDIX 4.1.B   Applicant and reviewer coproduction research proposal checklist

- Is a coproduction approach used to develop the proposal? Is it convincingly and adequately described?
- Is the applicants' definition of research coproduction clearly articulated and appropriate?
- Is a coproduction framework being used? Is it appropriate? How is it guiding the work described?
- Is the grant topic/issue/research question clearly articulated and its relevance, importance and potential benefit to the knowledge user partners clearly described?
- Is the description of the research coproduction process comprehensive and appropriate?
  ○ Does it include:
    - Identifying knowledge user partners
    - Coproduction principles and features
    - Coproduction activities
    - Project governance model that supports and embodies coproduction; study conflict resolution mechanisms
    - Specifics about the involvement of knowledge users in the research process. For example, when appropriate, knowledge user roles and involvement in: defining the research question; selecting study design, methods, study outcomes; data collection; data analysis and interpretation, disseminating the findings and co-authoring papers/ presentations; applying the findings; research ethics considerations and procedures related to the project

- Are the study research methods adequately described, taking into account adaptations required because of the coproduction approach?
- Is there demonstration of knowledge user commitment to the project, participating on the research team and potentially implementing the findings?
- Is there a letter of support from the knowledge user that has been tailored to this grant proposal?
- Is the team's experience with research coproduction described? Does the proposal demonstrate an ongoing relationship between the knowledge users and researchers? Is the team members' track record working together described?
- Are potential challenges to coproducing the research identified and mitigating strategies offered?
- Is the feasibility of conducting the study using a coproduction approach adequately described?
- Is knowledge user willingness and ability to move the study findings into action described?
- Is there a detailed dissemination plan included? Is it to be coproduced? Does the plan distinguish sharing research findings with the knowledge user partners and external audiences?
- Is the transferability of study findings discussed? If the study results are not transferrable, is this acknowledged and justified?
- When appropriate, is there an evaluation plan to assess the coproduction process?
- Is the budget appropriate for a coproduced project and are all additional costs related to coproduction included?
- Does the proposal address the aim of the funding call?
- Does the proposal address all of the funding call's evaluation criteria?

4.2 Coproduced Dissemination

Chris McCutcheon, Anita Kothari, Ian D. Graham, and Jo Rycroft-Malone

Key Learning Points

- There is an abundance of useful guidance on dissemination planning that can be adapted for coproduced dissemination. When adapting dissemination guidance it is important to adhere to coproduction principles, most importantly that power and decision-making is shared equally, and there is enough deliberation between researchers and knowledge users to discover new insights.
- Knowledge users and researchers can collaborate on every step of dissemination planning, but this is not always necessary. Agenda-setting about dissemination decisions should be made collaboratively, but the level of knowledge user involvement in the other steps will depend on their availability and the need for tailoring.
- Follow the principle of judicious knowledge translation and match the level of dissemination activity to the strength and relevance of the evidence. If we accept that coproduced dissemination will be more effective than researcher-driven dissemination, we should be prudent about when it is applied.

- Some of the most important decisions affecting the development of a coproduced dissemination plan occur before the planning stage.
- Coproduction aims to achieve knowledge use by changing the process of knowledge production. For this reason, research projects that were not coproduced at the outset should invite knowledge users to partner as early as possible if coproduced dissemination is desired and appropriate.
- There are important differences between a dissemination plan prepared for a grant proposal and one developed at the end of a project.

BACKGROUND

In an effort to improve the historically slow and limited impact of research on practice and policy, most health research funders now prioritize knowledge translation in their strategic planning (McLean et al. 2018) and require researchers to undertake knowledge translation activities (Tetroe et al. 2008). Researchers have become accustomed to dissemination planning, but in the early years of these requirements, some applicants and peer reviewers struggled with how to prepare and assess dissemination plans, leading to the development of multiple frameworks and instructional resources (Goering et al. 2010; Wilson et al. 2010). This material is also useful to research coproduction teams, but none of it offers guidance on how the coproduction approach applies to knowledge dissemination. This is understandable when we consider that research coproduction is itself a knowledge translation strategy, but one that emphasizes changes to the knowledge production process to achieve impact rather than activities at the end of a research project (Bowen and Graham 2013). Nonetheless, coproduction teams might aim for knowledge use beyond the knowledge users on their team if the findings are significant and generalizable. In theory, coproduction should transform the dissemination process in the same way that it transforms the research process, potentially achieving greater impact than standard approaches. This opens the possibility of a bridge between researcher-driven research and coproduction. Under the right circumstances, research projects that have not involved knowledge users could partner with them to coproduce at the dissemination phase. Drawing on the available guidance on dissemination planning, this chapter describes how to use the research coproduction approach to develop a coproduced dissemination plan.

WHAT IS COPRODUCED DISSEMINATION?

The knowledge translation field uses a lot of overlapping terminology (Graham et al. 2006), so clarifying some key terms is a good place to start. *Dissemination* is the planned and tailored communication of research findings to targeted audiences, usually knowledge users who can apply the evidence (Graham et al. 2013; Wilson et al. 2010). Lomas classifies dissemination as the middle term on a scale of "increasingly active and more focused intents" (Lomas 1993, p. 227) that begins with *diffusion* and ends with *implementation*. Dissemination occurs "somewhere between the generation and synthesis of knowledge and its application or use" (Gagnon 2011, p. 25). It attempts to connect knowledge to action. There are two different types of dissemination plans, those that investigators submit with grant proposals before they have started their research and those they prepare at the end of a project, based on research findings. As we will discuss later in the chapter, there can be important differences between the two, particularly when taking a coproduction approach.

When dissemination is coproduced, knowledge users and researchers work together to develop and execute dissemination plans according to the principles of coproduction (Hoekstra et al. 2020; Nguyen et al. 2020). These principles and other values are described in Chapters 2.1, 2.2, 2.3 and 3.3. All apply to co-produced dissemination, but the two most important elements are that power and decision-making is equally shared, and that there is adequate deliberation to combine the distinct knowledge user and researcher perspectives into new insights (Van de Ven and Johnson 2006). A research coproduction project could use a traditional, non-coproduced approach to dissemination if knowledge users are only involved in the research phase. Likewise, an researcher-driven research study could employ a coproduction dissemination strategy at the end of the project, as long as it is founded on an equitable and meaningful partnership with knowledge users.

Coproduced dissemination shares some of the features of *knowledge exchange*, but it is not the same concept. Knowledge exchange refers to any interactions between researchers and knowledge users that achieve knowledge translation goals. Sometimes it is viewed as a dissemination strategy and sometimes it is used to refer to the general philosophy underpinning coproduction (Gagnon 2011), but unlike coproduction, it does not typically speak to how interaction is managed. A distinction should also be made between coproduction and *engagement*. Engagement is an effective strategy for incorporating stakeholder or knowledge user perspectives and fostering buy-in. It certainly can and should be used in dissemination planning, but although engagement embraces many of the same goals and principles of coproduction, it falls short of full partnership (Boaz et al. 2018).

COPRODUCED DISSEMINATION: WHAT IS KNOWN FROM THE LITERATURE?

The literature on coproduction mostly focuses on how the approach applies to research, with little attention paid to dissemination. This is not to say that it goes completely unmentioned. Most discussions of research coproduction recommend that knowledge users and researchers collaborate on dissemination (Bowen and Graham 2013; Gagnon 2011; Redman et al. 2021), but unlike other aspects of the research process, how this is done is not covered in detail. We see a telling example in the Canadian Institutes of Health Research's *Guide to Knowledge Translation Planning at CIHR: Integrated and End-of-Grant Approaches* (Canadian Institutes of Health Research 2012). This document offers detailed guidance on how to conduct coproduced research studies and how to prepare standard dissemination plans, but there is no crossover other than to specify that dissemination planning is a part of research coproduction. Although the knowledge translation literature has little to say directly about coproduced dissemination, there are some themes in this literature that are relevant, specifically the theoretical compatibility of coproduction and dissemination; the role of knowledge exchange; the available guidance on dissemination planning; and the concept of judicious knowledge translation.

Compatibility of Coproduction and Dissemination

For some authors, research coproduction represents a paradigm shift away from an obsolete unidirectional model of knowledge translation, of which dissemination is a part (Bowen 2015; Bowen and Graham 2013; Davies et al. 2008, Greenhalgh and Wieringa 2011). In this account, dissemination efforts are unlikely to succeed because the research evidence is produced without any involvement from knowledge users, who may or may not be interested in, ready to receive, or capable of applying the findings. It is the idea that evidence is produced in one place and then transferred to another for application. Dissemination in this account is "too late if the questions that have been asked are not of interest to users" (Bowen 2015, p. 17). Research coproduction solves this problem of disconnectedness by enabling knowledge users to direct the research process to address topics they are already invested in and have responsibility for, what Gibbons et al. have called "discovery in the context of application" (Gibbons et al. 1994, p. 21). In principle, dissemination isn't required for knowledge use because the users are also the producers. However, the greater potential for relevance and application in research coproduction studies does not preclude the need to disseminate research findings to new audiences. Neither does it mean that there aren't aspects of the old paradigm that remain applicable. Ginsburg et al. (2007) argue that there are conditions when it may be more appropriate to involve knowledge users at the end of a researcher-driven project to collaborate on dissemination, specifically in large multi-stakeholder studies that may become politicized; replication studies that use fixed methods; and studies of high public interest, where there will already be strong demand for the findings among knowledge users.

Knowledge Exchange

Knowledge exchange is frequently discussed in the knowledge translation literature (Gagnon 2011; Lawrence 2006; Mitton et al. 2007; Ward et al. 2012), sometimes labeled as linkage and exchange (Lomas 2000) or the interaction model of knowledge translation (Ginsburg et al. 2007; Landry et al. 2001; Lomas 2000). Much of this work is theoretical, but there are some empirical studies showing that knowledge exchange increases the use of research evidence and builds relationships between researchers and knowledge users that provide a foundation for future knowledge translation activities (Huberman 1990; Landry et al. 2001; Rynes et al. 1999; Van de Ven 2018). The more that researchers and knowledge users interact, the more that knowledge users trust researchers as sources of knowledge and researchers become capable of providing contextually relevant evidence (Van de Ven 2018). To a large degree, research coproduction is the application of this mechanism in the research process, though it differs in the emphasis it places on specific principles and practices of partnership. In terms of dissemination, this scholarship supports the use of interactive activities, such as workshops or deliberative dialogues, to achieve knowledge use, but the importance of establishing trusting relationships suggests longer-term interactions could be more valuable. It would be worthwhile to invest in networks of knowledge users and researchers, as they provide a soft infrastructure for the circulation of new knowledge. We should also note that knowledge exchange among the members of a research team will be effective only for those individuals, and the effect will not extend to external audiences. When our focus shifts to external audiences, we need to look at creating opportunities for interaction between project team members and a broader range of knowledge users from other sectors and organizations.

Guidance on Dissemination Planning

There is a great deal of published and gray literature available to assist investigators with dissemination planning. In their 2010 scoping review, Wilson et al. (2010) identified 33 knowledge translation frameworks, of which 20 were designed specifically to guide dissemination planning. Many of these frameworks feature interaction or collaboration between researchers and knowledge users. However, like the CIHR guide mentioned earlier, when these frameworks align with a coproduction approach, the focus is on knowledge production, not dissemination to new audiences. Other frameworks espouse interaction between researchers and knowledge users as a general principle or specific strategy for dissemination, but they do not offer guidance on how to coproduce dissemination plans. In preparation for this chapter we conducted a systematic Google search to see what guidance is available in the gray literature and found 40 different dissemination guides. Thirty-three of these guides recommend knowledge user involvement, but again the emphasis is either on research collaboration or engagement of knowledge users when dissemination planning, not coproduced dissemination. A selection of these guides is provided in Table 4.2.1.

Judicious Knowledge Translation

Judicious knowledge translation is one of the most important concepts in all dissemination planning, whether coproduced or researcher-driven (Graham et al. 2013). It refers to the need to match the scale and intensity of dissemination

TABLE 4.2.1 Sample dissemination guides recommending knowledge user involvement.

Authors	Title	URL
AllerGen 2009	Knowledge Translation Planning Tools for Allergic Disease Researchers	https://allergen.ca/wp-content/uploads/2014/04/KTTool.pdf
Briggs et al. 2015	Questing Your Way to a Knowledge Mobilization Strategy	https://carleton.ca/communityfirst/wp-content/uploads/KMB-Questing Your Way to a KMb-Strategy-Jun-29-2015-3.pdf
Health Canada 2017	Knowledge Translation Planner	https://www.canada.ca/en/health-canada/corporate/about-health-canada/reports-publications/grants-contributions/knowledge-transfer-planner.html
Lyons & Warner 2005	Demystifying Knowledge Translation for Stroke Researchers: A Primer on Theory and Praxis	https://www.researchgate.net/publication/265658194_Demystifying_Knowledge_Translation_for_Stroke_Researchers_A_Primer_on_Theory_and_Praxis_Paper_by
Mathematica Policy Research 2015	PCORI Dissemination & Implementation Toolkit	https://www.pcori.org/sites/default/files/PCORI-DI-Toolkit-February-2015.pdf
Reardon, Lavis & Gibson 2006	From Research to Practice: A Knowledge Transfer Planning Guide	https://www.iwh.on.ca/tools-and-guides/from-research-to-practice-kte-planning-guide
Ward et al. 2010	Planning for knowledge translation: A researcher's guide	https://www.researchgate.net/publication/233591272_Planning_for_knowledge_translation_A_researcher%27s_guide & https://doi.org/10.1332/174426410X535882

efforts to the quality and significance of the research findings. Generally speaking, synthesized evidence merits the greatest investment of time and resources, and we should be more reserved when disseminating the results of single studies, which are more prone to bias (Grimshaw et al. 2012; Wilson et al. 2008). The word "judicious" is used because this decision is a matter of judgement. There may be moments when findings of single studies are very timely and significant, there is a paucity of evidence on the topic, findings are very action-oriented, or there is strong knowledge user interest. There is also an ethical imperative to share all research findings to at least some degree – to be transparent about how public funds were used, for example. When disseminating the results of single studies, it is important to contextualize the evidence, providing knowledge users with the information they need to understand the place of these findings in the existing literature and the relevance of the findings to their context (Davies et al. 2008). We can do more harm than good if there is broad uptake of findings that have yet to be replicated or that turn out to be incorrect or misinterpreted. For this reason, we need to be cautious about applying a coproduction approach to dissemination, just like we would with traditional dissemination. We posit that coproduction is more resource-intensive, time-consuming, and impactful than researcher-driven dissemination, so it should only be used when the effort is justified by the evidence.

DISSEMINATION PLANNING AT THE GRANT PROPOSAL STAGE

When describing the steps of coproduced dissemination planning in this chapter, we focus on the work that is done as findings emerge. These same steps apply when developing a plan for a grant proposal, but there are some important differences to keep in mind. First, when writing a grant proposal, the research findings are most often unknown. It isn't possible to assess the significance of the evidence or craft key messages for the identified audiences. Nonetheless, the overall research design will give the team a sense of what kind of evidence will be produced, and the knowledge users on the team can make a case for the importance of the research question in their context and for other knowledge users in their sector. The second major difference is the degree to which attention is paid to the resources needed for dissemination. Funding is required for effective dissemination, and the proposed dissemination activities need to be budgeted for in the grant proposal. At the grant proposal stage the dissemination plan is a loose framework that will be updated and refined as the project unfolds and shareable knowledge emerges. That said, the plan still has to be coherent and well justified, as is the case for the other components of the research proposal. CIHR's knowledge translation guide is one of the few guides that focuses on dissemination planning at the proposal stage (Canadian Institutes of Health

Research 2012). Although it does not advise users on how to apply coproduction to planning, it does a good job of addressing some of the subtleties of how a dissemination plan should be prepared for and evaluated in funding competitions. Readers will find detailed advice on preparing coproduction research proposals in Chapter 4.1.

FROM RESEARCH TO DISSEMINATION

The traditional depiction of dissemination portrays it as a distinct phase that begins when the research is complete and the findings are known. We suggest looking at it differently when taking a coproduction approach – that it is when the project team analyses and interprets the data that the transition from research to dissemination begins. As discussed throughout this book, the central premise of the coproduction approach is that knowledge use is achieved through changes to the research process. Knowledge users influence the development of the research question so that it addresses a problem they can act upon.[1] The data analysis stage is equally critical to the coproduction process. Findings do not automatically emerge from data, rather they are socially constructed through deliberation and interpretation, a process influenced by the unique perspectives of team members and the context in which they work (Cornish et al. 2013; Flicker 2014). At this stage the team is still tailoring the knowledge to the needs of the participating knowledge users. For research coproduction projects we would expect collaborative data analysis to be part of the project design, but of course this would not be the case for researcher-driven projects. In the latter case, if researchers are genuinely interested in coproduced dissemination, we recommend inviting knowledge users to partner at this stage or be open to reinterpreting or contextualizing the data if analysis is already done. Without the collaboration of knowledge users in at least this stage of the process, they have not participated enough in knowledge creation to describe the activity as coproduction.

As the project transitions to the dissemination phase, it is the time to answer key questions that will inform the development of the dissemination plan. It is when the team reflects on judicious knowledge translation, i.e., the amount of dissemination that is warranted by the findings. The right course of action might be for the team to moderate their ambition to achieve impact and lessen the level

---

[1] In the introduction we discuss the different categories of knowledge users and the nature of their involvement in research coproduction projects. A dissemination plan will usually target knowledge users outside of the project who would have some capacity to act on the findings. There will be potential audiences interested in, or potentially affected by, the findings. When these audiences are targeted, the key messages and dissemination strategies may have to be different.

of dissemination activity. Alternatively, have new insights emerged through the data analysis that suggest other audiences should be informed of the findings? If the team decides that broad reach to multiple different audiences is warranted, this stage presents an opportunity to expand the coproduction team to include new knowledge users. Although it is not strictly speaking a coproduction process, we see a model for this approach in the Patient-Centered Outcomes Institute's (PCORI) guidelines on dissemination and implementation. They recommend inviting all potential stakeholders to participate in pre-dissemination process that they call "evidence assessment" (Mathematica Policy Research 2015, p. 15). These stakeholders are engaged through meetings, focus groups, or surveys to evaluate the "usefulness, relevance, and value of evidence in the context of existing evidence and findings" (p. 15). This process helps PCORI to decide if the results of the study warrant dissemination, if so to what scale, and whether new research is needed to complement the evidence. This does not need to be an extensive or complicated process. The points to remember are: that there is a preparatory phase before dissemination planning begins; that important decisions about the content of the dissemination plan are made at this time; and it is an opportunity to collaborate with knowledge users new to the research team. The knowledge users on a coproduction team can be a critical resource when it comes to finding new partners, as they will usually have extensive networks to draw upon. For researchers, anticipation of opportunities for future dissemination collaborations is an argument for routinely participating in knowledge exchange activities and developing networks that include a variety of knowledge users.

THE STEPS OF COPRODUCED DISSEMINATION PLANNING

In 2017, three of the chapter authors developed a workshop entitled *Making an Impact: Using Integrated Knowledge Translation to Build KT Plans*. This was our first attempt to apply the coproduction approach to dissemination planning, and since that time we have run the workshop in three different countries, improving each iteration based on feedback from participants. The primary resource for these workshops was the *Guide to Knowledge Translation Planning at CIHR*. We are most familiar with the planning steps outlined in this guide, but we know there are many other guides available. The planning process we describe here integrates the core steps from the CIHR guide with guidance from other resources. Although we believe there is value in following these steps sequentially, we agree with the advice from Ward *et al.* that knowledge translation is a "dynamic, interactive and multidirectional process where elements of the process can occur simultaneously or in different sequences" (Ward et al. 2010, p. 532). This is especially true with coproduction, where many of the questions that need to be answered in developing a dissemination plan require dialogue with knowledge users. Moreover, in coproduced research it can be difficult to isolate a distinct phase at the end of a project when dissemination begins. Knowledge is continually created, shared, and re-created throughout the research coproduction process.

Set Dissemination Goals

To a large extent the goals of the dissemination plan will be determined at the data analysis and interpretation stage. However, in a coproduced research project many outputs will be generated for the knowledge user partners throughout the life of the project. Co-produced research projects can be real-time dissemination platforms, as the knowledge users may need information at multiple stages to promote the project within their organizations or assist with decision-making. The data analysis stage is when the scale of dissemination is matched to the strength and significance of the research findings. Like translating a research topic into a research question, setting dissemination goals is a direction-setting exercise. As such, it is very important that knowledge users participate. The team specifies in concrete terms what it seeks to accomplish with the dissemination plan. Is conceptual or instrumental knowledge use anticipated? Perceptions of how to use knowledge can vary among team members, especially if some knowledge users were involved from the start of the project and others were invited to collaborate later on. Is the goal of the plan to inform knowledge users of the ongoing project, of the research findings or apply the evidence in a way that changes practice or policy? The knowledge users on the team may want to implement the findings in their organization with the assistance of the researcher partners. It could be appropriate to have multiple goals, depending on the ambitions of the team and the number of potential audiences that have been identified. Have the goals of the dissemination plan changed since the grant proposal stage? Did anything during the data analysis suggest an expansion or reduction in scale? When setting the goals, remember that all other decisions about the dissemination plan should support them. Consider how progress in achieving the goals might be evaluated. The ideal is to define the dissemination goals as measurable outcomes for subsequent evaluation.

Assess Resources

At the end of a research project, assessing resources is so entwined with setting goals that it almost shouldn't be separated as a step. The goals of the dissemination plan will only be achievable if there are available resources to achieve the plan. This step is not a budgeting exercise, but an opportunity for the team to reflect on what it has to work with before getting too far into the development of the dissemination plan. The team will have budgeted for dissemination in their grant proposal, but there may have been overruns during the research stage that cut into these funds. Or, the official project time period might be coming to a close. If after reviewing its findings the team decides to be more ambitious in its dissemination goals, it may need to apply for new funding or a project extension. Some funding agencies offer dissemination grants to support completed research projects with high potential for impact. Perhaps some of the goals are achievable in the short term but others need to wait until new resources are acquired. Expanding activity in a coproduction project likely means there will be more interaction between the researchers and the knowledge users, which adds costs. This is especially true if new knowledge users will be brought onto the team for the dissemination phase. Assessment of resources should be considered when making decisions about the feasibility of possible dissemination strategies to use and revisited when the dissemination strategies are selected.

Identify and Learn about Your Audience(s)

Remember that dissemination targets specific audiences. As discussed, there is an opportunity at the data analysis stage to bring in new knowledge users to interpret the findings and collaborate on the development of the dissemination plan. These new knowledge users could be representative of a general audience, such as physicians or health system managers, or they could be invited to participate for the role they play within specific organizations. Bringing a knowledge user onto the team improves the potential for tailoring key messages, dissemination strategies and the nature of the outputs, and they should develop a personal and professional investment in using the findings of the project. Once the project team has identified all of their potential audiences they should try to learn as much as possible about how the research findings are relevant to them and could be used by them: their level of knowledge on the topic; their preferred channels of communication; their professional responsibilities and capacity to act on new knowledge; barriers and facilitators of knowledge use; and, the political climate that they work within. Another word for this gamut of audience information is context. Jacobson et al. (2003) have developed a very useful framework for evaluating knowledge user context. It includes a series of questions that cover multiple dimensions of how knowledge users receive and use information. In a coproduced dissemination plan these questions would ideally be answered collaboratively, but this information can also be gathered through other engagement methods, such as focus groups or interviews.

Develop Key Messages

Some dissemination guides recommend developing key messages prior to audience identification, but our view is that the messages can be more tailored if this work is informed by what has been learned about the knowledge user audiences through coproduction. The emphasis should not be on what the key messages *of* the project are but the key messages *for* each identified audience. Collaboration with knowledge users should help to shift this focus. Key messages should be based on the dissemination goals, and they should combine the findings from the research study with implications for policy or practice and recommendations on how to use the findings. Sometimes key messages just provide evidence to knowledge users without making recommendations. These are messages in search of audiences rather than messages tailored to and with audiences. The evidence should still be contextualized so that knowledge users understand how it changes their current understanding of an issue. If the evidence is strong enough and the project team has enough information about an audience's context, they might recommend specific actions. Sometimes researchers recommend actions that are not realistic because they are not founded on an understanding of the factors that influence decision-making in knowledge users' practice. When key messages are coproduced by researchers and knowledge users who represent an identified audience, recommendations will be more credible and applicable and therefore more likely to be applied.

Select Dissemination Strategies

The coproduction team has decided what it wants to accomplish with the dissemination plan; it knows its audiences and their needs; and it has started to tailor the messages from the research project for use. Now it is time for the team to select the strategies it will use for dissemination. The other guidance documents referred to in this chapter all present a wide range of dissemination strategies. The information learned about how the factors influencing how the audiences use knowledge should help the team to prioritize among the many different options. The team should also refer to the knowledge translation research literature to learn if there is evidence available about the effectiveness of the strategies for the population of interest. There are no specific coproduction dissemination strategies, though many do focus on interaction and knowledge exchange. Input from knowledge users at this stage will help the team to tailor the strategies to maximize their potential effectiveness. Any dissemination products, such as reports, policy briefs, or electronic applications, should be approved by the knowledge users representing the target audiences. Knowledge users can also provide insight into the best timing for dissemination activities and overall integration into the day-to-day practices of their organizations. As the team chooses its dissemination activities it should begin to create or update the dissemination budget.

Determine What Expertise Is Needed

Some dissemination strategies require specialist expertise. For example, programmers or developers are needed to build web sites or design mobile applications. Writers with journalism or communications training are often more adept than researchers at plain-language communication. If the dissemination plan calls for interactive strategies, should facilitators or knowledge brokers be recruited? Even if specialists are not needed, all dissemination plans require human resources for successful implementation. When writing a dissemination plan for a grant proposal it is important to demonstrate that the people involved can successfully implement the plan. It is not essential that all decisions about expertise are made collaboratively, but the project team may wish to consider if there are staff within the knowledge user audience organizations that could assist with the dissemination activities. Knowledge users will have insight into the human resource implications of specific dissemination strategies within their organizations. Remember that the knowledge users are themselves experts on how knowledge is used in their settings (i.e., how decisions about practice, programs, or policies are made and the role of research in these processes). Unlike a traditional dissemination plan, in a coproduced plan there is significant overlap between audience and expertise.

Evaluate

Evaluating the outcomes of the dissemination strategies will tell the project team if they have succeeded in meeting their knowledge translation goals and potentially reveal impacts resulting from evidence uptake. Not all dissemination plans have to include an evaluation. Again, this investment of time and resources must be appropriate for the scale of the dissemination plan. Process evaluation can help teams to manage complex, multi-stage dissemination strategies, ensuring that activities roll out as planned. Evaluation is also an opportunity to build the knowledge base on the effectiveness of different dissemination strategies. The decision to evaluate or not should be made collaboratively. The reasons for wanting to evaluate may differ between the knowledge users and researchers on the team. For example, the evaluation results could help knowledge users to justify to their organizations the amount of time they have invested in the project. Another benefit of evaluation could be the continuation of the researcher and knowledge user partnership. It extends and strengthens the shared investment in achieving the goals set out at the beginning of the plan.

FUTURE RESEARCH

Not enough research has been done on either the best practices in research coproduction or the effectiveness of dissemination strategies. We need to learn more about how research teams apply the theory of coproduction in practice. The Integrated Knowledge Translation Research Network's *How We Work Together* series of casebooks are beginning to pull back the curtain on how research coproduction is operationalized (McCutcheon et al. 2021). This work should be broadened to include how research teams apply coproduction to the dissemination of research findings. For the time being, the hypothesis that coproduced dissemination is more effective than researcher-driven dissemination is an untested one, even though by definition coproduction means a user-designed approach, where knowledge products are tailored to needs, expectations and context (Norman 2013). Dissemination planning has generally been under-emphasized in the coproduction literature. We certainly need to learn more about coproduction as a research approach, but the time has come to look at how coproduction can contribute to dissemination.

CONCLUSION

This chapter is a first attempt to apply the research coproduction approach to knowledge dissemination. In the knowledge translation field we have best practices for dissemination and detailed guidance is available to assist research teams to prepare dissemination plans. Applying coproduction to these practices has the potential to achieve greater impact than the standard researcher-driven approach. When coproducing dissemination plans, it is important to remember that coproduction achieves knowledge use by involving knowledge users in knowledge production. As is the case when coproducing research, knowledge users should have meaningful influence over the key decisions made when dissemination planning. Coproduction is a resource-intensive process, so it should only be applied in the dissemination of researcher-driven projects when the evidence is strong and there is a high potential for impact.

REFERENCES

1. Allergen. (2009). *Knowledge Translation Planning Tools for Allergic Disease Researchers*. Hamilton: Allergen NCE Inc. https://allergen.ca/wp-content/uploads/2014/04/KTTool.pdf
2. Boaz, A., Hanney, S., Borst, R., O'Shea, A., and Kok, M. (2018). How to engage stakeholders in research: design principles to support improvement.

Health Research Policy and Systems/BioMed Central 16: 60. doi: 10.1186/s12961-018-0337-6.

3. Bowen, S. (2015). The relationship between engaged scholarship, knowledge translation and participatory research. In: *Participatory Qualitative Research Methodologies in Health* (ed. G. Higginbottom and P. Liamputtong), 183–199. SAGE Publications Ltd.

4. Bowen, S. and Graham, I.D. (2013). Integrated knowledge translation. In: *Knowledge Translation in Health Care: Moving from Evidence to Practice* (ed. S.E. Straus, J. Tetroe, and I.D. Graham), 2e, 14–23. John Wiley & Sons.

5. Briggs, G., Briggs, A., Whitmore, E., Maki, A., Ackerley, C., Maisonneuve, A, and Yordy, C. (2015). *Questing Your Way to a Knowledge Mobilization Strategy*. Ottawa: Community First: Impacts of Community Engagement. https://carleton.ca/communityfirst/wp-content/uploads/KMB-Questing-Your-Way-to-a-KMb-Strategy-Jun-29-2015-3.pdf

6. Canadian Institutes of Health Research. (2012). *Guide to Knowledge Translation Planning at CIHR: Integrated and End-of-Grant Approaches*. Ottawa: Canadian Institutes of Health Research. https://cihr-irsc.gc.ca/e/documents/kt_lm_ktplan-en.pdf.

7. Cornish, C., Gillespie, A., and Zittoun, T. (2013). Collaborative analysis of qualitative data. In: *The Sage Handbook of Qualitative Data Analysis* (ed. U. Flick), 79–93. London: SAGE Publications Ltd.

8. Davies, H., Nutley, S., and Walter, I. (2008). Why "knowledge transfer" is misconceived for applied social research. *Journal of Health Services Research and Policy* 13: 188–190. doi: 10.1258/jhsrp.2008.008055.

9. Flicker, S. (2014). Collaborative data analysis. In: *The SAGE Encyclopedia of Action Research (Vols. 1–2)* (ed. D. Coghlan and M. Brydon-Miller), 122–124. London: SAGE Publications Ltd.

10. Gagnon, M.L. (2011). Moving knowledge to action through dissemination and exchange. *Journal of Clinical Epidemiology* 64: 25–31. doi: 10.1016/j.jclinepi.2009.08.013.

11. Gibbons, M., Limoges, C., Nowotny, H., Schwartzman, S., and Trow, M. (1994). *The New Production of Knowledge: The Dynamics of Science and Research in Contemporary Societies*. SAGE Publications.

12. Ginsburg, L.R., Lewis, S., Zackheim, L., and Casebeer, A. (2007). Revisiting interaction in knowledge translation. *Implementation Science: IS* 2: 34. doi: 10.1186/1748-5908-2-34.

13. Goering, P., Ross, S., Jacobson, N., and Butterill, D. (2010). Developing a guide to support the knowledge translation component of the grant application process. *Evidence & Policy: A Journal of Research, Debate and Practice* 6: 91–102. doi: 10.1332/174426410X483024.

14. Graham, I.D., Logan, J., Harrison, M.B., Straus, S.E., Tetroe, J., Caswell, W., and Robinson, N. (2006). Lost in knowledge translation: time for a map? *The Journal of Continuing Education in the Health Professions* 26: 13–24. doi: 10.1002/chp.47.

15. Graham, I.D., Tetroe, J., and Gagnon, M. (2013). Knowledge dissemination: end of grant knowledge translation. In: *Knowledge Translation in Health Care: Moving from Evidence to Practice* (ed. S.E. Straus, J. Tetroe, and I.D. Graham), 2e, 75–92. John Wiley & Sons.

16. Greenhalgh, T. and Wieringa, S. (2011). Is it time to drop the "knowledge translation" metaphor? A critical literature review. *Journal of the Royal Society of Medicine* 104: 501–509. doi: 10.1258/jrsm.2011.110285.

17. Grimshaw, J.M., Eccles, M.P., Lavis, J.N., Hill, S.J., and Squires, J.E. (2012). Knowledge translation of research findings. *Implementation Science: IS* 7: 50. doi: 10.1186/1748-5908-7-50.

18. Health Canada (2017). Knowledge Translation Planner. Ottawa: Health Canada. https://www.canada.ca/content/dam/hc-sc/documents/corporate/about-health-canada/reports-publications/grants-contributions/KT%20Planner-EN-2017-10-16.pdf

19. Hoekstra, F., Mrklas, K.J., Khan, M., McKay, R.C., Vis-Dunbar, M., Sibley, K.M., Nguyen, T., Graham, I.D., SCI Guiding Principles Consensus Panel, and Gainforth, H.L. (2020). A review of reviews on principles, strategies, outcomes and impacts of research partnerships approaches: a first step in synthesising the research partnership literature. *Health Research Policy and Systems / BioMed Central* 18: 51. doi: 10.1186/s12961-020-0544-9.

20. Huberman, M. (1990). Linkage between researchers and practitioners: a qualitative study. *American Educational Research Journal* 27: 363–391. doi: 10.3102/00028312027002363.

21. Jacobson, N., Butterill, D., and Goering, P. (2003). Development of a framework for knowledge translation: understanding user context. *Journal of Health Services Research and Policy* 8: 94–99. doi: 10.1258/135581903321466067.

22. Landry, R., Amara, N., and Lamari, M. (2001). Utilization of social science research knowledge in Canada. *Research Policy* 30: 333–349. doi: 10.1016/S0048-7333(00)00081-0.

23. Lawrence, R. (2006). Research dissemination: actively bringing the research and policy worlds together. *Evidence & Policy: A Journal of Research, Debate and Practice* 2: 373–384. doi: 10.1332/174426406778023694.

24. Lomas, J. (1993). Diffusion, dissemination, and implementation: who should do what? *Annals of the New York Academy of Sciences* 703: 226–237. doi: 10.1111/j.1749-6632.1993.tb26351.x.

25. Lomas, J. (2000). Using "linkage and exchange" to move research into policy at a Canadian foundation. *Health Affairs* 19: 236–240. doi: 10.1377/hlthaff.19.3.236.

26. Lyons, R., and Warner, G. (2005). Demystifying Knowledge Translation for Stroke Researchers: A Primer on Theory and Praxis. Halifax: Atlantic Health Promotion Research Centre. https://www.researchgate.net/publication/265658194_Demystifying_Knowledge_Translation_for_Stroke_Researchers_A_Primer_on_Theory_and_Praxis_Paper_by

27. Mathematica Policy Research. (2015). *PCORI Dissemination & Implementation Toolkit*. Patient-Centered Outcomes Research Institute. https://www.pcori.org/sites/default/files/PCORI-DI-Toolkit-February-2015.pdf.

28. McCutcheon, C., Reszel, J., Kothari, A., and Graham, I.D. (eds.) (2021). *How We Work Together: The Integrated Knowledge Translation Research Network Casebook*, Vol. 4. Ottawa: Integrated Knowledge Translation Research Network. https://iktrn.ohri.ca/projects/casebook.

29. McLean, R.K.D., Graham, I.D., Tetroe, J.M., and Volmink, J.A. (2018). Translating research into action: an international study of the role of research funders. *Health Research Policy and Systems/BioMed Central* 16: 44. doi: 10.1186/s12961-018-0316-y.

30. Mitton, C., Adair, C.E., McKenzie, E., Patten, S.B., and Waye Perry, B. (2007). Knowledge transfer and exchange: review and synthesis of the literature. *The Milbank Quarterly* 85: 729–768. doi: 10.1111/j.1468-0009.2007.00506.x.

31. Nguyen, T., Graham, I.D., Mrklas, K.J., Bowen, S., Cargo, M., Estabrooks, C.A., Kothari, A., Lavis, J., Macaulay, A.C., MacLeod, M., Phipps, D., Ramsden, V.R., Renfrew, M.J., Salsberg, J., and Wallerstein, N. (2020). How does integrated knowledge translation (IKT) compare to other collaborative research approaches to generating and translating knowledge? Learning from experts in the field. *Health Research Policy and Systems/BioMed Central* 18: 35. doi: 10.1186/s12961-020-0539-6.

32. Norman, D. (2013). *The Design of Everyday Things*. Cambridge: The MIT Press.

33. Reardon, R, Lavis, J., and Gibson, J. (2006). From Research to Practice: A Knowledge Transfer Planning Guide. Toronto: Institute for Work & Health. https://www.iwh.on.ca/sites/iwh/files/iwh/tools/iwh_kte_planning_guide_2006b.pdf

34. Redman, S., Greenhalgh, T., Adedokun, L., Staniszewska, S., and Denegri, S., and Co-production of Knowledge Collection Steering Committee. (2021). Co-production of knowledge: the future. *BMJ* 372: n434. doi: 10.1136/bmj.n434.

35. Rynes, S.L., Mcnatt, D.B., and Bretz, R.D. (1999). Academic research inside organizations: inputs, processes, and outcomes. *Personal Psychology* 52: 869–898. doi: 10.1111/j.1744-6570.1999.tb00183.x.

36. Tetroe, J.M., Graham, I.D., Foy, R., Robinson, N., Eccles, M.P., Wensing, M., Durieux, P., Legare, F., Nielson, C.P., Adily, A., Ward, J.E., Porter, C., Shea, B., and Grimshaw, J.M. (2008). Health research funding agencies' support and promotion of knowledge translation: an international study. *The Milbank Quarterly* 86: 125–155. doi: 10.1111/j.1468-0009.2007.00515.x.

37. Van de Ven, A.H. (2018). Academic-practitioner engaged scholarship. *Information and Organization* 28: 37–43. doi: 10.1016/j.infoandorg.2018.02.002.

38. Van de Ven, A.H. and Johnson, P.E. (2006). Knowledge for theory and practice. *Academy of Management Review* 31: 802–821. doi: 10.5465/amr.2006.22527385.

39. Ward, V., Smith, S., Foy, R., House, A., and Hamer, S. (2010). Planning for knowledge translation: a researcher's guide. *Evidence & Policy: A Journal of Research, Debate and Practice* 6: 527–541. doi: 10.1332/174426410X535882.

40. Ward, V., Smith, S., House, A., and Hamer, S. (2012). Exploring knowledge exchange: a useful framework for practice and policy. *Social Science & Medicine* 74: 297–304. doi: 10.1016/j.socscimed.2011.09.021.

41. Wilson, P., Petticrew, M., Medical Research Council's Population Health Sciences Research Network knowledge transfer project team, Calnan, M., and Nazareth, I. (2008). Why promote the findings of single research studies? *BMJ* 336: 722. doi: 10.1136/bmj.39525.447361.94.

42. Wilson, P.M., Petticrew, M., Calnan, M.W., and Nazareth, I. (2010). Disseminating research findings: what should researchers do? a systematic scoping review of conceptual frameworks. *Implementation Science: IS* 5: 91. doi: 10.1186/1748-5908-5-91.

4.3 Evaluating Research Coproduction

Research Quality Plus for Coproduction (RQ+ 4 Co-Pro)

Robert K.D. McLean, Ian D. Graham, and Fred Carden

Key Learning Points

- Mainstream methods of research evaluation are poorly aligned to the values and objectives of research coproduction. This undermines the potential of coproduction and coproducers.

- Reviews of frameworks for doing and managing research coproduction suggest these frameworks have limited success in supporting rigorous evaluation. Moreover, they lack scientific validation and grounding for evaluative application.

- The validated Research Quality Plus (RQ+) approach holds three tenets that present opportunities to strengthen coproduction evaluation. These are: 1) context matters, 2) quality is multi-dimensional, and 3) judgements must be empirical and systematic.

Research Coproduction in Healthcare, First Edition. Edited by Ian D. Graham, Jo Rycroft-Malone, Anita Kothari, and Chris McCutcheon.

- In this chapter, the three tenets are tailored for evaluating coproduction specifically. The result is a novel *RQ+ 4 Co-Pro* evaluation framework. The authors outline the framework components, describe potential uses and users, and how it will be trialed with an international sample of coproduction projects.
- Establishing legitimate methods of coproduction evaluation will require collective action and the participation of many. *RQ+ 4 Co-Pro* is a promising and practical starting place. Try it out and share your experience.

INTRODUCTION

Research coproduction offers great promise for science and society. The meaningful integration of people into research can lead to ethical science (Lavery 2018; NESTA 2018; Wicks et al. 2018), rigorous science (Chambers 2015; Crocker et al. 2018; Duncan and Oliver 2017; Rose 2004), the translation of scientific results into action (McLean and Tucker 2013), and the scaling of science-informed actions into optimal impacts for people and society (Gargani and McLean 2017; McLean and Gargani 2019).

This book raises many important arguments and proposals for doing and improving coproduction research. But with these contributions come an equal number of questions and challenges for coproducers and those who study it. How will we know methods of coproduction are meaningful to both researchers and knowledge users? That they welcome and accept different types of knowledge users? That they empower the researchers and knowledge users who participate? That they uphold the same scientific standards as methods that don't engage users? How can we be sure they value local knowledge and ways of knowing? Do they generate desirable impacts? And ultimately, how do we address confidence in the quality of coproduction research?

We add to the agenda raised in the other chapters of this book, with a critical approach to addressing these questions. The *Research Quality Plus for Coproduction (RQ+ 4 Co-Pro)* framework we present builds upon the work of the International Development Research Centre (IDRC) to develop and validate the Research Quality Plus (RQ+) approach (McLean et al. 2021). As Boaz suggests, there is a significant opportunity for coproducers to learn from the experience of international development where participatory and engaged approaches to knowledge generation have been employed, promoted, and valued for some time (Boaz 2021). Here, we take up Boaz's challenge and we adapt RQ+ for coproduction; and in doing so, articulate a unique and practical evaluation framework. Our initial focus is placed on its use for evaluation because, in our view, rigorous evaluation is an essential component of achieving the promise of coproduction. Later in the chapter, we illustrate how RQ+ 4 Co-Pro might hold similar value for research design and management.

We argue that *RQ+ 4 Co-Pro* will be of value to researchers, funders, journals, universities, and research organizations who teach, hire, and institutionalize what counts as good science. To this end, we highlight uses and users to exemplify the framework's potential. It is our hope that it helps build the evidence base for coproduction as a valid and valued form of knowledge generation.

Roadmap

The next section sketches the research evaluation landscape. It is not a complete review of the research evaluation field. For recent reviews see: Curry et al. (2020) and Aubert Bonn and Bouter (2021, July 19). Our purpose is to provide a snapshot of the broad research evaluation domain and the challenges specific to coproduction. In the following section we introduce the RQ+ approach, highlight the potential it presents for improving coproduction evaluation, and then introduce the tailored adaptation, the *RQ+ 4 Co-Pro* framework. Finally, we describe a planned field test of *RQ+ 4 Co-Pro* with the Integrated Knowledge Translation Research Network, while inviting readers to rethink and transform how we judge the quality of research coproduction.

OVERVIEW OF THE RESEARCH EVALUATION LANDSCAPE

The shortcomings of the mainstream methods of research evaluation are well known, and the critique is well documented in the literature (Aubert Bonn and Bouter 2021, July 19; Curry et al. 2020; Hicks et al. 2015). At the highest level, the critique is not that research is under-evaluated, it is that research is poorly evaluated. In this section, we address the domain as a whole and then cast light on the specific challenges for research coproduction. We take aim at the broad field of research evaluation, mostly because our understanding of the literature and our practical experience as evaluators indicates an overview of these systemic challenges requires demonstration.[1] Specifically, we hope to initiate collective momentum against a deeply ingrained stumbling block for our practice: coproduction and coproducers are being judged inappropriately and ineffectively.

---

[1] Two recent reviews conclude that frameworks that might support the evaluation of engaged research exist, however, use of these frameworks is fragmented and limited, and, is not related to the theoretical strength or evidence-base underpinning the framework (Boivin et al. 2018a; Greenhalgh et al. 2019). Here we outline challenges in the mainstream research evaluation system in order to make the case for concerted uptake and experimentation with coproduction tailored frameworks. In Annex 4.3.A, we outline how we have structured RQ+ 4 Co-Pro to build on the lessons of these reviews, and other major advances in the literature.

Research Evaluation at Large

Global science systems[2] are layered with gatekeeping and assessment. The deliberative peer review method is most widely entrenched – as our scientific peers make decisions about what research is funded, ethically acceptable, and published. Next, these assessments are aggregated using the analytic approach of metrics (most common being biblio-, alt-, innovation-metrics). These metrics are gathered and interpreted by those seeking simplified and comparable indicators, and rest on the arithmetic manipulation of peer review processes on large scales. Their simplicity and clarity have granted them a position of relative authority in declaring the importance of a researcher, a journal, a university or research institution, or even the work of an entire country, to be in a certain domain. Today, these metrics are used to make decisions about who gets hired and promoted, what gets funded, university rankings, and how governments make science and innovation investments. The latest development in research evaluation is the research impact assessment, or RIA (Russell et al. 2020). The rise of RIA has been driven by the desire of governments, universities, funders, and researchers, to demonstrate the social and environmental benefits of their work (Penfield et al. 2014). Accordingly, methods of RIA look beyond the scientist and their productivity, and utilize frameworks such as the Canadian Academy of Health Sciences' (CAHS) Preferred Framework on Investment in Health Research to identify areas of late-stage benefit that categorize the value of research into concepts of economic impact (such as drug sales) and health impact (such as reduced disease burden) (Canadian Academy of Health Sciences 2009). In some settings, such as the United Kingdom, RIA is now a central component of public research accounting via the Research Excellence Framework and is collected and reported for individuals and institutions across the country (Higher Education Funding Council for England 2021).

In summary, whether by deliberative, analytic, or long-term impact assessment approaches, research evaluation is a widespread and deep-rooted component of the global science system. But critiques of the status quo in research evaluation are mounting. Around the world an interdisciplinary response is taking form and aims to push the global science system to rethink our approaches to how research quality is defined and evaluated (Belcher and Halliwell 2021; Belcher et al. 2016; Curry et al. 2020; DORA 2021; Hicks et al. 2015; Kraemer-Mbula et al. 2020).

---

[2] With the term science system, we refer to the collection of actors, institutions, and ideas that together comprise the dynamic sphere of scientific activity. This follows from the notions of László (1972) who refers to science as a "natural cognitive system." Using the systems thinking classifications of Checkland (1999) science may be best described as a "designed abstract system".

Challenges for Research Coproduction Evaluation

Next, we summarize how research evaluation is poorly constructed for coproduction specifically. To do so, we use the three-paradigm categorization of deliberative, analytic, and impact evaluation. We recognize these are not discrete categories and that the terminology across each is divergent in different fields, disciplines, and geographies.

Deliberative Paradigm – Coproduction Limitations?

The deliberative peer review paradigm relies on researchers, not users or beneficiaries, to judge a proposal or a project in terms of scientific criteria. With few exceptions,[3] coproduction proposals are assessed by scientific peers not knowledge users. Further, they use scientific criteria to determine whether a study is ethical for participants on behalf of participants and if a study contains publishable results, not actionable results. In our view, scientists' expertise can identify the knowledge gaps the work aims to fill and critique the strength of the methods that will be used to produce it. But without including knowledge users and other stakeholders, significant gaps persist, as knowledge users are best placed to assess the relevance, significance, utility, and potential impact of the research.

Analytic Paradigm – Coproduction Limitations?

Metrics are biased toward fields of research in which productivity in creating output is paramount, largely via the scholarly paper published in a peer-reviewed, indexed journal. Metrics and their aggregations tell us little, if anything, about the quality of the engagement of users in a project. Neither do they speak to the policy or practice relevance of a research topic, or the actual implications of the work for intended beneficiaries. Moreover, they are largely blind to research results that fall outside the indices of mainstream, English-language, academic journal publishing. Similarly, real-world impact resulting from coproduction typically goes uncounted with the analytic paradigm.

RIA Paradigm – Coproduction Limitations?

For coproducers whose aim is knowledge uptake and use, the RIA paradigm seems welcome at first glance. In some cases, the RIA may even privilege research coproduction which can be well positioned to accelerate the uptake

---

[3] See for example the work of PCORI (www.PCORI.org) or the former Knowledge Translation Funding Program at Canadian Institutes of Health Research (CIHR) (McLean et al. 2012; McLean and Tucker 2013) for examples of "Merit Review" in practice.

and impact of research by knowledge users. However, RIA is not a comprehensive solution for coproduction quality evaluation. RIA may provide a meaningful measure for funders and organizations whose primary concern is amplifying the magnitude of impact they can demonstrate and communicate, but it does not systematically recognize and study the process of user engagement and how it can set a course, and even create social change *during* study design and implementation (Greenhalgh and Fahy 2015; Russell et al. 2020). Furthermore, the mismatch between research funding trajectories (typically one to five years) and research impact trajectories (typically 10–20 years) leaves a significant gap in our knowledge of how to do better coproduction.[4]

In response to these challenges, those doing coproduction have initiated the search for more meaningful ways of judging the quality and impact of their work. Boivin et al. (2018b) suggest the international literature investigating the benefits of partnered research has more than tripled in the past 10 years. Moreover, reviews of coproduced research have regularly called for the development and trial of new means of coproduction evaluation (for example, Beckett et al. 2018; Domecq et al. 2014; Greenhalgh et al. 2019; Hoekstra et al. 2020; Jagosh et al. 2012; Jenkins et al. 2016; Jull et al. 2019).

However, the most recent of these reviews indicate how uptake, validation, and scaling of coproduction-specific evaluation frameworks has been fragmented and limited (Boivin et al. 2018a; Greenhalgh et al. 2019). For practicing research evaluators and coproduction specialists this is not a surprise. Despite the imminent need, it is challenging to construct new frameworks for evaluating the quality of coproduction, but more challenging still to have frameworks stick in the already busy domain of research evaluation that – as our three-paradigm model has outlined – largely overlook and undervalue coproduction. Addressing this challenge is essential if research coproduction is to realize its full potential.

In the next section, we introduce a possible solution, *RQ+ 4 Co-Pro*, and invite coproducers and coproduction scientists to experiment and improve it. Responding to the reviews of Greenhalgh et al. (2019) and Jull et al. (2019), *RQ+ 4 Co-Pro* offers a flexible approach and a menu of transferable options for different users and uses. We hope this will facilitate viable and responsible scaling. Responding to Russell et al.'s (2020) salient research agenda for evaluating public involvement in research, *RQ+ 4 Co-Pro* shines a light specifically on power, potentially negative consequences, and encourages adaptation for the different rationales and values that underpin different coproduction efforts. Annex 4.3.A summarizes how *RQ+ 4 Co-Pro* builds on these and other recent developments in the coproduction literature related to evaluation.

---

[4] It is possible the RIA approaches will facilitate experiments that will help to prove or disprove claims about the value of coproduction. And if so, this will be a welcome contribution.

ANNEX 4.3.A   *RQ+ 4 Co-Pro* can learn, benefit from, and build on existing frameworks, lessons from experience, and systematic reviews.

Article/ Framework and Theoretical Lens	Recommendation/ Lesson	Lesson for RQ+ 4 Co-Pro
Kreindler (2018) *Integrated Knowledge Translation (IKT) lens*	Accept context as inseparable component of a causal chain Use a realist evaluation approach to highlight context in evaluations of IKT	RQ+ 4 Co-Pro makes context a framework component Use the three contextual factors of the framework to categorize and study context-mechanism interactions
Ward et al. (2018) *Community-based Participatory Research (CBPR) lens*	Equity is critical to understanding CBPR process and impact for communities, and thus, should be in the foreground of evaluations and informed by various methods and instruments	RQ+ 4 Co-Pro names sub-dimensions that prioritize and critically interrogate equity: 2.1. Inclusion of Local Knowledge and Ways of Knowing; 2.2. Trust, Power and Mutually Beneficial Partnerships; 2.3. Intersectionality 2.4. Negative Consequences
Beckett et al. (2018) *Coproduction lens*	Recognize social and transformational effects of coproduction, including both those that occur as a part of the research process (as a result of productive interactions) and those related to research results	RQ+ 4 Co-Pro sheds light on the process of engagement and utility of results, by naming both elements in specific quality dimensions of the framework (2 and 3), and by doing so, highlights "the hidden" relational and at times transformational benefits of coproduction
Boivin et al. (2018a) *Patient and Public Engagement lens*	Increase scientific rigor of framework development Include stakeholders in framework development. Improve accessibility of frameworks (understandability/ readability)	RQ+ 4 Co-Pro is derived from the validity and reliability tested, theory informed, RQ+ approach RQ+ 4 Co-Pro will be tested in the IKTRN trial described, which will be a stakeholder inclusive IKT effort. Ensure simple, clear, accessible publication in various formats and a well-developed sharing strategy.

Article/ Framework and Theoretical Lens	Recommendation/ Lesson	Lesson for RQ+ 4 Co-Pro
Greenhalgh et al. (2019) *Patient and Public Involvement lens*	A single, one-sized fits all framework is unlikely to emerge. Instead, co-develop frameworks for local contexts, principles, and objectives.	RQ+ 4 Co-Pro is a modular construct, whereby new users can adapt and re-shape the framework components to match their values and objectives, while keeping in-tact the three tenets that address the shortcomings of status quo deliberative, analytic, and RIA evaluation approaches when applied to coproduction.
Russell et al. (2020) *Public Involvement lens*	Acknowledge: 1) the different rationales for public involvement, 2) that there may be negative impacts, 3) the role of power relations	RQ+ 4 Co-Pro embraces sub-dimensions that platform and will help the field to learn about power and potentially negative consequences of coproduction.

THE RESEARCH QUALITY PLUS (RQ+) APPROACH AND THE NOVEL RESEARCH QUALITY PLUS FOR COPRODUCTION (RQ+ 4 CO-PRO) FRAMEWORK

To construct a framework for evaluating research coproduction we begin with the work of the IDRC and the RQ+ Approach (Lebel and McLean 2018; McLean et al. 2021). RQ+ offers a validity and reliability tested, theory-informed approach to research assessment that has proven capable of mitigating challenges associated with the prevalent evaluation methods. Several of these advantages are particularly compelling for coproduction research, and we will unpack this logic next. A full exploration of the RQ+ Approach and its use at the IDRC is available in McLean et al. (2021).

We propose an adaptation of RQ+ while keeping intact the three central tenets of the approach. To our knowledge, this chapter presents the first adaptation of RQ+ for a particular field of research. This is presented in three subsections. We address the three tenets of the RQ+ Approach and how they apply to the coproduction field specifically. Second, we present the coproduction adaptation, *RQ+ 4 Co-Pro*, outlining a set of contextual factors and quality dimensions that together present a novel framework for coproduction evaluation. Third, we suggest possibilities for the framework in designing, managing, and evaluating research coproduction.

Three Tenets of the Research Quality Plus (RQ+) Approach

RQ+ is an approach for holistic and systems-oriented research quality evaluation. As McLean and Sen (2019, p. 124) state:

> RQ+ moves beyond traditional measures of scientific research rigor, to capture the multiple objectives that underpin the greater potential of research for society, such as research uptake and use, capacity strengthening of researchers and/or research institutions, and the legitimacy of the research to local knowledge and demand.

To accomplish this, the RQ+ Approach holds three tenets: 1) context matters, 2) accept a multi-dimensional view of quality aligned to the specific values for the work, and 3) utilize a systematic and empirical evaluation design (McLean and Sen 2019). Here we summarize each tenet and note the implications and importance for coproduction.

Tenet 1 – Context Matters

Context can inhibit or enable the success of research. Rather than isolating or blinding a research output, project, program, etc. from its context during evaluation, strive to understand the contextual factors that cultivate its strengths and weaknesses. Contextual factors may be internal to the research effort such as capacity or team environments, or they may be external, such as political environments or maturity of the research domain in which the study is situated.

Why Does This Matter for Coproduction?

When research is coproduced, it opens the science to new stakeholders and their working environments and cultures, to new political or commercial pressures, and to a variety of challenges and opportunities related to data, methods, and epistemology. In simplest terms, research coproduction is influenced by the context, giving rise to the research questions, the operating context of both the knowledge users and the researchers involved, and the context in which the findings will be used.

Tenet 2 – Research Quality Is Multi-Dimensional

Design, manage, and evaluate, using a multidimensional view of research quality that is aligned to the values and objectives of the research effort being assessed. Scientific rigor is essential, but it should be balanced alongside all objectives for the work. In the case of coproduction this likely includes its legitimacy, salience, and/or utility. The dimensions that are selected will highlight the components of the project that are a priority to the research and help the evaluation appraise the complex notion of research quality holistically.

Why Does This Matter for Coproduction?

With attention to equity and fairness, coproducers are required to embrace the ways knowledge is produced, interpreted, and shared with users as they are central actors in the process and product. Accordingly, a robust and reliable evaluation of coproduction research must embrace the multiple dimensions that underpin and drive coproduction quality.

Tenet 3 – Judgement of Research Quality Must Be Grounded in Empirical Evidence and Its Systematic and Transparent Appraisal

To truly understand the value of science, mixed and multiple sources of evidence are needed, and these must be weighed against one another to inform assessment. Rather than drawing judgements based only on opinion, evaluators might ask the principal investigator (PI), the knowledge users, trainees, or the intended beneficiary of the effort how they assess its value; then weigh this against the bibliometrics and their own review of the project.

Why Does This Matter for Coproduction?

Assessments of coproduction quality require multiple sources of evidence and, in particular, the experience/perspective of the knowledge user.

The Research Quality Plus for Coproduction (RQ+ 4 Co-Pro) Framework

Here we introduce a means of putting the RQ+ tenets into practice. The *RQ+ 4 Co-Pro* Framework articulates specific contextual factors and quality dimensions which bring the first two tenets of the RQ+ Approach to the experience of research coproduction (Figure 4.3.1). The third tenet – empirical and systematic data collection and appraisal – will be tailored and published in the protocol for the field test we outline in Section 4 of this chapter.

Here we present the framework as though it were an evaluation tool for completed coproduction research. After its initial presentation, we outline how it may be applied before, during and after coproduction to design, manage, and evaluate the coproduction process.

RQ+ 4 Co-Pro is not a static construct. While keeping intact the three tenets, we encourage readers to select contextual factors that best describe their research environments, and to re-imagine the quality dimensions to align with the values and mission of their coproduction agenda. Framework fluidity is

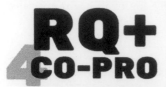

Research Quality Plus for Coproduction

RQ+ 4 Co-Pro is an approach to defining and evaluating the quality of coproduction. It allows tailoring to context, values, and purpose. It can support planning, management and learning across the lifecycle of a coproduction project, program or organization.

The RQ+ 4 Co-Pro Framework

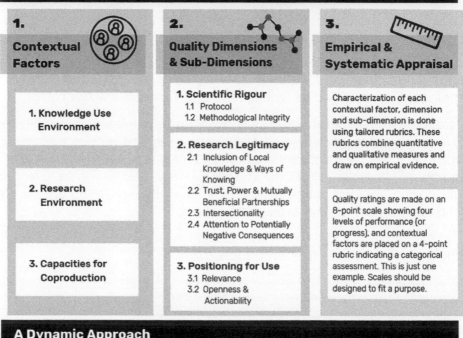

1. Contextual Factors

1. Knowledge Use Environment

2. Research Environment

3. Capacities for Coproduction

2. Quality Dimensions & Sub-Dimensions

1. Scientific Rigour
1.1 Protocol
1.2 Methodological Integrity

2. Research Legitimacy
2.1 Inclusion of Local Knowledge & Ways of Knowing
2.2 Trust, Power & Mutually Beneficial Partnerships
2.3 Intersectionality
2.4 Attention to Potentially Negative Consequences

3. Positioning for Use
3.1 Relevance
3.2 Openness & Actionability

3. Empirical & Systematic Appraisal

Characterization of each contextual factor, dimension and sub-dimension is done using tailored rubrics. These rubrics combine quantitative and qualitative measures and draw on empirical evidence.

Quality ratings are made on an 8-point scale showing four levels of performance (or progress), and contextual factors are placed on a 4-point rubric indicating a categorical assessment. This is just one example. Scales should be designed to fit a purpose.

A Dynamic Approach

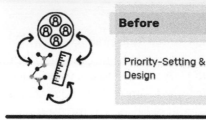

Before	**During**	**After**
Priority-Setting & Design	Management & Development	Reporting Results, Evaluation & Teaching

Authors: Robert McLean, Ian Graham, Fred Carden

FIGURE 4.3.1   RQ+ 4 Co-Pro (Infographic).

essential if we hope to co-develop a more rigorous and critical means of measuring and managing quality. As our contexts and values evolve, so too must our evaluative frameworks. So we name framework components (contextual factors and quality dimensions) that we hope inspire uptake, experimentation, and improvement.

1. Contextual Factors

Research always occurs in political, economic, sociological, and natural settings. This is particularly true in the case of coproduction (Kreindler 2018). We identify three contextual factors that can be monitored and categorized in a coproduction project or program evaluation. By studying these factors, users of *RQ+ 4 Co-Pro* can learn, share experience, and cultivate enabling environments for coproduction work. In the more immediate term, categorizing research context can help project coordinators, funders, or managers understand risk factors and identify mitigation strategies for individual projects or for monitoring project portfolios. Classifications of context are done independently of ratings against the quality dimensions, and they are not intended to modify project quality ratings. One categorization is not meant to imply "better than" another categorization. The three *RQ+ 4 Co-Pro* contextual factors are: 1) Knowledge Use Environment; 2) Research Environment; 3) Capacities for Coproduction.[5]

1.1 Knowledge Use Environment

This contextual factor addresses the absorptive capacity of the knowledge use environment. This typically stems from the broad environment and culture of the knowledge user partner and then manifests for the coproduction team. The knowledge use environment may be highly empowering, with a strong appetite for research and evidence to inform policy, program, practice, or product improvement. Here, resources and incentives will encourage and reward the use of evidence in decision-making. Alternatively, the political environment may be restrictive, and the coproduction team faces significant barriers, even professional risks, to research evidence vis-à-vis alternative decision-making approaches. In a restrictive environment, resources and incentives do not support research uptake and use.

1. Restrictive   2. Unsupportive   3. Supportive   4. Empowering

1.2 Research Environment

This contextual factor addresses the environment in which the researcher partner(s) in the coproduction team works. In some circumstances the environment may empower coproduction as a valid means of knowledge

---

[5] In the 2021 IDRC RQ+ Framework there are five contextual factors. Three are closely aligned to those here, given some tailoring to match these to coproduction specifically. The additional two contextual factors, "Data Environment" and "Maturity of the Research Field" are not included in *RQ+ 4 CO-Pro* as they were determined to have less immediate alignment with the aims of coproduction.

generation and provide researchers incentives, resources, and rewards for good practice. Alternatively, coproduction may be an undervalued or diminished means of conducting science where researchers may be explicitly or implicitly discouraged from undertaking coproduction and thus put career progression and peer acceptance at risk by engaging knowledge users in their research.

1. Restrictive   2. Unsupportive   3. Supportive   4. Empowering

1.3 Capacities for Coproduction

This factor categorizes the extent to which the research places focus on training and developing coproduction practice and/or theory amongst researchers and knowledge users. We track this contextual factor because coproduction is a new and emerging field, and nurturing the next generation is required for future acceptance and sustainability. When the focus is strong, a considerable amount of time and resources are devoted to purposefully and consciously developing the skills of junior team members and aptitude for coproduction is envisaged as a positive result of the effort (amongst both researchers and knowledge users). Alternatively, capacity building in coproduction may not be a deliberate part of the research effort. This is identified when no discernible resources are devoted to it, and the only viable skill development opportunity for researchers or knowledge users will come from learning by doing. This may be the case with a highly experienced or beginner coproduction team. Unlike the other contextual factors, Capacities for Coproduction does not denote a measure of risk. This is not an outcome measure. It is a measure of the intensity of the effort.

1. No Focus   2. Minimal focus   3. Significant focus   4. Strong focus

2. Quality Dimensions and Sub-Dimensions

Any judgement of research quality should reflect the values underpinning that research effort. We articulate three dimensions, and eight corresponding sub-dimensions of quality that reflect broad values for partnered research.

Coproduction research must be scientifically robust, thus we begin with Scientific Rigour, a non-negotiable component of any coproduction effort. The second dimension of *RQ+ 4 Co-Pro*, Research Legitimacy, highlights four sub-dimensions that together measure the fidelity of the research effort to the environment in which it occurs and the results it will produce for intended beneficiaries. The third dimension, Positioning for Use, examines the relevance of the research to the needs of users and the openness and actionability of the process and results.

In the *RQ+ 4 Co-Pro* Framework, these dimensions are not independent variables, they are interrelated. Yet, by disaggregating and allowing focus on each component, *RQ+ 4 Co-Pro* highlights and brings importance to the alternative and diverse qualities that ultimately underpin excellence in coproduction. For our purposes the dimensions hold equal weight. Other users may choose to weigh dimensions differently in order to increase focus on challenging or significant components of their work. Table 1 presents an eight-point rubric for assessing dimensions in the frameworks:

Insufficient information to assess	Unacceptable	Less than acceptable	Good		Very good	
IIA	1	2	3	4	5	6	7	8

2.1 Scientific Rigor

The first dimension of research coproduction quality addresses the technical merit and demonstrable excellence of the research. This requires an examination of the project vis-à-vis the standards and expectations of the methodological approach (qualitative research, clinical trials, statistical methods, ethnographic immersion, for example). Meaningful coproduction partnerships are considered across any and all fields. Yet, this part of the assessment must be considered vis-à-vis the intentions of the work and the fair expectations of the knowledge user partners. In some circumstances engagement will be necessary from start to finish, in other cases knowledge users and researchers will have negotiated mutually beneficial terms, and these idiosyncrasies should be considered and examined here. The dimension is represented with two distinct sub-dimensions.

2.1.1 Protocol

This measure of quality addresses the design of the research project using the accepted best practices of the field. It examines how the study is framed in the current knowledge, reproducibility of the design, how methodological standards are met or exceeded with viable innovations, and the overall design openness. This dimension also considers the coproduction process, including when and how engagement is built in.

2.1.2 Methodological Integrity

Refers to the technical fidelity of protocol implementation and research management decisions. This will include how principles of working practice are established and navigated by the full coproduction team. How partnerships are managed is essential throughout each part of the process, which will typically examine issues such as: (i) research questions are pursued rigorously, (ii) adequate and appropriate data collection is conducted, (iii) relevant analysis frameworks are selected and applied according to best practice and knowledge user needs, (iv) conclusions are grounded in data collected, (v) and clear and accurate presentation of results in light of knowledge user contexts and needs.

2.2 Research Legitimacy

Legitimacy addresses the fidelity of the research to the context in which it is or will be implemented. In the context of coproduction, legitimacy includes sub-dimensions related to fairness and meaning in knowledge generation, diversity, equity and inclusion, and meaningful relationships being created and/or sustained between all partners involved in the coproduction effort. Specifically, Research Legitimacy is represented in four sub-dimensions.

2.2.1 Inclusion of Local Knowledge and Ways of Knowing

This sub-dimension addresses the degree to which the research is grounded in the reality and knowledge base of the intended users and beneficiaries of the work. Exemplary projects will ensure scientific methods embrace and empower the realities of local ways of knowing, existing cultures, and norms or expectations about knowledge. These could be cultural, commercial, organizational, or political knowledge localities, depending on the aims and context of the project. Attention must be paid to decolonizing local standards from predominant scientific standards surrounding knowledge and evidence, and appropriately weighing all partners' perspectives.

2.2.2 Trust, Power, and Mutually Beneficial Partnership

This sub-dimension examines the underlying power dynamics of the research process, specifically examining how power was created, shared, and sustained. It also interrogates if/how the coproduction effort is designed and managed to address the needs and desires of all parties throughout the research process. A mutually beneficial partnership does not mean all tasks and resources are shared equally; it means decisions about how tasks and resources are utilized are mutually endorsed.

2.2.3 Intersectionality

This sub-dimension addresses the degree to which the research takes account of the varied perspectives underpinning the work and produces equitable processes and outcomes for different intersectional connections with the work. Issues of diversity, equity, and inclusion are considered here. For a discussion of how these issues should be considered in the research coproduction process, see Chapter 2.2. Very good research will be sensitive to the social environment in which the research takes place and cognizant of the potential biases the coproduction team bring to the work. Intersectionality is a critical element in each of the design, conduct and implementation components of the work. The assessment should focus on the extent to which intersectionality is considered and built into each phase of the project. In the case of an impact assessment, it may examine outcomes for varied intersectional groups. In the case of a needs assessment, it may examine whose needs are being considered and whose are not, or how they are being valued and why. No coproduction project should be blind to intersectional considerations.

2.2.4 Attention to Potentially Negative Consequences

This sub-dimension refers to the strategies employed in the coproduction project to minimize and mitigate any negative consequences of the work, whether expected or unexpected. Negative consequences could include damages to individual partners or their organizations, damages to participants, adverse outcomes for beneficiary communities, or damages to the natural environment. Evidence of exemplary performance is found in ethics adherence through the research coproduction, but also in the way user/beneficiary relationships are managed and how these perspectives are valued in how decisions about project progress are made.

2.3 Positioning for Use

Positioning for Use addresses the extent to which the coproduction process enhanced the likelihood of research uptake and impact. A first critical element is how relevant the research objectives and questions are for the intended beneficiaries and/or users of the work. Second is the creation of audience-friendly and open access research outputs and results. User engagement as a means of facilitating knowledge translation is a matter of scientific rigor in coproduction: thus, it is assessed specifically under quality dimension one.

2.3.1 Relevance

This sub-dimension reflects the extent to which the research takes on existing and predominant societal or practical problems of relevance to knowledge users. The measure examines how the research was prioritized, who it serves, and how widely endorsed the needs and challenges it addresses are by coproducers and impacted organizations or communities.

2.3.2 Openness and Actionability

This sub-dimension addresses how research is conducted and how results are tailored into outputs, products, and results that are useful, attractive, and understandable for knowledge users. The usability of the solution generated is considered, and so is the presentation of the solution in an engaging format. This includes how openly available (open access), applicable, tailored, and timely the conduct and results are for action.

3. Empirical Evidence and Systematic Appraisal

The third tenet of the RQ+ Approach is the systematic and empirical design of the quality assessment.

In section four we introduce the first planned application of this framework. During this application, the team will coproduce the specific data collection and valuation strategy. Keeping in line with the RQ+ Approach, this application will utilize empirical data and systematic assessment using transparent rubrics. In the above sections, we have provided quantitative rubrics to align to each Contextual Factor and Quality Dimension in order to provide a simplified image of how the issue can be assessed. In the first stage of the pilot application, we will co-develop the components with our user group, the Integrated Knowledge Translation Research Network, and create qualitative criteria related to each score on the rubric to support holistic and rigorous assessment. Accordingly, we will not present a specific proposal for data collection and appraisal here; this is beyond the scope of this chapter.

How, When, and by Whom Might RQ+ 4 Co-Pro Be Applied?

RQ+ 4 Co-Pro has the potential to support the design, management and post-hoc evaluation of a coproduction research effort. In other words, it can be applied before, during and after research coproduction. It may be used to support a research project, program, or organization interested in improving coproduction. Figures 4.3.2 and 4.3.3 outline examples of potential uses and users.

PUTTING THE FRAMEWORK INTO ACTION

Field Test

Over the course of 2021–22 the *RQ+ 4 Co-Pro* framework will undergo a trial implementation using a sample of Integrated Knowledge Translation Research Network (IKTRN) coproduced health research projects. The IKTRN is an

RQ+ 4 CO-PRO

Applying RQ+ 4 Co-Pro

RQ+ 4 Co-Pro can support the design, management and evaluation of research coproduction. It can be used before, during and after coproduction.

When	Use	Motive
Before	Establishing expectations, priorities and meaningful partnerships Developing principles and shared values Coproduction research design Grant application review	RQ+ 4 Co-Pro can provide an agenda for fair and transparent terms of engagement. The contextual factors and quality dimensions can and should be adapted to the needs of the effort at hand. When they are set, they identify/define clear priorities and parameters for what is considered good in the work. This priority-setting exercise can be used to communicate objectives and values of importance to the user.
During	Monitoring and managing progress Formative or developmental evaluation Sharing and reporting protocols and processes	RQ+ 4 Co-Pro presents an approach for regularly revisiting shared values and objectives as well as course correcting when needed. Whether RQ+ 4 Co-Pro is applied as a self-assessment checklist, as a formative evaluation framework, or in any mid-term format, the approach can provide a clear learning agenda and systematic means of risk management for the user.
After	Publication review Summative evaluation of a project or portfolio of projects Support impact assessment Teaching, capacity strengthening and field-building	RQ+ 4 Co-Pro provides a retrospective assessment approach that can shine new light on the benefits, limitations, and areas for improvement in/of research coproduction. By selecting evaluative criteria that reflect the values coproducers prioritize, and observing how these play out under different contexts, there is much that can be learned. Some possibilities include better advocacy, teaching, and capacity strengthening of proven practice. In addition, systematic application of the approach will provide data on context and qualities that impact assessors can use to explain the determinants of societal and environmental impact.

Authors: Robert McLean, Ian Graham, Fred Carden

FIGURE 4.3.2   RQ+ 4 Co-Pro (Uses).

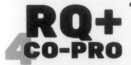

RQ+ 4 Co-Pro can be used by a variety of actors. These include researchers and knowledge-users partnering in a research effort, but also the numerous individuals, organisations, and institutions that play stewarding roles for coproduction. Here we provide four illustrative cases. This list is not exhaustive.

Case #1

Coproducers

A coproduction team uses RQ+ 4 Co-Pro from start to finish of a research project. At the outset, researchers and knowledge-users apply the approach to develop and clarify a shared understanding of goals for the work. As the project progresses, the team uses the framework to assess progress, and identify areas for project improvement. When the research is completed, the team evaluates their effort against the framework components and shares successes and failures.

Case #2

Funders

A research funder launches a call for coproduction research projects. To send a clear message to its community about what will be valued and assessed, the funder articulates its quality dimensions in the call. When peer-reviewers are assessing applications received, they systematically apply the framework to each application ensuring consistent and transparent reviews. Years later, the funder revisits this portfolio of projects, and assesses their quality using the same framework as a post-hoc evaluation tool.

Case #3

Publishers

A journal that specializes in publishing research coproduction works with its editorial board and representatives of its community to build an RQ+ 4 Co-Pro framework that represents the mission and values it wants to espouse. The journal then puts RQ+ 4 Co-Pro to work in its peer-review and editorial decision-making processes. Because it keeps a record of individual reviewer assessments, at year end the journal's editorial board commissions a meta-analysis of results against the contextual factors and quality dimensions it assessed in every paper received and published, learning much about the strengths, weaknesses, and opportunities ahead for its field.

Case #4

Universities

A university faculty decides to re-think how it supports, rewards, and teaches coproduction. Using RQ+ 4 Co-Pro as an evaluative framework it begins to assess and reward faculty based on the components of quality that matter for this type of research. This sets clear and meaningful goalposts for staff who have felt coproduction work was under-valued using traditional research evaluation metrics. At the same time, the faculty draws on RQ+ 4 Co-Pro as a teaching device, to share case studies and highlight critical components of coproduction quality to students and staff.

Authors: Robert McLean, Ian Graham, Fred Carden

FIGURE 4.3.3   RQ+ 4 Co-Pro (Users).

international network of health researchers and knowledge users who aim to advance the science and practice of research coproduction (Graham et al. 2018). Seeing promise in *RQ+ 4 Co-Pro* as a means of assessing their work, but also, in the importance of advancing new methods of valuing coproduction, the IKTRN has committed to fund and participate in this field test, and to share the experience.

The objectives of the project are to test the components of the *RQ+ 4 Co-Pro* Framework, understand the viability of its implementation, and identify and document the strengths and weaknesses of using it. The study will be a coproduction research project itself, engaging knowledge users from the IKTRN management and others, such as research funders, who may wish to better evaluate funded coproduction; journal editors interested in exploring the approach for manuscript review; university leaders who evaluate and promote research staff; and trainee's learning about coproduction theory and practice.

The study will use the framework described in this chapter. The study protocol and results will be prepared for open access publication and in simplified user-oriented formats.

Join Us

Our hope is that the *RQ+ 4 Co-Pro* Framework presented in this chapter inspires adaptations and implementation trials amongst researchers, funders, publishers, universities, and other science systems actors with interest in better understanding and critically evaluating coproduction work.

For coproduction research to meet its potential, it must be evaluated accurately for what it sets out to do, but also, systematically and scientifically. *RQ+ 4 Co-Pro* is a starting place. It too requires critical assessment and development. Join us and help to advance a more meaningful way of assessing coproduction research.

REFERENCES

1. Aubert Bonn, N. and Bouter, L. (2021, July 19). Research assessments should recognize responsible research practices – narrative review of a lively debate and promising developments (Preprint). [Online]. MetaArXivPreprints. https://osf. io/preprints/metaarxiv/82rmj (accessed 29 September 2021).

2. Beckett, K., Farr, M., Kothari, A., Wye, L., and le May, A. (2018). Embracing complexity and uncertainty to create impact: exploring the processes and transformative potential of coproduced research through development of a social impact model. *Health Research Policy and Systems / BioMed Central* 16: 118. doi: 10.1186/s12961-018-0375-0.

3. Belcher, B. and Halliwell, J. (2021). Conceptualizing the elements of research impact: towards semantic standards. *Humanities and Social Sciences Communications* 8. doi: 10.1057/s41599-021-00854-2.

4. Belcher, B.M., Rasmussen, K.E., Kemshaw, M.R., and Zornes, D.A. (2016). Defining and assessing research quality in a transdisciplinary context. *Research Evaluation* 25: 1–17. doi: 10.1093/reseval/rvv025.

5. Boaz, A. (2021). Lost in coproduction: to enable true collaboration we need to nurture different academic identities. https://blogs.lse.ac.uk/ impactofsocialsciences/2021/06/25/lost-in-coproduction-to-enable-true-

collaboration-we-need-to-nurture-different-academic-identities (accessed 21 September 2021).

6. Boivin, A., L'Esperance, A., Gauvin, F.P., Dumez, V., Macaulay, A.C., Lehoux, P., and Abelson, J. (2018a). Patient and public engagement in research and health system decision making: a systematic review of evaluation tools. *Health Expectations* 21: 1075–1084. doi: 10.1111/hex.12804.

7. Boivin, A., Richards, T., Forsythe, L., Gregoire, A., L'Esperance, A., Abelson, J., and Carman, K.L. (2018b). Evaluating patient and public involvement in research. *BMJ* 363: k5147. doi: 10.1136/bmj.k5147.

8. Canadian Academy of Health Sciences. (2009). *Making an Impact: A Preferred Framework and Indicators to Measure Returns on Investment in Health Research*. Ottawa: CAHS. https://cahs-acss.ca/making-an-impact-a-preferred-framework-and-indicators-to-measure-returns-on-investment-in-health-research.

9. Chambers, R. (2015). Inclusive rigour for complexity. *Journal of Development Effectiveness* 7: 327–335. doi: 10.1080/19439342.2015.1068356.

10. Checkland, P.B. (1999). *Systems Thinking, Systems Practice*. Chichester: John Wiley & Sons, Ltd.

11. Crocker, J.C., Ricci-Cabello, I., Parker, A., Hirst, J.A., Chant, A., Petit-Zeman, S., Evans, D., and Rees, S. (2018). Impact of patient and public involvement on enrolment and retention in clinical trials: systematic review and meta-analysis. *BMJ* 363: k4738. doi: 10.1136/bmj.k4738.

12. Curry, S., de Rijcke, S., Hatch, A., Pillay, D. (Gansen), van der Weijden, I., and Wilsdon, J. (2020). *The Changing Role of Funders in Responsible Research Assessment: Progress, Obstacles and the Way Ahead*. Research on Research Institute. doi: 10.6084/m9.figshare.13227914.v1.

13. Domecq, J.P., Prutsky, G., Elraiyah, T., Wang, Z., Nabhan, M., Shippee, N., Brito, J.P., Boehmer, K., Hasan, R., Firwana, B., Erwin, P., Eton, D., Sloan, J., Montori, V., Asi, N., Dabrh, A.M., and Murad, M.H. (2014). Patient engagement in research: a systematic review. *BMC Health Services Research* 14: 89. doi: 10.1186/1472-6963-14-89.

14. DORA. (2021). *Read the declaration – DORA*. [Online]. https://sfdora.org/read (accessed 21 September 2021).

15. Duncan, S. and Oliver, S. (2017). Editorial: motivations for engagement. *Research for All* 1: 229–233. doi: 10.18546/RFA.01.2.01.

16. Gargani, J. and McLean, R. (2017). Scaling science. Stanford Social Innovation Review, Fall Issue. https://ssir.org/articles/entry/scaling_science.

17. Graham, I.D., Kothari, A., and McCutcheon, C., and Integrated Knowledge Translation Research Network Project Leads. (2018). Moving knowledge into action for more effective practice, programmes and policy: protocol for a research programme on integrated knowledge translation. *Implementation Science: IS* 13: 22. doi: 10.1186/s13012-017-0700-y.

18. Greenhalgh, T. and Fahy, N. (2015). Research impact in the community-based health sciences: an analysis of 162 case studies from the 2014 UK Research Excellence Framework. *BMC Medicine* 13: 232. doi: 10.1186/s12916-015-0467-4.

19. Greenhalgh, T., Hinton, L., Finlay, T., Macfarlane, A., Fahy, N., Clyde, B., and Chant, A. (2019). Frameworks for supporting patient and public involvement in research: systematic review and co-design pilot. *Health Expectations* 22: 785–801. doi: 10.1111/hex.12888.

20. Hicks, D., Wouters, P., Waltman, L., de Rijcke, S., and Rafols, I. (2015). Bibliometrics: the Leiden Manifesto for research metrics. *Nature* 520: 429–431. doi: 10.1038/520429a.

21. Higher Education Funding Council for England. (2021). *What is the REF? – REF 2021*. [Online]. https://www.ref.ac.uk/about/what-is-the-ref (accessed 21 September 2021).

22. Hoekstra, F., Mrklas, K.J., Khan, M., McKay, R.C., Vis-Dunbar, M., Sibley, K.M., Nguyen, T., Graham, I.D., SCI Guiding Principles Consensus Panel, and Gainforth, H.L. (2020). A review of reviews on principles, strategies, outcomes and impacts of research partnerships approaches: a first step in synthesising the research partnership literature. *Health Research Policy and Systems / BioMed Central* 18: 51. doi: 10.1186/s12961-020-0544-9.

23. Jagosh, J., Macaulay, A.C., Pluye, P., Salsberg, J., Bush, P.L., Henderson, J., Sirett, E., Wong, G., Cargo, M., Herbert, C.P., Seifer, S.D., Green, L.W., and Greenhalgh, T. (2012). Uncovering the benefits of participatory research: implications of a realist review for health research and practice. *The Milbank Quarterly* 90: 311–346. doi: 10.1111/j.1468-0009.2012.00665.x.

24. Jenkins, E.K., Kothari, A., Bungay, V., Johnson, J.L., and Oliffe, J.L. (2016). Strengthening population health interventions: developing the CollaboraKTion Framework for Community-Based Knowledge Translation. *Health Research Policy and Systems/BioMed Central* 14: 65. doi: 10.1186/s12961-016-0138-8.

25. Jull, J.E., Davidson, L., Dungan, R., Nguyen, T., Woodward, K.P., and Graham, I.D. (2019). A review and synthesis of frameworks for engagement in health research to identify concepts of knowledge user engagement. *BMC Medical Research Methodology* 19: 211. doi: 10.1186/s12874-019-0838-1.

26. Kraemer-Mbula, E., Tijssen, R.J.W., Wallace, M.L., and Mclean, R. (2020). *Transforming Research Excellence: New Ideas from the Global South*. Cape Town, South Africa: African Minds. https://www.africanminds.co.za/transforming-research-excellence-new-ideas-from-the-global-south.

27. Kreindler, S.A. (2018). Advancing the evaluation of integrated knowledge translation. *Health Research Policy and Systems / BioMed Central* 16: 104. doi: 10.1186/s12961-018-0383-0.

28. László, E. (1972). *Introduction to Systems Philosophy: Toward a New Paradigm of Contemporary Thinking*. Gordon & Breach Science Publishers.

29. Lavery, J.V. (2018). Building an evidence base for stakeholder engagement. *Science* 361: 554–556. doi: 10.1126/science.aat8429.

30. Lebel, J. and McLean, R. (2018). A better measure of research from the global south. *Nature* 559: 23–26. doi: 10.1038/d41586-018-05581-4.

31. McLean, R. and Gargani, J. (2019). *Scaling Impact: Innovation for the Public Good.* Routledge. https://www.idrc.ca/en/book/scaling-impact-innovation-public-good.

32. McLean, R., Ofir, Z., Etherington, A., Acevedo, M., and Feinstein, O. (2021). *Research Quality Plus (RQ+) Evaluating Research for Global Sustainable Development.* Ottawa: International Development Research Centre.

33. McLean, R.K., Graham, I.D., Bosompra, K., Choudhry, Y., Coen, S.E., Macleod, M., Manuel, C., McCarthy, R., Mota, A., Peckham, D., Tetroe, J.M., and Tucker, J. (2012). Understanding the performance and impact of public knowledge translation funding interventions: protocol for an evaluation of Canadian Institutes of Health Research knowledge translation funding programs. *Implementation Science: IS* 7: 57. doi: 10.1186/1748-5908-7-57.

34. McLean, R.K.D. and Sen, K. (2019). Making a difference in the real world? A meta-analysis of the quality of use-oriented research using the Research Quality Plus approach. *Research Evaluation* 28: 123–135. doi: 10.1093/reseval/rvy026.

35. McLean, R.K.D. and Tucker, J. (2013). *Evaluation of CIHR's Knowledge Translation Funding Program.* Canadian Institutes of Health Research. https://cihr-irsc.gc.ca/e/documents/kt_evaluation_report-en.pdf.

36. NESTA. (2018). *Seven principles for public engagement in research and innovation policymaking.* [Online]. https://www.nesta.org.uk/report/seven-principles-public-engagement-research-and-innovation-policymaking (accessed 21 September 2021).

37. Penfield, T., Baker, M.J., Scoble, R., and Wykes, M.C. (2014). Assessment, evaluations, and definitions of research impact: a review. *Research Evaluation* 23: 21–32. doi: 10.1093/reseval/rvt021.

38. Rose, D. (2004). Telling different stories: user involvement in mental health research. *Research and Policy Planning* 22: 23–30.

39. Russell, J., Fudge, N., and Greenhalgh, T. (2020). The impact of public involvement in health research: what are we measuring? Why are we measuring it? Should we stop measuring it? *Research Involvement and Engagement* 6: 63. doi: 10.1186/s40900-020-00239-w.

40. Ward, M., Schulz, A.J., Israel, B.A., Rice, K., Martenies, S.E., and Markarian, E. (2018). A conceptual framework for evaluating health equity promotion within community-based participatory research partnerships. *Evaluation and Program Planning* 70: 25–34. doi: 10.1016/j.evalprogplan.2018.04.014.

41. Wicks, P., Richards, T., Denegri, S., and Godlee, F. (2018). Patients' roles and rights in research. *BMJ* 362: k3193. doi: 10.1136/bmj.k3193.

CHAPTER 5

Capacity-Building and Infrastructure

5.1 Researcher Coproduction Competencies and Incentives

Christopher R. Burton and Tone Elin Mekki

Key Learning Points

- Research coproduction requires researchers to have some degree of competency in stakeholder engagement and creating real-world impact from collaborative research.
- Stakeholder engagement and creating impact complement the foundational theoretical, methodological and technical grounding in a professional or academic discipline.
- Research coproduction competences also build on transferable skills, such as communication, engagement and leadership, which research training funders are increasingly interested in.
- Stakeholder engagement is a defining feature of coproduction, highlighting that there are requirements of other stakeholders in research.

Research Coproduction in Healthcare, First Edition. Edited by
Ian D. Graham, Jo Rycroft-Malone, Anita Kothari, and Chris McCutcheon.
© 2022 John Wiley & Sons Ltd. Published 2022 by John Wiley & Sons Ltd.

INTRODUCTION

Our starting point for this chapter is that there are competencies for research coproduction required of researchers, and which augment those competencies associated with any disciplinary or methodological tradition. We provide an overview of what these competencies are, drawing on themes of mastery of research, personal effectiveness, patient and public involvement, and the generation of impact. These themes point to a broad base of competencies of research coproduction which have yet to be fully integrated within policies, systems and incentives to drive capability building. Although research coproduction should not be limited to a healthcare context, we have drawn predominantly on literature from this sector, and some of our ongoing work, to develop our thinking about what these competencies are, and how they are sustained with career development strategies and frameworks.

We focus on the ambitions of research coproduction as they relate to increasing the impact of investment in research which, particularly in the health and care sectors is consistently framed as a global priority. If research coproduction has stakeholder engagement at its core, then its raison d'être has to be increasing the relevance, utility and therefore impact of the coproduced research.

Research impact is associated with the use of knowledge in practice and policy in different ways, such as professional behavior change or policy development, but has been consistently problematized in terms of a gap between knowledge generation and use. This gap has been presumed to result largely from differences between knowledge producers (e.g., researchers) and knowledge users (e.g., policy makers and practitioners) (Nutley et al. 2003). This position neglects the fact that many medical and health researchers are indeed practising clinicians, and the renewed interest in developing structures, such as researchers-in-residence and clinical academic careers, that support working across service and university settings. More fundamentally it is challenged both through the emergence of a more socially constructed view of the "knowledge gap" in which knowledge is coproduced with and between stakeholders to maximise its impact (Rycroft-Malone et al. 2016b). Research coproduction provides a new lens on the issue of impact by foregrounding this throughout the knowledge production lifecycle through the engagement of stakeholders and the systems in which they live and work. This change may, of course, be the application of new knowledge in discourse, practice and professional behavior change, politics and policy as research progresses (Weiss 1979), and is implicitly linked to the improvement of processes and outcomes.

GUIDING FRAMEWORKS

An established framework describing the competencies for knowledge coproduction is lacking. However, we can draw on frameworks that have been developed in research policy areas that are aligned with research coproduction (see Figure 5.1.1).

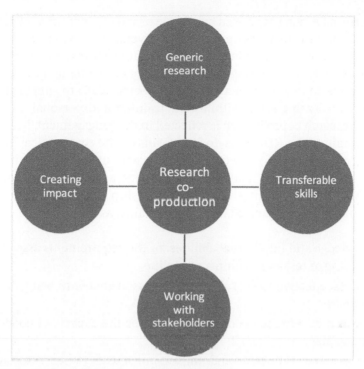

FIGURE 5.1.1 Competencies for research coproduction.

Research Competence

Research coproduction builds on a foundation that melds the methodological and technical aspects of knowledge production, or research more generally. However, thresholds for knowledge and technical competence may resonate differently across a wide range of stakeholders. For example, the peer academic community may have a collective view about threshold knowledge and skills for research; other stakeholders may have different perspectives on this issue. Policy makers and service managers may be willing to draw on more pragmatic investigations, or those which meld different research designs. In these situations, research coproduction may be best served by a broader methodological knowledge and skillsbase. This does not necessarily negate the need for deep expertise as making appropriate trade-offs between methodological purity and pragmatism requires additional insight and understanding.

Transferable Skills

Alongside the development of a researcher within a given field, there is an increasing focus on the growth of transferable skills required to sustain a career as a researcher, some of which are relevant to research coproduction.

Concerns have been expressed by a range of stakeholders about the ability of postdoctoral staff to thrive as employees in diverse and dynamic employment contexts which require a combination of technical and transferable skills. Within the United Kingdom for example, doctoral research students have access to a Researcher Development Framework (RDF) (Vitae 2010) to support the development of transferable skills within their training and personal development programs. Research coproduction is reflected in the "engagement, influence and impact" domain of the RDF. This domain spans (i) the communication and dissemination of research, (ii) aspects of working with others (e.g., team working, influence and leadership), and (iii) engagement and impact, framed across teaching, public engagement, enterprise, citizenship, and policy work.

The framework is organized into four domains, as follows:

- Knowledge and intellectual abilities, or the requirements associated with the doing of research within a discipline
- Personal effectiveness, or the qualities associated with being an effective researcher
- Research governance and organization, or the aspects of good research management
- Engagement, influence and impact, or those issues associated with building impact from research.

The framework is presented as a generic framework for development as researchers develop from novice to more experienced and expert within their field, and is now well embedded within the training offered by many higher education institutions across the globe.

Working with Stakeholders

An essential element which must be foregrounded within research coproduction is stakeholder engagement. Health policy research requires researchers to (i) demonstrate the involvement of patients and the public in many, if not all aspects of their research, and (ii) increase the impact of knowledge through its implementation in practice and policy. Training programs tend to focus on the appropriateness of involvement of patient and public stakeholders in research as the "right thing" to do (see for example INVOLVE (2012)), reflecting a range of perspectives including, ethical dimensions, the publicly funded nature of research, and the potential of generating better quality research with more impact (Boivin et al. 2018; Wilson et al. 2015).

However, research coproduction requires engagement with a much wider group of stakeholders and groups, each of whom need consideration in terms of the nature of their engagement with the focus of research. Within healthcare, these may include service users, professionals, managers, commissioners, payers and policy makers, in addition to broader public representatives. Methods such as system mapping can be used to identify stakeholders from across different constituencies, and many applied health research designs focus on the proximity or otherwise between stakeholders and the healthcare practice. Damschroder's et al.'s (2009) Consolidated Framework for Implementation Research locates stakeholders in either an inner or outer context. Inevitably some stakeholders may only emerge during research coproduction as knowledge emerges of the context in which the research is being conducted. In addition to being able to identify important stakeholders, research coproduction requires their effective engagement, drawing on the communication and relational skills referred to above, as the basis for partnership working.

Creating Impact

The thesis developed within this chapter is that meaningful engagement of stakeholders in coproduction generates impact. Increasing the impact of research is at the core of a range of movements which share a common goal within health and care policy and practice: ensuring that knowledge is as close as possible to the points of decision-making. These include evidence-based healthcare, implementation (knowledge translation, knowledge mobilization), improvement science to name three. The competencies for each movement reflect its particular interests and provide different perspectives on some of the competencies that may be relevant for research coproduction.

For example, evidence-based approaches prioritize the use of best available evidence from research alongside service user preferences and other parameters such as cost. Competencies for development generally relate to evidence retrieval, critical appraisal and practical decision-making (Albarqouni et al. 2018).

From the perspective of implementation, there is interest in both the synthesis of evidence from research, and the strategies available to ensure its use within practice and policy. Strategies include the development of knowledge products; for example, clinical guidelines and decision aids, which meet different stakeholder needs, dissemination, education and training, the facilitation of change, and system-related incentives. The literature demonstrates both considerable variation in the competencies addressed through education and training, and the lack of an evidence base to underpin the development and delivery of capability-building programs (Davis and D'Lima 2020).

In the United Kingdom, Gabbay et al. (2014) have written extensively on the types of impact-related knowledge and skills from an improvement science perspective. Impact in this sense is usually associated with the effectiveness, reliability, or acceptability of healthcare processes. Drawing together evidence from several studies across the United Kingdom, they conclude that effective improvers possess and apply an assortment of knowledge. This ranges from the possession of "local knowledge" which enables an improver to gauge the context and understand the values, priorities, concerns, and practices of a population; to an awareness of the psychological and emotional consequences of change; knowledge of the research process, qualitative and quantitative methods and data analysis; in addition to aspects of sociology, including the role of professional identities and organizational structure and hierarchies. Competencies linked to the improvement science literature also concentrate on the use of an array of technical processes and tools designed to deliver improvement-related impact associated with their particular "brand," including Total Quality Management (Brannan 1998), Lean (Toussaint and Berry 2013), Six Sigma (Schroeder et al. 2008) and the Model for Improvement (Langley et al. 2009) to name but a few. The "Habits of Mind" provides a new lens on competencies for improvement work, linked to operating within the contexts of complex systems (Lucas and Nader 2015). In addition to a positive approach to learning and influencing others, dimensions of systems thinking, creativity, and resilience point to attributes which are linked to dealing with complexity. Lucas and Nader's model focuses on the capabilities of individual improvers, including tolerating uncertainty, accepting of change, connection-making, and generating ideas.

In summary, competencies for research coproduction can be drawn from different conceptual and policy areas, inevitably leading to the development of a comprehensive mix of potential core, general, and specific domains. The translation of these into a curriculum framework to support competency development is outlined in the following project.

EUROPEAN IMPLEMENTATION SCIENCE EDUCATION NETWORK

Improving patient and service user outcomes and increasing citizen participation in the use of knowledge continues to gain momentum across health and social care. The European Implementation Science Education Network (EISEN) was funded by the European Union through its Erasmus+ program to identify associated competencies. These have directed the development of EISEN training programs that increase capacity and capability in aspects of research coproduction and the impact of research-based knowledge more broadly.

The program commenced with focused reviews of the literature, research policy evaluation, and stakeholder engagement within and across European nations to identify an overarching curriculum framework. As the purpose of the scoping literature review was to inform the development of educational programs, the review analysis was organized around three major areas, knowledge, skills, and attitudinal capabilities. The task of elucidating items which specifically related to what a research student on the EISEN program needs to know was made more difficult by the way in which many of the subjects naturally overlapped into other domains of skills and attitudes; for example, knowledge of research methods, and principles and practice of coproduction. Those competencies which relate to research coproduction are summarized below.

Knowledge-Related Competencies

Alongside collaboration with stakeholders, appreciating and being able to work with different knowledge types, and recognizing that these are associated with different rules, processes, and potential impacts, is key to research coproduction. Hidden knowledge, such as stakeholder experience and professional wisdom, can emerge from the contexts in which research is coproduced. Different strategies are required to surface different knowledge types, paying attention to their authenticity and credibility, and to synthesize these with other forms of relevant knowledge.

Knowledge-related capabilities identified through our scoping review work related to a wide range of formal, stakeholder, and context-related knowledge types which emerge within research coproduction (Table 5.1.1). Although psychology and sociological thinking dominates, the knowledge base is increasingly influenced by a diverse range of academic disciplines, theories, and approaches. The inclusion of perspectives from the design sciences, arts, and humanities provides (i) new opportunities to revisit long-standing practical and policy challenges which have otherwise been resistant to change, and (ii) new opportunities to engage stakeholders within the knowledge work. For example, the analysis process in a recent evidence synthesis focusing on the adoption of low-value health interventions drew on the design sciences to explain how information displays can make low-value options difficult to select. Thinking about cults from religious studies was considered to understand the emotional connection that clinicians may have with some ineffective interventions (Burton et al. 2021).

Research coproduction also extends thinking about context beyond the backdrop to the design and conduct of research, and the mix of barriers and enablers that can shape the implementation of knowledge. Whilst these are important, knowledge creation should also be "negotiated," influencing, and being influenced by, the context in which it is situated. Although context is multifactoral and multi-dimensional, the systems which provide structure and function to health and care services include multiple stakeholder groups with competing interests and varying degrees of power. Being able to work within these complex systems requires at least some insider knowledge, credibility, and the personal skills and reserves to navigate these complex systems successfully.

TABLE 5.1.1 Indicative knowledge-based capabilities.

Knowledge capabilities	Description	Relevance to Research Coproduction
Interdisciplinary knowledge	An appreciation of the research paradigms, theories and frameworks from disciplines that can be used within research coproduction.	Research coproduction requires that threshold indicators of the quality of the research itself are maintained.
Health Services Research	A multidisciplinary field of inquiry that provides a framework to examine healthcare organization and delivery and produce new knowledge and improvements for individuals and populations.	Within healthcare, the purpose of research coproduction is to generate solutions to problems and to improve health and wellbeing.
Systems knowledge	The configurations of services and activities with a purpose to promote, restore or maintain health, operating within a broader political, social, and geographical context.	Research coproduction requires insight into the systems which provide a content for the understanding of a research challenge, and the engagement of stakeholders
Public and lay knowledge	Experiential knowledge and expertise that generates different insights for research coproduction.	Research coproduction generates and values different sources and types of knowledge.
Local knowledge	Contextualized, insider knowledge of organizations and the behaviors and beliefs, cultural values, priorities, and norms of stakeholders.	Research coproduction generates and values different sources and types of knowledge.
Implementation	Theories, models and frameworks that summarise understandings about how knowledge, usually research-based, can have the greatest impact in policy and practice.	Research coproduction draws on knowledge of Implementation to shape and enhance impact.

Skills-Related Competencies

There is consensus that those working in coproduction require honed interpersonal skills including high-level communication skills, agility across different policy, organizational and professional boundaries, and the ability to engage relevant stakeholders in authentic ways (Table 5.1.2) to drive coproduction and

TABLE 5.1.2 Indicative skills-based capabilities.

Skills capabilities	Description	Relevance to Research Coproduction
Working with multiple communities	The ability to work across disciplinary, organizational, professional, and political boundaries to engage relevant stakeholders.	Requires navigating and bridging boundaries, including research and practice, different organizations, professions, groups, and other social entities.
Leadership and political skills	Understanding the system, managing vested interests, navigating and exploiting power bases, shrewd timing of interventions, listening to, and taking into account other people's views	Embedded within stakeholder perspectives, research coproduction is a political act requiring negotiation and establishing common ground.
Research and analytical skills	Critical thinking, creative thinking, collectively learning how to improve healthcare.	Within any research framework, research coproduction requires skills to collect, analyse and interpret data in ways which generate new insights into improvement.
Communication skills	Conveying information to another person or groups effectively to help facilitate the sharing of information and knowledge between people.	Requires the ability the communicate different types of information effectively with multiple audiences.
Facilitation of change	Change agency, knowledge brokerage, championing, influencing, facilitation, and mobilizing resources for change.	Research coproduction should generate different impacts over time, which need supporting as part of the coproduction process.

embedded impacts. Negotiation skills are encompassed in the skill set described as "soft skills." The emphasis is that this descriptor is soft in name rather than nature, as working through *"the leadership, structures and political wrangles involved in achieving genuine and lasting improvements can call for real toughness'* (Gabbay et al. 2014). Navigating multiple boundaries can have implications for individuals in terms of encountering conflict, which requires resilience to work towards reconciliation, negotiation, and progress.

Leadership is key both to the creation of a learning culture and receptive context of organizations and systems in which knowledge is used, and as a deliberate strategy to support the facilitation of research impact. Whilst leadership can be viewed as a set of practices or skills which can be taught, it also infers a characteristic or quality possessed by an individual who leads by example, and develops personal influence to galvanize individuals, communities, and resources around partnership working and research coproduction.

The practice of research coproduction is inherently interdisciplinary. Overall, there is a consensus that embedding an interdisciplinary ethos and fostering the boundary spanning skills of those engaged in facilitating research impact is key (Kislov 2018). Leadership skills and attitudes are also the hallmark of knowledge champions, knowledge translation brokers, mentors, and other change agents who play a crucial role in motivating and sustaining engagement in research coproduction activities. The role of leadership as a desirable and beneficial quality of those who succeed in generating change, sustaining improvement and cultivating a culture of knowledge impact is well-documented, and is strongly linked to traits including personal influence, supporting the learning of others through mentoring relationships, and the possession of well-developed networks and relationships.

Possessing an understanding of the influence of contextual factors, including the ability to identify and assess barriers and enablers to impact, is widely recognized as an essential researcher skill for research coproduction. Aligned to this is the ability to tailor knowledge to local needs, engage relevant stakeholders, and work with multiple communities. These skills dovetail with the ability to synthesize and translate knowledge into appropriate formats, tailor it to the needs of specific target audiences, mobilize the necessary resources to initiate and sustain change, and ultimately support the impact of knowledge.

Attitude-Related Competencies

The third dimension of competency relates to the affective domain: the attitudes that should be demonstrated by those engaged in research coproduction. This domain determines the way in which an individual should "be" in terms of behavior and value (Table 5.1.3). The literature is less specific about this domain.

Possessing a spirit of inquiry and being willing and able to learn, through reflection, learning from others, and by participating in learning communities or communities of practice, is also core. Gabbay et al. (2014) identified assertiveness as a characteristic of those involved in creating impact from research; similarly, Pereira and Creary (2018) highlight personal resilience as a necessary attribute. Being orientated to service user or stakeholder perspectives and taking

TABLE 5.1.3 Indicative attitude-based capabilities.

Attitude capabilities	Description	Relevance to Research Coproduction
Values-driven	Being motivated and driven by core social, emotional, psychological or beliefs, qualities and opinions that are important to individual, shared, collective or organization concerns.	Research coproduction can be set within multiple and competing contexts which need reflecting and honoring.
Person-centered	Placing patient and people at the center of decision-making, planning, designing, delivering, coproducing interventions, ideas, tools, products, services, policies etc.	Research coproduction requires a willingness to engage with the concerns of others.
Committed to impact	A spirit of inquiry closely linked with the motivation and desire to change and improve issues for individuals and society, possessing an approach and disposition that motivates and support others to change and achieve.	Research coproduction is concerned primarily with change and the resolution of health-related challenges.
Commitment to personal development	Commitment to developing the skills and mechanisms for learning and self-care in stressful or demanding situations.	Research coproduction can be messy, requiring a willingness to tolerate uncertainty, learn, and persevere.

a value-driven approach are also recognized as important features of those who undertake research coproduction.

Whilst capturing the knowledge and skills in which proficiency is expected has been comparatively straightforward, defining the qualities for coproduction is less clear cut. This is due in part to the way in which those items identified as representing the affective often overlap. For example, the concept of leadership occupies both the skills domain (it can be taught), and the attitudes domain (it is a quality recognized as important in those who lead by example and influence the thinking and behavior of others). Likewise, being multidisciplinary in one's approach to research coproduction could be described as a state of mind, whereas it overlaps with possessing the skills to work across boundaries and professions. As it currently stands there is no definitive set of qualities or traits that have been proposed and this domain remains under-explored and under-articulated; more work is required to develop and define what is the qualitative hallmark of a competent coproductive researcher.

DEVELOPING RESEARCH COPRODUCTION COMPETENCIES

Drawing the EISEN curriculum themes together points to some key consider-ations for the development of competencies for researchers engaging in copro-duction. Research coproduction, through its engagement in the worlds of multiple stakeholders, is messy. It may bring some degree of uncertainty associ-ated with different stakeholder agenda, the personal demands of affecting change through negotiation, and persuasion engagement in policy and practice. From a methodological perspective, it requires a willingness to balance the need for research rigour within the more turbulent and less controlled contexts in which research coproduction will occur.

Our thinking points to a generalist profile of research-related competencies and theoretical insights research, but with greater focus on the political and per-sonal skills to create impact. Supporting the development of research coproduc-ers will inevitably challenge the ways in which research training is organized, how and where it is provided, and the criteria that govern access to that training. In addition to exposure to credible training in research methodology, students will need to develop a sufficient degree of credibility with different stakeholders, probably best obtained through immersion in different aspects of the health sys-tem. If this is the case, there should be the potential for trainees to have refined some of these personal and political skills, or at the very least be able to demon-strate the potential to build these through professional development programs.

Typically, entry to research training programs has been dependent on the student's curiosity towards their topic; indeed, this would seem to be key to help-ing students deal with inevitable problems they will encounter along the way. A more coproductive context for research training will inevitably mean some degree of flexibility in students' underpinning research programs, as these will need to be responsive to different stakeholder perspectives and interests. Those supporting capability building will need to draw on different strategies to sup-port students' perseverance. The preparation for our EISEN programs indicates that research coproduction is rarely the guiding framework in which research training programs are organized; there are, of course, some that have potential, and which have been aligned with integrated knowledge translation in Canada (Sim et al. 2019). Less use of didactic teaching methods and opportunities for students to work together to explore the different contexts in which their research coproduction is located seem to be key through; for example, the use of problem-based learning and reflection, with facilitation of interprofessional and interdisciplinary solutions (Carlfjord et al. 2017).

Although there is renewed interest in interdisciplinary health research, research methodology, methods and practices are generally set within a broader disciplinary tradition. Research capability building approaches have essentially consisted of a doctoral apprenticeship in which students are immersed within the tradition in a supervisory relationship with a more experienced academic. Although knowledge and technical competencies will have an element of specificity, the aim of an apprenticeship is a sufficient degree of independence on which a career within the discipline can be built.

Universities have traditionally held research at the core of frameworks and processes for academic promotion. The degree to which these frameworks value particular types of research will be dependent on national research policy, and the weighting attached to different factors such as journal rankings and / or methodological quality. More recently, some national funders have raised the visibility of impact as an indicator of research quality. It is inevitable, then, that universities are likely to pay less attention to academic or professional scholarship, enterprise, or knowledge-exchange activities as vehicles for academic promotion. Some academic staff, of course, have dual roles in services; for example, as a clinical academic. Here, it can be more complicated to navigate the pathways to financial rewards and academic promotion, as service organizations may place greater value on the generation of more specific and local knowledge and impact.

The clinical academic role is well established in some professional disciplines, most notably medicine. However, policy efforts to focus attention on maximizing the return on investment in applied research have generated a wide range of roles and opportunities which support working across practice and research boundaries. Examples include fellowship and similar programs that provide specific boundary spanning opportunities, often linked to defined and time-limited projects, and "in-residence" roles (Marshall et al. 2016). Here, an individual with typically very different worldviews and skills spends time within a host organization to challenge thinking and practices, and to support change. Although additional benefits for researchers appear less clear, evaluations of programs to bridge research and practice through shared organizational architectures have indicated the potential for positive emotional rewards and opportunities for career progression (Rycroft-Malone et al. 2016a).

CONCLUSION

Knowledge coproduction provides a new lens on the issue of impact by foregrounding this throughout the knowledge production cycle through the engagement of stakeholders and the systems in which they live and work. This change may, of course, be the application of new knowledge in discourse, practice and professional behavior change, politics and policy as research progresses (Weiss 1979), and is implicitly linked to the improvement of processes and outcomes.

There is a distinct set of competencies for research coproduction which cover a range of core, common, and specific issues relating to knowledge work.

Coproduction should not be associated with any one research methodology, but competence within the methodologies used is core. Other competencies reflect two key dimensions of coproduction, including engagement with stakeholders in their systems, and building impact from research. These competencies are broader than common transferable skills, which are often aligned with traditional research training programs, and which seek to ensure that research postgraduates have a sufficient degree of "rounding" to thrive in the workplace and broader economy. Specific competencies are associated with the ability to effect change and impact in the contexts of research implementation; we argue that these competencies can also be useful for research coproduction efforts. Implementation research is generating an evidence base for some of these competencies; for example, facilitation. However, the wider change management literature points towards inter-disciplinarity, cross-boundary working, creativity, systems thinking, and political and emotional intelligence as essential competencies for research coproduction. Embedding coproduction within the systems that sustain training and careers in research requires a refreshed suite of curricula, and the development of incentive systems which prioritize real-world impact.

FUTURE RESEARCH

There are broader research priorities which will focus on the relative merits of research coproduction, and which will highlight conceptual and methodological difficulties to be resolved. From the perspective of the competencies proposed for research coproduction within this chapter, these require investigation within the real world, and across the academic and policy domains in which a coproductive stance on research is developing. Are there specific thresholds of competence, and what combinations of competence are most appropriate for research coproduction challenges of different scope and scale? How may competence best be developed over time, and over the course of coproduction programs? The development of researchers' competencies for research coproduction will require a fresh analysis of researcher training programs and systems, alongside the rewards and incentives that promote these across research, policy and practice contexts.

REFERENCES

1. Albarqouni, L., Hoffmann, T., Straus, S., Olsen, N.R., Young, T., Ilic, D., Shaneyfelt, T., Haynes, R.B., Guyatt, G., and Glasziou, P. (2018). Core competencies in evidence-based practice for health professionals: consensus statement based on a systematic review and Delphi survey. *JAMA Network Open* 1: e180281. doi: 10.1001/jamanetworkopen.2018.0281.

2. Boivin, A., Richards, T., Forsythe, L., Gregoire, A., L'Esperance, A., Abelson, J., and Carman, K.L. (2018). Evaluating patient and public involvement in research. *BMJ* 363: k5147. doi: 10.1136/bmj.k5147.

3. Brannan, K.M. (1998). Total quality in health care. *Hospital Materiel Management Quarterly* 19: 1–8. https://www.ncbi.nlm.nih.gov/pubmed/10178544.

4. Burton, C.R., Williams, L., Bucknall, T., Fisher, D., Hall, B., Harris, G., Jones, P., Makin, M., McBride, A., Meacock, R., Parkinson, J., Rycroft-Malone, J., and Waring, J. (2021). Theory and practical guidance for effective de-implementation of practices across health and care services: a realist synthesis. *Health Services and Delivery Research* 9. doi: 10.3310/hsdr09020.

5. Carlfjord, S., Roback, K., and Nilsen, P. (2017). Five years' experience of an annual course on implementation science: an evaluation among course participants. *Implementation Science: IS* 12: 101. doi: 10.1186/s13012-017-0618-4.

6. Damschroder, L.J., Aron, D.C., Keith, R.E., Kirsh, S.R., Alexander, J.A., and Lowery, J.C. (2009). Fostering implementation of health services research findings into practice: a consolidated framework for advancing implementation science. *Implementation Science: IS* 4: 50. doi: 10.1186/1748-5908-4-50.

7. Davis, R. and D'Lima, D. (2020). Building capacity in dissemination and implementation science: a systematic review of the academic literature on teaching and training initiatives. *Implementation Science: IS* 15: 97. doi: 10.1186/s13012-020-01051-6.

8. Gabbay, J., le May, A., Connell, C., and Klein, J.H. (2014). *Skilled for improvement? Learning communities and the skills needed to improve care: an evaluative service development*. London: The Health Foundation. https://www.health.org.uk/sites/default/files/SkilledForImprovement_fullreport.pdf. Accessed January 11 2022.

9. INVOLVE. (2012). *Briefing Notes for Researchers: Involving the Public in NHS, Public Health and Social Care Research*. Eastleigh, UK: INVOLVE. https://www.invo.org.uk/wp-content/uploads/2014/11/9938_INVOLVE_Briefing_Notes_WEB.pdf. Accessed January 11 2022.

10. Kislov, R. (2018). Selective permeability of boundaries in a knowledge brokering team. *Public Administration* 96: 817–836. doi: 10.1111/padm.12541.

11. Langley, G.J., Moen, R., Nolan, K.M., Nolan, T.W., Norman, C.L., and Provost, L.P. (2009). Changes that result in improvement. In: *The Improvement Guide: A Practical Approach to Enhancing Organisational Performance*, 2e. San Francisco, CA: Jossey-Bass.

12. Lucas, B. and Nader, H. (2015). *The habits of an improver. Thinking about learning from improvement in healthcare*. London: The Health Foundation. https://www.health.org.uk/sites/default/files/TheHabitsOfAnImprover.pdf. Accessed January 11 2022.

13. Marshall, M., Eyre, L., Lalani, M., Khan, S., Mann, S., de Silva, D., and Shapiro, J. (2016). Increasing the impact of health services research on

service improvement: the researcher-in-residence model. *Journal of the Royal Society of Medicine* 109: 220–225. doi: 10.1177/0141076816634318.

14. Nutley, S., Walter, I., and Davies, H.T.O. (2003). From knowing to doing: a framework for understanding the evidence-into-practice agenda. *Evaluation* 9: 125–148. 10.1177/1356389003009002002.

15. Pereira, P. and Creary, N. (2018). *Q: The journey so far. Connecting improvement across the UK – insights and progress three years in.* London: The Health Foundation. https://www.health.org.uk/sites/default/files/upload/publications/2018/Q-Journey-So-Far-Report-180924.pdf. Accessed January 11 2022.

16. Rycroft-Malone, J., Burton, C.R., Bucknall, T., Graham, I.D., Hutchinson, A.M., and Stacey, D. (2016a). Collaboration and co-production of knowledge in healthcare: opportunities and challenges. *International Journal of Health Policy and Management* 5: 221–223. doi: 10.15171/ijhpm.2016.08.

17. Rycroft-Malone, J., Burton, C.R., Wilkinson, J., Harvey, G., McCormack, B., Baker, R., Dopson, S., Graham, I.D., Staniszewska, S., Thompson, C., Ariss, S., Melville-Richards, L., and Williams, L. (2016b). Collective action for implementation: a realist evaluation of organisational collaboration in healthcare. *Implementation Science: IS* 11: 17. doi: 10.1186/s13012-016-0380-z.

18. Schroeder, R.G., Linderman, K., Liedtke, C., and Choo, A.S. (2008). Six sigma: definition and underlying theory. *Journal of Operations Management* 26: 536–554. doi: 10.1016/j.jom.2007.06.007.

19. Sim, S.M., Lai, J., Aubrecht, K., Cheng, I., Embrett, M., Ghandour, E.K., Highet, M., Liu, R., Casteli, C.P., Saari, M., Ouedraogo, S., and Williams-Roberts, H. (2019). CIHR health system impact fellows: reflections on "driving change" within the health system. *International Journal of Health Policy and Management* 8: 325–328. doi: 10.15171/ijhpm.2018.124.

20. Toussaint, J.S. and Berry, L.L. (2013). The promise of Lean in health care. *Mayo Clinic Proceedings* 88: 74–82. doi: 10.1016/j.mayocp.2012.07.025.

21. Vitae. (2010). *Researcher Development Framework.* https://www.vitae.ac.uk/vitae-publications/rdf-related/researcher-development-framework-rdf-vitae.pdf/@@download/file/Researcher-Development-Framework-RDF-Vitae.pdf. Accessed January 11 2022.

22. Weiss, C.H. (1979). The many meanings of research utilization. *Public Administration Review* 39: 426–431. doi: 10.2307/3109916.

23. Wilson, P., Mathie, E., Keenan, J., McNeilly, E., Goodman, C., Howe, A., Poland, F., Staniszewska, S., Kendall, S., Munday, D., Cowe, M., and Peckham, S. (2015). ReseArch with Patient and Public invOlvement: a RealisT evaluation – the RAPPORT study. *Health Services and Delivery Research* 3. doi: 10.3310/hsdr03380.

5.2 Trainees and Research Coproduction

Christine Cassidy, Emily Ramage, Sandy Steinwender, and Shauna Best

Key Learning Points

- Many research trainees do not receive formal training in research coproduction.
- Research coproduction offers several benefits to trainees, knowledge users and supervisors, including valuable experiential learning opportunities and more relevant and useful research findings.
- Despite these benefits, particular attention should be paid to the potential challenges in research coproduction related to partnership structure and function, level of engagement, and resources.
- Facilitators of trainee research coproduction include being flexible and adaptable to knowledge user needs and context, building trusting relationships, and leveraging existing research partnerships.
- Developing research coproduction skills is not a simple, linear process; research coproduction is an iterative, continuous learning cycle where trainees move through different stages of expertise to become true partners in research coproduction.
- Further research is needed to understand the most effective way to prepare trainee researchers for coproduction and the effect coproduction training has on trainees' professional development, knowledge user outcomes, research impact, and health system outcomes.

Research Coproduction in Healthcare, First Edition. Edited by
Ian D. Graham, Jo Rycroft-Malone, Anita Kothari, and Chris McCutcheon.
© 2022 John Wiley & Sons Ltd. Published 2022 by John Wiley & Sons Ltd.

- To address these questions and contribute to the growing literature on the science of research coproduction, we encourage trainees to monitor and evaluate their coproduction approach, including strategies, activities, level of engagement, and knowledge user involvement on thesis committees.

INTRODUCTION

This chapter focuses on the trainee experience in research coproduction and is written from the perspective of trainees, knowledge users, and early career researchers. There continues to be limited guidance to enable researchers and knowledge users to develop expertise in relationship building needed to establish meaningful partnerships (de Moissac et al. 2019). As a result, researchers often lack an understanding of the health system context and skills to engage in research coproduction. This can affect the development of positive, mutually beneficial research partnerships (Bowen et al. 2019).

A lack of knowledge and skills (among trainees and researchers) needed to co-produce research is a critical gap in the literature. A survey of PhD-prepared researchers highlighted unmet learning needs related to collaboration in research during their training (Kyvik and Olsen 2012). Further, previous research explored Canadian health system leaders' perspectives on research collaborations and found that researchers often lack an understanding of how to work collaboratively within the health system context. Participants from this study identified the need to improve academic preparation for researchers engaging in health services research partnerships (Bowen et al. 2019). Most researchers do not have the opportunity to learn how to participate in research coproduction, yet they are expected to establish effective collaborative relationships with knowledge users (Nyström et al. 2018). Similarly, most graduate students do not receive formal training in collaborative health research approaches (Bornstein et al. 2018). As a result, graduate students and postdoctoral trainees who conduct research coproduction are self-directed and must seek experiential learning opportunities or receive mentorship from established researchers with coproduction expertise (Cassidy et al. 2020).

This chapter aims to address this gap by describing the trainee (graduate student and/or postdoctoral fellow) experience in research coproduction and identifies key considerations for trainees, their supervisors, and knowledge users partners for undertaking research coproduction. We begin by providing an overview of the literature on the trainee experience in research coproduction. Next, we discuss our experiential knowledge, as trainees and knowledge users, of engaging in research coproduction in graduate thesis work, postdoctoral fellowships, and using research coproduction to launch a research career. We offer practical advice and guidance to other trainees, their supervisors, and knowledge users interested in or currently engaged in research coproduction. Finally, this chapter ends with implications for future research and practice in research coproduction.

TRAINEES AND RESEARCH COPRODUCTION: WHAT IS KNOWN FROM THE LITERATURE?

In an effort to understand the experience of research coproduction among trainees, our larger team of trainees and early career researchers conducted a scoping review that aimed to map and characterize the available evidence related to using research partnership approaches from the perspectives of trainees in thesis and/or postdoctoral work (Cassidy et al. 2021) (C. Cassidy, work in preparation). As outlined below, preliminary findings from this review highlight the range of research coproduction approaches, benefits, and impacts to the trainee and knowledge user partners, as well as challenges and potential solutions.

Types of Knowledge Users and Research Context

The literature outlines a wide range of knowledge user partners engaged in research coproduction with trainees. Depending on the study context, knowledge users include healthcare consumers, members of the public, community leaders, healthcare providers, and senior leadership in healthcare organizations. Trainees have engaged with these knowledge users in research coproduction in a variety of contexts, including community and public health, Indigenous health, rural health, acute and chronic care, school health, and mental health. While a variety of different terms are used to describe the research coproduction approach (i.e., integrated knowledge translation, collaborative research, coproduction, participatory action research), trainees are engaged in partnership research globally, including Canada, the United States, the United Kingdom, and Australia, to name a few (C. Cassidy, work in preparation).

Research Coproduction Approach

Knowledge users play important roles throughout the research process from project inception through to knowledge dissemination. With trainee-led research described in the literature, the level of knowledge user involvement exists on a continuum of passive involvement to extensive collaboration (C. Cassidy, work in preparation). At one end, knowledge users are engaged as co-researchers, whereby they assist with identification and validation of relevant research questions, develop recruitment and data collection approaches, interpret findings, and develop knowledge translation (KT) strategies (Boland 2018; Hilario 2018). Second, knowledge users may be engaged through an advisory council, whereby they provide higher-level feedback throughout the research process (Cammer 2018; Sanderson et al. 2020). Lastly, ad hoc stakeholder engagement is also common, whereby knowledge users are not involved consistently throughout the research process but at specific decision points (Gowan 2017). Despite the involvement of knowledge users throughout the research process, it is not clear how knowledge users have been involved in the trainees' thesis committee structure and the impact this has on formal thesis guidelines.

Barriers and Challenges

The barriers to engaging in research coproduction as a trainee are well documented in the literature (C. Cassidy, work in preparation). Knowledge users may have many competing priorities; it can be challenging for trainees to find the right balance of communication to keep knowledge users informed and engaged in the process, without overloading them with information (Boland et al. 2020). Further, for trainees partnering with knowledge users within the health system, there is often a high level of turnover in healthcare organizations (Sanderson et al. 2020). There can be challenges with continued engagement and having to restart partnership development with new staff members (Boland et al. 2020; Sanderson et al. 2020). Time is consistently reported as a significant barrier for trainees engaging in research coproduction. As a result, challenges may arise related to scope of the research project and anticipated timelines (Sanderson et al. 2020; van der Meulen 2011). Studies report difficulties in developing a research proposal that meets the needs of knowledge users, but also the timelines and graduate study requirements (Boland et al. 2020; Khobzi and Flicker 2010; Sanderson et al. 2020).

Facilitators

To address the barriers to research coproduction, trainees need to be adaptable and flexible to address key health system issues and maintain relevance of the research. Pre-existing, well-established, and trusting relationships are key facilitators to success (Cassidy et al. 2019; van der Meulen 2011). However, it can take considerable time and effort to develop meaningful partnerships and encourage efficient collaborative research (Boland et al. 2020). Supporting and maintaining knowledge user engagement can be facilitated by creating feedback loops (e.g., staff meetings, presentations, newsletters, web-based discussion platforms) whereby knowledge user input in decision-making can be actively sought and included in the decision-making process (Sanderson et al. 2020).

Impact/Outcome of Partnerships

Despite evidence of the positive impact of research coproduction, there is limited empirical evidence on the effect of research coproduction for research trainees and their knowledge user partners (C. Cassidy, work in preparation). Although not formally evaluated, some trainees have described their experiences with research coproduction in the literature (Haywood et al. 2019; Nadimpalli et al. 2016). Trainees report that coproduction with knowledge users: (i) facilitates the research process, (ii) provides insight and contextual knowledge of organizational policies and procedures in the health system, and (iii) facilitates buy-in from key members of the organization (Boland et al. 2020). Furthermore, this level of knowledge user engagement helps support the project's acceptability within organizations and facilitates recruitment and data collection (Boland et al. 2020). At the data analysis stage, trainees have also described that research coproduction adds richness and relevance to their research findings. By cultivating meaningful partnerships throughout the research process, a coproduction approach supports the sustainability of changes in the healthcare system or community beyond the trainee's project (C. Cassidy, work in preparation). Trainees report research coproduction to be a worthwhile and rewarding experience that increases a trainee's confidence and skills, improves access to organizational and community resources, and likelihood of impact on the knowledge user context (Boland et al. 2020; Khobzi and Flicker 2010). Lastly, engaging in research coproduction as a trainee may increase likelihood of applied health research career opportunities. Preliminary reports from an evaluation of a Canadian health system-academic training program for doctoral and postdoctoral trainees has shown early indicators of successful career transitions into traditional academic and applied health system settings (McMahon et al. 2019).

Implications and Recommendations from the Literature

Key implications and recommendations for trainees interested or engaged in research coproduction include developing proposals that allow for an emergent design, adaptability, and flexibility (C. Cassidy, work in preparation). Further, previous research highlights the importance of identifying and working with knowledge users early in the process and consider their comments and contributions as being equal to those received by researchers (Bengle and Schuch 2018). It is important for trainees to practice humility during research coproduction by acknowledging their positionality as an outsider and take the time to learn about the context and culture of an organization or community (Bowen 2020; Cassidy et al. 2019). Lastly, a key recommendation is to develop a memorandum of understanding or document to clarify roles and responsibilities, co-authorship, copyright, and ownership of study findings (Bengle and Schuch 2018).

TRAINEE RESEARCH COPRODUCTION EXPERIENCE

Building on the existing literature, the following section further describes the research coproduction process from our collective experience as trainees (doctoral and postdoctoral trainees) and knowledge users (manager of a pediatric clinical unit).

Rewards and Benefits

Research coproduction offers many rewards and benefits for research trainees throughout their graduate studies, postdoctoral fellowships, and when launching a career in an academic or non-academic setting. Similarly, there are additional rewards and benefits for knowledge users and supervisors who support trainees in research coproduction.

Experiential Learning Opportunity

From our experience, engaging in research coproduction at the outset of academic training offers trainees a rich experiential learning opportunity to form partnerships early in one's academic careers. Trainees are able to build confidence in developing, nurturing, and sustaining research partnerships and facilitating the research coproduction process (Gagliardi et al. 2016). It is challenging to read about building confidence in collaboration from a textbook or journal article. However, experiencing the research coproduction process gives trainees the lived experience and opportunity to grow their own knowledge, skills, and confidence.

For most trainees undertaking a coproduction process, this is their first introduction to applied research and collaborating with knowledge users. Supervisors provide trainees with mentorship and "real-life" experiential learning opportunities. These non-traditional academic skills, related to relationship building, collaboration, negotiation, facilitation, and leading and working with teams are crucial in preparing trainees to make a meaningful contribution to applied health research.

Beneficial learning opportunities are not restricted to trainees. While knowledge users contribute to trainee skill development by providing space for experiential learning, there is mutual learning that occurs. Research coproduction offers knowledge users the opportunity to build their own capacity related to the research process and evidence-informed decision-making (Gagliardi et al. 2016). These mutual gains are a strong incentive for all members to engage in research coproduction with trainees.

Relevant and Useful Research Findings

Research coproduction generates relevant, timely, and useful research findings for knowledge users (Hoekstra et al. 2020; Jull et al. 2019). From our experience, there is increased acceptance when trainees use common language to tailor information to knowledge user's unique priorities and normative practices. Knowledge users and researchers are able to share relevant research findings that directly apply to practice and decision-making. By being involved in the research coproduction process, knowledge users are more likely to adopt the evidence and sustain its use in practice. Trainees and supervisors also develop a deeper understanding of the knowledge user's perspective on the topic. In turn, trainees co-produce more meaningful findings and can see the direct impact or implications of their work. Further, supervisors can support efforts to decrease research waste and guide trainees towards making meaningful contributions to their discipline and knowledge user partners.

Advance Research Partnerships

Research coproduction helps to develop lasting relationships and networks that may extend beyond the research project (Sibbald et al. 2019). As a trainee, taking time to cultivate meaningful research coproduction partnerships can lead to future career opportunities beyond your training period that may inform your future research agenda. In our own experiences, new research questions stem from coproduction projects and have led to postdoctoral fellowship projects and collaborative programs of research as independent scientists. In doing so, this may take you down a path of inquiry that you could not identify in the literature and may be more relevant in the *real-world* context.

For knowledge users, research coproduction with trainees provides benefits to developing strong networks and formal partnerships with researchers. Knowledge users are investing in working relationships with future researchers. For supervisors, involving trainees in your research is beneficial as it assists progression of your existing research partnerships and may catalyze new research coproduction projects.

Expectations vs. Reality

The realities of coproduction do not always match initial expectations of shared partnership and collaboration. As outlined below, trainees should consider the pragmatic realities of engaging in research production during their training.

Partnership Structure and Function

Research partnerships with strong working relationships are critical to the success of coproduction. Ideally, trainees are embedded in a partnership and working collaboratively with knowledge users throughout the research process. However, in reality, research coproduction is not always smooth and linear. Successful partnerships take time and humility to develop (Bowen 2020; Gagliardi et al. 2016). Significant preparation is required to build the trust required to support shared decision-making in these partnerships. Research coproduction aims to have all perspectives and expertise represented and valued equally.

However, the reality of shared decision-making means there will not always be total agreement within the partnership. Such conflict can be challenging for trainees to navigate while maintaining working relationships and ensuring decisions are made and prioritized appropriately.

Supervisors play an important role in guiding trainees through the some-times "messy" realities of coproduction. The reliance on experiential learning to develop coproduction skills means trainees are often learning as they go. Supervisors should role-model facilitation, humility, and conflict resolution skills. Trainees need direction and guidance on how to engage knowledge users and navigate decision-making, conflicts, and differing opinions. In reality, a research coproduction process for trainees involves many discussions and debriefs with supervisors to discuss how the research partnership is working and what to do differently to support partnership structure and function.

From the knowledge user perspective, clearly defining roles at the beginning of a project is not always realistic due to the iterative, evolving nature of copro-duction, particularly if knowledge users have not been involved in research pro-jects before. In reality, knowledge users need individualized and sometimes substantial preparation to understand the research coproduction process to allow them to adequately and more accurately identify their role within the team. Similarly, clear role definition is needed for trainees; knowledge users may provide more task-focused roles, as opposed to treating students as "researchers-in-training" and supporting them to learn while also making important contri-butions. Differences in power (or perceived power) can make shared decision-making challenging. Often the knowledge user may perceive a power differential from the lead researchers in the project and effort needs to be made to facilitate sharing of power and empowerment of knowledge users (e.g., by reinforcing the coproduction approach, providing adequate training prepara-tion). Knowledge users may not be aware of the power differential and leader-ship roles between supervisors and trainees which may lead to increased responsibility placed on the trainee.

Engagement

Knowledge users should be involved throughout the coproduction process; how-ever, there are factors that could constrain their engagement. Knowledge users are often immersed in their own commitments and priorities; participating in a research study may be seen as an "extra" project, if the time and resources allow. As a result, not all knowledge users are able to contribute the time to the project that would be optimal (Gagliardi et al. 2016). Constraints specific to the individual project will likely be experienced and efforts should be made to understand these early in the process so they can be addressed to ensure genuine partnership is still achieved. Trainees should work closely with their supervisors to explore the right fit with a knowledge user. Collectively, the research team should clearly define roles and engagement strategies at the beginning of a partnership and discuss the professional development focus for trainees. To sustain engagement, trainees can aim to provide tangible outputs (evidence briefs, project summaries) for knowledge users throughout the project.

Unpredictability

Unlike many other approaches to research, some aspects of coproduction are inherently unpredictable due the iterative nature of the process, hence the need for a flexible and adaptable approach to coproduction.

Some knowledge users may be more comfortable with unpredictability due to the nature of fast-paced decision-making in their workplace. Other knowledge users unfamiliar with the demands of research may require more time and support to optimize their experience and input in the collaborative research process (Gagliardi et al. 2016). It is important for knowledge users to understand that there is a certain level of structure needed for trainees. Marrying the expectations of knowledge users and trainees can be challenging due to their differing priorities, motivation, or other work or personal commitments (e.g., thesis completion vs. managing a clinical caseload). The reality is there may need to be compromises made by the knowledge user and trainee to adapt expectations of the project (e.g., timelines, outputs, etc.).

Although trainees are expected to develop their independence, the unpredictability of engaging in research coproduction can be high-risk for supervisors. Knowledge user relationships that are monitored and maintained by supervisors helps to prevent any negative impact on the overarching research program partnership and subsequent research studies. It is the role of the supervisor to maintain open lines of communication between the trainee, supervisor, and knowledge user to troubleshoot unanticipated challenges with the project.

Barriers and Facilitators

Team Structure and Decision-Making

Research coproduction requires a supportive and motivated team. It is critical that thesis and postdoctoral supervisors support the coproduction process and value the involvement of stakeholders throughout the research study. Ideally, trainees can set themselves up for success by seeking out supervisors with experience in research coproduction and are committed to the epistemology of coproduction and true shared decision-making. Trainees should work closely with their supervisor early in the relationship to identify the role coproduction will play in the trainee's work and the level of supervisor expertise with this research approach. If the supervisor is not supportive of coproduction, trainees may benefit from a co-supervisor or committee member with coproduction experience to offer important mentorship in this area. If a supervisor actively discourages a partnership approach, trainees may need to have an honest, frank discussion about the philosophical differences in their research approaches. In these cases, it is likely best to seek out a supervisor with research coproduction experience.

Similarly, there may be barriers with finding the appropriate knowledge user for the thesis or postdoctoral project. Often, trainees have limited networks or pre-established relationships with knowledge users. This speaks to the importance of research program partnerships, whereby supervisors have ongoing working relationships with knowledge users and students can easily fit into existing partnerships. Supervisors can support effective team structure by helping to formalize these partnerships between trainees and knowledge users.

Different knowledge users have different preferences for how they like to receive information and provide input into decisions. This can be challenging for trainees to accommodate while working towards genuine joint decision-making. It is important to spend the time at the outset of a project to explore how all team members prefer to engage. From there, co-develop an engagement strategy (i.e., recurring meetings, brief huddles, email summaries, in-person, or teleconference meetings). Identifying the group's preferred consensus building strategies at the beginning of a partnership can help to prevent conflict and support an efficient decision-making process. For example, teams may decide to use a rank and scoring approach, discussing strengths and weaknesses, or independent voting on key decision items.

Time and Resources

The time required to develop and maintain research partnerships can have a significant impact on trainee's timeline to thesis, dissertation, or fellowship completion. Academic programs have explicit guidelines for completion of masters and doctoral studies. These graduate study guidelines are often rigid when it comes to timelines and required components to graduate. This can cause significant stress for trainees who are trying to meet their requirements for graduation, while also applying a flexible research coproduction approach to generate relevant and useful findings for their knowledge users. The supervisor plays an important role in helping trainees to find a balance in following the iterative path that allows for adaptability to meet knowledge users' needs, while also following the structured thesis guidelines and meeting the requirements for successful completion. Further, the supervisor needs to develop clear lines of communication with knowledge users to help them understand the learning component of a trainee's academic journey. Frequent communication between the trainee, supervisor, and knowledge users to assess the trainee's academic progression is needed to ensure timely completion, while also meeting key project deliverables.

Sufficient resources also play a critical role in research coproduction (Gagliardi et al. 2016). Unfortunately, most trainees have little to no funding to support knowledge users on their teams, which impacts their ability to compensate knowledge users for their time and contributions (i.e., providing honorarium to patient partners on their research team). Supervisors can support their students with funding, if available, to provide to knowledge users. Trainees can also apply for small grants to support their partnership work. If funds are not feasible, further discussions around role clarity and engagement expectations should be had to develop a plan that meets the time and resources available to knowledge users and ensure adequate engagement in the research process. In the end, the project scope and outcomes will be limited by the constraints of the project (e.g., time, money); trainees need to ensure they prioritize the project to deliver key outcomes based on resources available.

Meeting Knowledge User Needs

Trainees primarily focus on completing their thesis or dissertation and submitting a manuscript for publication. That is often the extent of their knowledge dissemination activities. However, with research coproduction, it is important for the team to identify and develop appropriate knowledge translation products that target the relevant knowledge users and address knowledge user needs. Some knowledge users have tight deadlines and are involved in fast-paced decision-making. Additional guidance is needed to support students with meeting the short-term needs of these knowledge users but ensuring scientific rigor is maintained throughout the research process. It is helpful for trainees to have an understanding of this context and identify time efficient outputs to support knowledge translation throughout the project. These types of dissemination activities could be in the form of presentation slides, findings tables, or infographics as opposed to a completed manuscript at the end of a study.

CONSIDERATIONS FOR THE DEVELOPMENT OF RESEARCH COPRODUCTION SKILLS

Developing research coproduction skills is not a simple process that begins and ends with reading this textbook. While our intent is for this chapter to be a valuable starting point for trainees, we recognize that research coproduction is an iterative, continuous learning cycle where trainees move through different stages of expertise to become true partners in research coproduction. The practice of research coproduction is evolving – new literature and empirical evidence is constantly being developed and disseminated. It is important for novice and more experienced researchers to continuously read, reflect, and practice the principles of research coproduction. Figure 5.2.1 depicts a continuous research coproduction development process of learning, doing, and becoming.

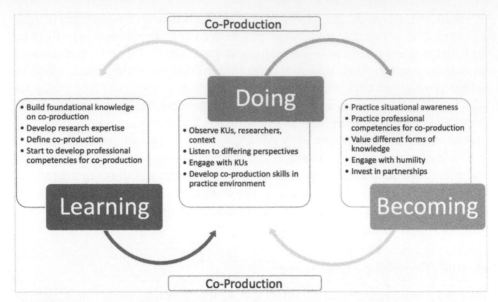

FIGURE 5.2.1   Learning process for research coproduction skill development.

Learning

Developing skills in research coproduction begins with *learning* the foundational knowledge related to coproduction. This includes exploring the literature on the history, approaches, values, and meanings behind coproduction. The other chapters in this book are a good starting point for this foundational reading. The *learning* stage also includes discussions with your supervisor and actively defining what coproduction means to you. This upfront work is essential before diving into a partnership with a knowledge user. If omitted, the partnership and subsequent research projects could be negatively affected.

The *learning* stage should also focus on the development of research coproduction skills. Previous research has identified key competencies that trainees need for applied health research. In 2015, the Canadian Health Services and Policy Research Alliance (CHSPRA) developed a set of ten enriched core competencies (professional and traditional competencies) for health services and policy research training to increase student preparedness and potential impact in a variety of workplace settings (Bornstein et al. 2018). The six professional core competencies relate directly to research coproduction skills, including: Leadership, mentorship, and collaboration; Change management and implementation; Interdisciplinary work; Project management; Dialogue and negotiation; and Networking (Bornstein et al. 2018). A baseline self-assessment on these professional core competencies is a helpful starting point for trainees interested in developing their research coproduction skills. As you move through the *doing* and *becoming* stages, you will have opportunities to practice these skills and further develop your expertise in research coproduction.

Doing

The next step in this journey is starting to do the work of research coproduction and practicing your coproduction knowledge and skills. *Doing* research coproduction is gradual; this is not the time to rush into a partnership with a knowledge user. We know building effective and meaningful relationships takes time. It is important in this stage of *doing* to start observing dynamics and conversations between knowledge users, researchers, and the context that the knowledge user is situated in. This can happen by attending meetings with your supervisor and knowledge user or observing staff meetings and patient advisory committee meetings. Active listening is critical to develop an understanding of the context and factors influencing knowledge user practice and decision-making. It is at this *doing* stage that trainees can start to engage with knowledge users and plant the seeds for relationship development, including trust-building, and have opportunities to develop their professional core competencies in a safe, supportive environment.

Becoming

As trainees develop the building blocks for research coproduction, they reach the stage of *becoming* a true research partner. This involves practicing situational awareness, whereby you understand the contextual factors (i.e., competing priorities, organizational culture, knowledge user needs) and how these factors play a role in the research coproduction process. Further, you have opportunities to foster your leadership, mentorship, dialogue, negotiation, and interdisciplinary skills. In the *becoming* stage, trainees must practice with humility, and understand the different forms of expertise and the role of each partner in the decision-making process (Cassidy et al. 2020). This prevents researchers from seeking knowledge user input but disregarding it when it comes time for decision-making. Humility goes beyond simply communicating research methods and findings; it speaks to the need for respecting diverse perspectives that are needed to address complex problems and being responsive to what is relevant to knowledge users (Bowen 2020). This requires developing skills and confidence in group facilitation and leadership in order to incorporate differing opinions, expand on critical issues, explore the nuances of the practice or policy context, and be flexible to respond to the iterative nature of research coproduction. (Cassidy et al. 2019). This is not easy; however, in the *becoming* stage, trainees practice their facilitation skills and enable participation from all partners.

This cycle is a continuous development process of learning, doing, and becoming. Depending on the knowledge user or research project, you may find yourself at different stages of development. It is important to be aware of the skills and approach needed for different groups of knowledge users. Even experienced researchers return to the learning and doing stages to further develop their ability to foster meaningful and sustainable research partnerships with knowledge users.

Training Programs

Several training programs exist to provide trainees with experiential learning opportunities to move through the stages of *learning, doing*, and *becoming*. For example, the Canadian Institutes of Health Research (CIHR) Health System Impact (HSI) Fellowship was designed to modernize doctoral and postdoctoral training to better equip researchers with the professional and research skills needed to address complex health system challenges (Canadian Institutes of Health Research 2018). HSI doctoral and postdoctoral research fellows are embedded in health system organizations to develop enriched core competencies (i.e., project management, dialogue and negotiation, change management, interdisciplinary work) (Bornstein et al. 2018), understand the intricacies of health system delivery, and partner with members of the health system to support relevant research efforts (Canadian Institutes of Health Research 2018). Similarly, Mitacs is a Canadian, not-for-profit organization that provides research training opportunities to develop trainee's research networks, experience and professional skills. Mitacs works closely with industry partners and academic institutions to pair trainees with partner organizations on a collaborative-research project (Mitacs 2021). In the United States, Academy Health developed the Delivery System Science Fellowship to provide experiential learning and professional development opportunities for postdoctoral trainees (Kanani et al. 2017). These types of training programs offer formalized experiences that focus on the development of professional skills not currently emphasized in health services doctoral training. An evaluation of the CIHR HSI Fellowship program found enhanced core competencies for many HSI fellows included developing aptitude in change management, leadership and collaboration, and dialogue and negotiation (McMahon et al. 2019). Trainees may wish to consider these types of formalized training programs to further their research coproduction skills development and better support the use of a coproduction approach in their graduate or postdoctoral research.

IMPLICATIONS FOR THE PRACTICE OF RESEARCH COPRODUCTION

Research coproduction is primarily relational work focused on understanding a different worldview and working together to solve a problem. Due to its complexity, there may be risks in attempting to provide guidance in simple resources such as a "How to" checklist. Table 5.2.1 provides practical advice and recommendations for trainees, supervisors, and knowledge users engaged in research coproduction through the stages of *learning, doing*, and *becoming*. While these tangible strategies may be helpful to support research coproduction, we reiterate the importance of self-reflection throughout the process.

TABLE 5.2.1 Tips for coproduction from Trainee and knowledge user perspectives.

	Tips for Research coproduction		
	Learning (Developing Skills)	Doing (Experiential Learning)	Becoming (Engage in coproduction)

Trainees	• Conduct a self-assessment on non-traditional academic skills, including: facilitation, communication, collaboration, conflict resolution, negotiation, project management.
	• Explore resources for your own skills development, including:
	  • Webinars, online course
	  • Empirical literature
	• Review reference lists of germinal coproduction papers.
	• Read trainee examples of coproduction (IKTRN casebooks)
	• Discuss coproduction with supervisors, including best practice approaches to engagement.
	• Network with other trainees who are engaged in coproduction.
	• Familiarize yourself with the knowledge user context.
	• Build committee structure that includes expertise in research coproduction.
		• Meet with knowledge users.
		• Consider knowledge user comments and contributions as being equal to those received by researchers.
		• Sit in on meetings between supervisor and knowledge user.
		• Observe supervisor in action on their coproduction projects.
		• Build rapport with knowledge users through formal and informal meetings/debriefs.
		• Examine the context and culture.
		• Practice identifying context/cultural factors influencing decision-making and/or practice.
		• Discuss overall goals and priorities of project.
		• Identify what preparation is needed to start project (i.e., orientation, planning, priority setting).
			• Map out roles, responsibilities and expectations.
			• Facilitate coproduction process.
			• Apply consensus building approaches.
			• Ensure situational awareness.
			• Practice a sense of humility with engaging with knowledge users.
			• Check in with knowledge users regularly (informal and formal check-ins).
			• Provide tangible outputs for knowledge users along the way.
			• Breakdown key deliverables throughout the project.
			• Take time to reflect on progress and coproduction approach (keep journal of log).
			• Ensure your project design allows for an emergent design, adaptability and flexibility.
			• Acknowledge positionality as an outsider and take the time to learn about the context and take the culture of an organization or community.
			• Develop a memorandum of understanding or document to clarify roles and responsibilities, co-authorship, copyright, and ownership of study findings.

(Continued)

Tips for Research coproduction

	Learning (Developing Skills)	Doing (Experiential Learning)	Becoming (Engage in coproduction)

Knowledge Users	• Work with research team to understand the role of research evidence in practice and decision-making.
	• Ensure you feel adequate preparation for the research process and training context (researchers should provide orientation to meet your learning needs).
	• Examine practice issues and their potential for a research approach.
	• Develop a clear understanding of:
	  • Training/academic context and requirements.
	  • Project team's roles (including trainee vs. supervisor).
	  • Limitations imposed by the project forming part of a thesis and/or fellowship project.
		• Create a group of knowledge users, including champions or individuals invested in the success of the research outcome, to build credibility within the broader team, and facilitate buy-in with organization/community.
		• Identify the right types of influences to include on team (e.g., team level, different stages of administrators, interprofessional colleagues).
		• Develop clear lines of communication with supervisor to discuss trainee progress and project challenges.
		• Discuss the context of practice issues (i.e., the history of the issue, what efforts have been made to date).
			• Facilitate connections between trainee and key stakeholders.
			• Value and appreciate trainee's professional development and contributions.
			• Promote buy in from your own context.
			• Support trainee in exploring the context and its impact on research process and outcomes.
			• Lead the team through organizational challenges and barriers.
			• Provide constructive feedback throughout the project, including ways to improve process, engagement, decision-making.
			• If within scope of work, facilitate open and honest conversations to allow for reframing and re-prioritizing objectives to address unanticipated challenges.
			• Invest in partnership to enhance potential for ongoing collaboration.

Tips for Research coproduction

	Learning (Developing Skills)	Doing (Experiential Learning)	Becoming (Engage in coproduction)
Supervisors	• Support trainee through the three stages and highlight when it is important to loop back to learning stage (i.e., identify gaps in skills or knowledge). • Encourage self-reflection on learning needs. • For supervisors will limited knowledge or experience in research coproduction, partner with co-supervisor or committee members with coproduction expertise to advance own skills to support trainees.	• Facilitate experiential learning opportunities (formal or informal). • Role-model the coproduction process. • Provide opportunities for trainees to observe effective coproduction partnerships and processes. • Initiate trainee and knowledge users working relationships, including introductions. • Provide leadership role in the beginning as trainee builds knowledge and skills. • Ensure clear roles and responsibilities are identified at outset of project and return to these often. • Develop clear lines of communication with knowledge users to discuss trainee progress and challenges. • Navigate thesis/degree requirements.	• Provide a safety net to let trainee try to fly on their own but ready to catch them before they crash (support trainees to practice their coproduction skills but be available to address issues). • Provide feedback on the trainee's development of skills necessary for coproduction, including facilitation, situational awareness, humility. • Review progress towards key deliverables for knowledge user and thesis fellowship/completion. • Step in if challenges arise and steer the project back on course. • Facilitate challenging discussions between trainees and knowledge users. • Facilitate debriefs with trainees and knowledge users to discuss strengths and areas for improvement related to project progress and trainee development. • Build a research program partnership with knowledge users to facilitate trainees' engagement with knowledge user in their projects.

FUTURE RESEARCH

Training Preparation for Research Coproduction

We have been fortunate to stumble upon research coproduction in our graduate training and developed valuable skills and appreciation for coproduction through experiential learning opportunities. Similar to our experience, most of the trainee research coproduction described in the literature are one-off projects, whereby students and fellows learn about coproduction as they move through their programs. Based on our experience in "learning as we go," we recognize the critical importance of tailored training efforts to prepare trainees to engage in research production. While some training programs exist, efforts are needed to formalize graduate training in coproduction to reap its benefits on trainees, the research process, and the health system.

To move the needle forward in academic training, several gaps in our understanding of coproduction need to be addressed. For instance, what is the most effective way to prepare trainee researchers for coproduction? Further work is needed to understand what coproduction skills should be taught versus what skills can only be learned through experience. From our collective experience, we believe trainees in the *learning* stage can review existing literature on key competencies for collaborative research; however, the importance of experiential learning opportunities for coproduction skills development should not be underestimated. Trainees that are exposed to experienced researchers working in a coproduction approach with knowledge users can observe coproduction in action and practice skills related to facilitation, negotiation of challenging conversations, conflict resolution, and sharing power. Providing safe learning environments for trainees to practice with humility are needed to foster this important coproduction skill (Bowen 2020; Cassidy et al. 2020). Currently, many applied health research training programs are optional and not formalized in the traditional academic training. Are there opportunities to embed the key coproduction competencies into academic curriculum? Addressing these gaps will help prepare trainees to understand *how* to engage in an effective, respectful and efficient way with knowledge user.

Build the Empirical Knowledge Base on Research Coproduction

In addition to academic training, there is a need to build the empirical scientific base on trainees using a research coproduction approach. What effect does coproduction training have on trainee's professional development, knowledge user outcomes, research impact, health system outcomes, etc.? To address these questions, empirical studies are needed to describe the strategies, approaches, and interventions on how to effectively engage knowledge users with trainees and effects of this coproduction process. The use of reporting guidelines (e.g., the GRIPP2 which is designed to improve reporting of patient and public involvement in research) (Staniszewska et al. 2017) within dissertations and trainee-led manuscripts would help strengthen the quality of reporting and provide a detailed understanding of the partnership process. Additional questions remain on how to find the right balance between adaptability and research rigor. What research designs support this adaptable approach to health services research while effectively supporting trainee skill development and program completion? What types of formal knowledge user-academic partnership structures facilitate the trainee coproduction experience? What are the most effective ways to navigate a supervisor relationship or academic environment that is not supportive of research coproduction? To address these questions and contribute to the growing literature on the science of research coproduction, we encourage trainees to monitor and evaluate their coproduction approach, including strategies, activities, level of engagement, and knowledge user involvement on thesis committee. This will be critical as we advance the field of coproduction to generate more relevant and useful research findings.

CONCLUSION

This chapter provides trainees with a blueprint for engaging in research coproduction in their graduate and/or postdoctoral training. Building on the existing literature on this topic, we describe our experiences as trainees and knowledge users in using a research coproduction approach. Throughout this chapter we detail the benefits and impacts, barriers and enablers, as well as pragmatic realities for trainees interested in or engaged in research coproduction. Relationship building and approaching research coproduction with a sense of humility and appreciation for knowledge user's context is critical for successful research coproduction. When developing the skills to engage in research coproduction, trainees move through stages of learning, doing, and becoming an effective research partner. This is a continuous learning cycle for all researchers from beginners to more experienced coproduction researchers. While this chapter is a starting point for trainees involved in research coproduction, further work is needed to advance academic training and better equip trainees to be effective research partners.

REFERENCES

1. Bengle, T. and Schuch, C. (2018). Integrating participatory action research into graduate geography studies: a tale of two dissertations. *Journal of Geography in Higher Education* 42: 617–629. doi: 10.1080/03098265.2018.1514589.
2. Boland, L. (2018). Implementation of shared decision making in pediatric clinical practice. PhD Thesis. University of Ottawa. doi: 10.20381/ruor-22436.
3. Boland, L., Reszel, J., McCutcheon, C., Kothari, A., and Graham, I.D. (eds.) (2020). *How We Work Together: The Integrated Knowledge Translation Research*

Network Casebook. Vol. 3. Ottawa: Integrated Knowledge Translation Research Network. https://iktrn.ohri.ca/projects/casebook.

4. Bornstein, S., Heritage, M., Chudak, A., Tamblyn, R., McMahon, M., and Brown, A.D. (2018). Development of enriched core competencies for health services and policy research. *Health Services Research* 53 (Suppl 2): 4004–4023. doi: 10.1111/1475-6773.12847.

5. Bowen, S. (2020). *Should We Be Teaching Researchers Humility? Literature Review and Reflection.* Ottawa, ON: Integrated Knowledge Translation Research Network.

6. Bowen, S., Botting, I., Graham, I.D., MacLeod, M., Moissac, D., Harlos, K., Leduc, B., Ulrich, C., and Knox, J. (2019). Experience of health leadership in partnering with University-based researchers in Canada – A call to "Re-imagine" research. *International Journal of Health Policy and Management* 8: 684–699. doi: 10.15171/ijhpm.2019.66.

7. Cammer, A.L. (2018). Nutrition care for long-term care residents with dementia in urban and rural contexts: an evidence based practice examination of the role of care aides and registered dietitians. PhD Thesis. University of Saskatchewan. http://hdl.handle.net/10388/8636.

8. Canadian Institutes of Health Research. (2018). *The health system impact fellowship.* [Online]. https://cihr-irsc.gc.ca/e/51211.html (accessed 31 August 2021).

9. Cassidy, C.E., Beck, A.J., Conway, A., Demery Varin, M., Laur, C., Lewis, K.B., Ramage, E.R., Nguyen, T., Steinwender, S., Ormel, I., Stratton, L., and Shin, H.D. (2021). Using an integrated knowledge translation or other research partnership approach in trainee-led research: a scoping review protocol. *BMJ Open* 11: e043756. doi: 10.1136/bmjopen-2020-043756.

10. Cassidy, C.E., Bowen, S., Fontaine, G., Cote-Boileau, E., and Botting, I. (2020). How to work collaboratively within the health system: workshop summary and facilitator reflection. *International Journal of Health Policy and Management* 9: 233–239. doi: 10.15171/ijhpm.2019.131.

11. Cassidy, C.E., Burgess, S., and Graham, I.D. (2019). It's all about the IKT approach: three perspectives on an embedded research fellowship comment on "CIHR Health System Impact Fellows: reflections on 'Driving Change' Within the Health System." *International Journal of Health Policy and Management* 8: 455–458. doi: 10.15171/ijhpm.2019.31.

12. de Moissac, D., Bowen, S., Botting, I., Graham, I.D., MacLeod, M., Harlos, K., Songok, C.M., and Bohemier, M. (2019). Evidence of commitment to research partnerships? Results of two web reviews. *Health Research Policy and Systems / BioMed Central* 17: 73. doi: 10.1186/s12961-019-0475-5.

13. Gagliardi, A.R., Berta, W., Kothari, A., Boyko, J., and Urquhart, R. (2016). Integrated knowledge translation (IKT) in healthcare: a scoping review. *Implementation Science: IS* 11: 38. doi: 10.1186/s13012-016-0399-1.

14. Gowan, D.M. (2017). Exploring patient safety issues in massage therapy and understanding patient safety incidents (adverse events). Phd Thesis. University of Saskatchewan. http://hdl.handle.net/10388/8036.

15. Haywood, C., Martinez, G., Pyatak, E.A., and Carandang, K. (2019). Engaging patient stakeholders in planning, implementing, and disseminating occupational therapy research. *The American Journal of Occupational Therapy: Official Publication of the American Occupational Therapy Association* 73: 7301090010p1–7301090010p9. doi: 10.5014/ajot.2019.731001.

16. Hilario, C.T. (2018). Applying integrated knowledge translation to address mental health among young immigrant and refugee men in Canada. PhD Thesis. University of British Columbia. doi: 10.14288/1.0368796.

17. Hoekstra, F., Mrklas, K.J., Khan, M., McKay, R.C., Vis-Dunbar, M., Sibley, K.M., Nguyen, T., Graham, I.D., SCI Guiding Principles Consensus Panel, and Gainforth, H.L. (2020). A review of reviews on principles, strategies, outcomes and impacts of research partnerships approaches: a first step in synthesising the research partnership literature. *Health Research Policy and Systems/BioMed Central* 18: 51. doi: 10.1186/s12961-020-0544-9.

18. Jull, J., Graham, I.D., Kristjansson, E., Moher, D., Petkovic, J., Yoganathan, M., Tugwell, P., and Welch, V.A., Members of the CONSORT-Equity, and Boston Equity Symposium. (2019). Taking an integrated knowledge translation approach in research to develop the CONSORT-Equity 2017 reporting guideline: an observational study. *BMJ Open* 9: e026866. doi: 10.1136/bmjopen-2018-026866.

19. Kanani, N., Hahn, E.E., Gould, M.K., Brunisholz, K.D., Savitz, L.A., and Holve, E.C. (2017). AcademyHealth's Delivery System Science Fellowship: training embedded researchers to design, implement, and evaluate new models of care. *Journal of Hospital Medicine* 7: 570–574. doi: 10.12788/jhm.2776.

20. Khobzi, N. and Flicker, S. (2010). Lessons learned from undertaking community-based participatory research dissertations: the trials and triumphs of two junior health scholars. *Progress in Community Health Partnerships: Research, Education, and Action* 4: 347–356. doi: 10.1353/cpr.2010.0019.

21. Kyvik, S. and Olsen, T.B. (2012). The relevance of doctoral training in different labour markets. *Journal of Education and Work* 25: 205–224. doi: 10.1080/13639080.2010.538376.

22. McMahon, M., Brown, A., Bornstein, S., and Tamblyn, R. (2019). Developing competencies for health system impact: early lessons learned from the Health System Impact Fellows. *Healthcare Policy = Politiques de Santé* 15: 61–72. doi: 10.12927/hcpol.2019.25979.

23. Mitacs. (2021). *Mitacs Programs*. [Online]. https://www.mitacs.ca/en/programs (accessed 31 August 2021).

24. Nadimpalli, S.B., Van Devanter, N., Kavathe, R., and Islam, N. (2016). Developing and conducting a dissertation study through the community-based participatory research approach. *Pedagogy in Health Promotion* 2: 94–100. doi: 10.1177/2373379915616646.

25. Nyström, M.E., Karltun, J., Keller, C., and Andersson Gare, B. (2018). Collaborative and partnership research for improvement of health and social

services: researcher's experiences from 20 projects. *Health Research Policy and Systems / BioMed Central* 16: 46. doi: 10.1186/s12961-018-0322-0.

26. Sanderson, V., Vandyk, A., Jacob, J.D., and Graham, I.D. (2020). Engaging knowledge users with mental health experience in a mixed-methods systematic review of post-secondary students with psychosis: reflections and lessons learned from a Master's thesis. *International Journal of Health Policy and Management*. doi: 10.34172/ijhpm.2020.138.

27. Sibbald, S.L., Kang, H., and Graham, I.D. (2019). Collaborative health research partnerships: a survey of researcher and knowledge-user attitudes and perceptions. *Health Research Policy and Systems/BioMed Central* 17: 92. doi: 10.1186/s12961-019-0485-3.

28. Staniszewska, S., Brett, J., Simera, I., Seers, K., Mockford, C., Goodlad, S., Altman, D.G., Moher, D., Barber, R., Denegri, S., Entwistle, A., Littlejohns, P., Morris, C., Suleman, R., Thomas, V., and Tysall, C. (2017). GRIPP2 reporting checklists: tools to improve reporting of patient and public involvement in research. *BMJ* 358: j3453. doi: 10.1136/bmj.j3453.

29. van der Meulen, E. (2011). Participatory and action-oriented dissertations: the challenges and importance of community-engaged graduate research. *Qualitative Report* 16: 1291–1303. doi: 10.46743/2160-3715/2011.1299.*(Continued)*

5.3 The Role of Funders

Bev Holmes and Chonnettia Jones

Key Learning Points

- Funders should support coproduction through programming, and advocate for systemic change to support coproduction.
- Funders need to be clear on the requirements for, and their commitment, to coproduction.
- Funders should be sensible and strategic in what they ask and expect from coproduction participants.
- Funders should consider equity, diversity, inclusion in all coproduction work.
- Funders should evaluate their coproduction programs and activities.
- Funders should contribute to the literature on coproduction.

INTRODUCTION

There is increasing evidence to suggest that research coproduction, a collaborative approach that enables a closer working relationship between researchers and those who will use the evidence produced (knowledge users), can enable

Research Coproduction in Healthcare, First Edition. Edited by
Ian D. Graham, Jo Rycroft-Malone, Anita Kothari, and Chris McCutcheon.
© 2022 John Wiley & Sons Ltd. Published 2022 by John Wiley & Sons Ltd.

more innovative and relevant science, improve research quality, and result in better impact (Campbell and Vanderhoven 2016; Moser 2016; Pain et al. 2015).

With this recognition, interest in research coproduction is high. Many will argue, and rightly so, that there is nothing new in the fundamental premise of partnership in research: it has existed for decades in such traditions as participatory action research (Holmes et al. 2018). What does seem new is the attention of the broader scientific community, which increasingly sees the potential of coproduction to solve complex societal problems in an era of constrained budgets and increased calls for accountability and impact (Arnott et al. 2020a; Durose et al. 2012).

Despite this increased interest, the global scientific ecosystem largely continues to separate science from society (Arnott et al. 2020b). If coproduction is to achieve its potential, institutional changes are needed to reflect the embeddedness of science within – not apart from – society. Among these institutions are research funders, which can play a much stronger role in linking research to action (Cooper et al. 2017; Cordero et al. 2008; Holmes et al. 2012; Matso and Becker 2014; Riley et al. 2011; Smits and Denis 2014; Tetroe et al. 2008).

This topic – how funders can embrace and support coproduction – is the focus of this chapter. We write from the perspective of a government-funded health research agency in British Columbia, Canada that is committed to knowledge translation, which is broadly defined as activities that increase the use of evidence in policy and practice (Holmes et al. 2012, 2014). Funders can play an important role in knowledge translation not only through the programs they offer, but through active influence on the systems in which they operate (Holmes et al. 2012; Smits and Denis 2014). Coproduction is one knowledge translation activity that holds great promise for what Arnott et al call actionable science (Arnott et al. 2020b).

We discuss funders and their role in evidence use generally, before reviewing some of the literature on funders and coproduction specifically. Examples of how five funders are supporting coproduction come next, followed by a discussion on where we see opportunities for funders to enhance their work in this area.

SETTING THE SCENE: FUNDERS AND THEIR ROLE IN THE USE OF EVIDENCE

In writing about funders – in this case health research funders – we acknowledge their great diversity. They include government and other publicly funded agencies; donor-supported hospital foundations; private foundations with endowments; community-based philanthropic organizations; and charities focused on specific health conditions. Funding programs include researcher salary support, fellowships, and operating grants for a spectrum of research traditions and methodologies, from basic or laboratory-based, to clinical trials, to population and public health studies, to research about health services and systems. Finally, funders' work varies in its focus – the topics or areas they support, as well as the wide range of stakeholders they serve, including researchers, patients and the public, communities, healthcare providers and policymakers (Cordero et al. 2008).

Given the variety among funders, their roles in evidence use will also vary. Some have an explicit mandate to connect evidence and action; for example, funders of community-based research. Others – for example, large publicly funded organizations that support basic or discovery research, based on formal peer review of scientific excellence – largely consider knowledge dissemination and utilization separate from scientific pursuits (Riley et al. 2011) and leave knowledge translation activities to the researchers. It has been noted that basic or early translational applied research is particularly challenging for coproduction (Tembo et al. 2019).

Regardless of the type of funder, it is acknowledged that not enough science links to decisions, and it is increasingly argued that funders can and should play a more active role to see that knowledge produced from research is actually used (Cooper et al. 2017; Holmes et al. 2012, 2014; Matso and Becker 2014). Indeed, interest is growing for funders around the world (Arnott et al. 2020b; Cordero et al. 2008; McLean et al. 2018; Sibbald et al. 2014): they are becoming more active in the space between knowledge produced from research and impact (Cooper et al. 2017; Holmes et al. 2012; Smits and Denis 2014).

Funders' actions in knowledge translation vary – from encouraging, requiring or supporting funded researchers to develop and implement knowledge translation plans, to offering knowledge translation-specific grants, to forming coalitions to study and improve their own participation in knowledge translation (see, for example, the Research on Research Institute (2021) and Transforming Evidence for Policy and Practice (2021)). The literature on funders and knowledge translation, however, is sparse. There are some studies on how funders can enhance knowledge translation through different approaches to funding calls and application review (Arnott et al. 2020b; Cooper et al. 2017; Scarrow et al. 2017; Smits and Denis 2014). A few funders are publishing on their own knowledge translation work (e.g., McLean et al. (2012)), including our own funding agency, which developed a model to guide funders' knowledge translation work (Holmes et al. 2012) in five areas: advancing knowledge translation science; building knowledge translation capacity; managing knowledge translation projects; funding knowledge translation activities; and advocating knowledge translation. Finally, despite what seems to be increased interest and activity among funders, studies by Tetroe et al. (2008) and McLean et al. (2018) suggest that their knowledge translation activities are not often evaluated, and do not appear to be evidence-based.

FUNDERS AND COPRODUCTION IN THE LITERATURE

As noted, coproduction is one approach in the spectrum of knowledge translation activities to increase the use of evidence in practice in various types of
research. Although different terms for coproduction are used (Arnott et al.
2020a; Sibbald et al. 2014), each refers to a model of collaboration that explicitly
responds to the needs of knowledge users in order to produce findings that are
useful, useable and used (Graham et al. 2019). This definition differentiates
coproduction from "partnership," whose definition is broad and does not necessarily involve, as coproduction models do, shared power and decision-making
between knowledge users and researchers.

Though the literature on coproduction as a research approach is rich – if
diverse, given the varied terminology used – as with knowledge translation generally, there is little focused on funders and coproduction. What exists, however,
is promising, including several large-scale studies on funders of environmental research.

Riley et al. (2011), in a case study of 130 projects funded by the US Cooperative
Institute for Coastal and Estuarine Environmental Technology between 1997 and
2006, explored what factors increased the likelihood of the application of produced
evidence. Through an analysis of surveys, interviews with principal investigators
and intended users of the evidence, focus groups and progress reports, the authors
determined that funders can increase the likelihood of application by: being
explicit about definitions of research use, changing resource allocation methods,
ensuring funded science is relevant to users, directly connecting scientists and
decision-makers, and considering a longer duration of funding for projects to
allow for both meaningful user involvement and demonstration of results. Arnott
et al. (2020a) reviewed 180 research projects funded by the US National Estuarine
Research Reserve System from 1998 to 2014, over which time the program
increased requirements for collaboration between researchers and knowledge
users. Their analysis included interviews and documents, such as requests for proposals and reports; they found that funding program design led to significant
changes in research practice, and that more intensive interaction between
researchers and knowledge users significantly increased the likelihood of use.

Also in the environmental research field, Matso and Becker (2014) investigated the short-term impacts of a funding process with a focus on societal outcomes, as opposed to only evidence generation. Their qualitative cross-case
analysis, including interviews and observations, focused on three projects funded
by the US Cooperative Institute for Coastal and Estuarine Environmental Technology. Resulting recommendations were that funders should: ensure that problems are robustly defined with potential knowledge users; allocate more resources
and attention to communicating effectively with knowledge users throughout projects; and, demand more engagement of knowledge users during projects.

Moving to health research, Campbell and Vanderhoven (2016) presented
findings from a program funded by the UK Economic and Social Research

Council on benefits and challenges associated with generating knowledge coproductively. A main finding from the program, which included five coproduction pilot projects, was that coproduction poses challenges for existing research practices: it requires flexibility, a non-linear research process, the blurring of boundaries, specific leadership capabilities, and a new understanding of research itself. Among the authors' recommendations for funders were to: examine research impact, support the development of capacity and training, consider the merits of more hands-on approaches, review ethical and financial procedures and rules in relation to coproduced research, and build a network of research funders to support learning. Sibbald et al. (2014), using the term "research-funder-required-research-partnerships," investigated the experiences, perceived barriers, successes, and opinions of researchers and knowledge users funded by the Canadian Institutes of Health Research. They concluded that funders could play a bigger role in helping facilitate the partnerships to which they award grants. Specific recommendations included considering coproduction in grant adjudications, providing support for partnerships (for example, matching researchers and users) and considering planning grants and term of awards.

The related literature on funders of global health research uses the term "partnership," but does reflect the tenets of coproduction as defined in this book. One such study (Fransman et al. 2018), conducted on behalf of UK Research and Innovation, aimed to improve research collaboration through learning exchanges and resources for research collaboration by academics and practitioners based in the global South and UK based international brokers. Recommendations for funders were to: ensure global representation of partners in research agenda-setting and governance, incentivize equitable partnerships, monitor partnerships and provide support when things go wrong, invest in partnership, and promote a learning culture by encouraging researchers to reflect on failure. Another article by Dodson (2017) summarized 11 models of North–South research programs based on interviews with funders and a survey of Global South science funders and ministries about their perspectives on these programs. The authors' recommendations for funders included supporting inclusive agenda-setting, funding new research questions and valuing complementary skills and knowledge, setting equitable budgets, widening participation, investing for the long-term, and working closely with other funders and agencies to streamline processes and reduce duplication.

COPRODUCTION IN ACTION – EXAMPLES OF FUNDERS' ACTIVITIES

To complement the literature on funders' roles in coproduction, we consulted five funders of healthcare research to uncover more examples. We selected these organizations to illustrate the range of coproduction activities supported by funders of health research; they vary depending on their mandate and global, national, or regional context. The examples from these funders, which are presented below from the global to regional level, also illustrate the range of knowledge users involved in the coproduction of research, including policymakers, communities, health practitioners, patients and the public. Common observations were: the integration of coproduction into funding streams on the premise that coproduction would benefit the research; the critical role that funders play in relationship-building between researchers and knowledge users; and, shared interest by funders for the need for more empirical evidence on what works in coproduction, as well as the impacts.

Research in Action | Stakeholder Engagement

International Development Research Centre, Canada

As part of Canada's international assistance efforts, the International Development Research Centre (IDRC) invests in knowledge and innovation, and mobilizes alliances to respond to challenges in five areas: global health, climate-resilient food systems, education and science, democratic and inclusive governance, and sustainable inclusive economies (International Development Research Centre 2021b).

Coproduction is supported by IDRC in different ways, depending on factors such as scientific discipline, research objectives, and the region of the world. As one example, the Innovating for Maternal and Child Health in Africa (IMCHA) initiative – jointly funded by IDRC, the Canadian Institutes of Health Research, and Global Affairs Canada – put coproduction into action to improve maternal, newborn, and child health outcomes (International Development Research Centre 2021a). IMCHA funded research teams, led by an African researcher principal investigator (PI) working in collaboration with a Canadian researcher co-PI and an African co-PI decision-maker (knowledge user). IMCHA required the engagement of a decision-maker as co-PI, from the design stage and through the project, to emphasize the importance of the translation of evidence into policy and practice. Furthermore, IMCHA supported two regional entities to coproduce with the teams to make research evidence available to high-level decision-makers not usually accessible to researchers. Throughout the research process, teams also engaged key stakeholders (e.g., community members and health service providers). Successful projects designed and implemented solutions that were practical and culturally acceptable to overcome barriers, increase use of services, and improve health outcomes.

Recognizing how easily jeopardized coproduction relationships can become; for example, due to personnel turnover or personality clashes, the funders devoted time and resources to regular group meetings, close project follow-ups, or fostering collaboration between the three core members of each team. IMCHA's final evaluation noted grantees' appreciation for the unique support and technical expertise provided to them by IMCHA staff.

Strong coproduction processes are expected to contribute to ownership, scaling impact and sustainability. This requires ongoing problem-solving, and nurturing of open and frank discussions on the part of all actors, including funders.

Evidence Leaders in Africa | Policymaking

The African Academy of Sciences, Africa

The African Academy of Sciences (AAS) is a non-profit pan-African organization whose vision is to transform lives on the African continent through science (The African Academy of Sciences 2021). The AAS achieves this by: recognizing African excellence through fellowships and awards to African research leaders; providing advice and think tank functions to shape African Science, Technology and Innovation (STI) strategies and policies; and implementing STI programs through a coordinating research platform in partnership with The African Union and Global Partners.

The AAS sees collaboration and relationships as key to enabling coproduction that can inform policymaking. For example, the AAS partnered with the African Institute for Policy Development (AFIDEP) to launch Evidence Leaders in Africa (African Institute for Policy Development (AFIDEP) 2021). The aim of this initiative is to build and sustain relationships between African research leaders and policymakers to enable the use of evidence in policy formulation and implementation by African governments.

Evidence Leaders in Africa empowers AAS scholars to proactively engage policymakers and champion evidence-informed decision-making by governments. Training workshops equip African researchers with the skills and capacity to effectively communicate with audiences particularly in the policymaking space. Fellows benefit from sessions that cover various aspects of research communication and policy-engagement strategies. Workshop discussions present the opportunity for African researchers and policymakers to share their respective perspectives as a foundation for relationship building.

Evidence Leaders in Africa also facilitates regular discussions of evidence on policy issues among African policymakers and AAS researchers. The AAS and AFIDEP convened an Evidence Leaders in Africa Virtual Conference to facilitate sharing of lessons among Africa researchers, policymakers and practitioners in Africa on researchers' roles and experiences in strengthening evidence use in government decision-making. Conference themes included research and knowledge translation, and relationship-building.

Coordinating Center | Research Partnerships

National Health and Medical Research Council, Australia

The National Health and Medical Research Council (NHMRC) is an independent agency within the portfolio of the Australian Government that funds health and medical research for the Australian community (National Health and Medical Research Council (NHMRC) 2021). NHMRC supports the creation of knowledge about the mechanisms underlying health and disease and in the development of better ways to prevent and treat ill health.

The Australian Prevention Partnership Centre was one of three Partnership Centres for Better Health established by the NHMRC in 2013 (The Australian Prevention Partnership Centre 2021). The Prevention Centre is the only one of these centres that continues today. The Prevention Centre is a national collaboration of leading academics, policymakers, practitioners, and research organizations from across Australia working together to build an effective, efficient, and equitable system to prevent lifestyle-related chronic disease.

The Prevention Centre was established to try a new approach to research partnerships that granted the time, resources, and flexibility to ensure a greater impact on policy and practice. Their work goes beyond simply putting academics in touch with policymakers. All funded projects involve research that is coproduced by teams of researchers and policymakers. Priority topics are set by funding partners but the research questions and priorities are co-developed by the academics and policy partners. Partner involvement ranges from defining research questions or priorities, to participating as research investigators involved throughout the course of the research projects.

The Coordinating Centre manages the business of the Prevention Centre, including project oversight, funding and accountability, and delivers a number of strategies to support the research partnerships to increase the uptake of evidence in policy and practice. They find that the most effective way for researchers to learn coproduction is by doing it. The centre facilitates coproduction by providing access to a network of academics and policymakers in the prevention space; through formal processes, such as requiring policy–practice partnerships in research proposals and approvals and requesting regular progress reports; and through governance arrangements that ensure research is guided by partners.

The Coordinating Centre also facilitates introductions between researchers and knowledge users and works with research teams on knowledge mobilization strategies. They support an online research network for early- and mid-career researchers – initially, researchers funded by the centre, but expanded to include other prevention researchers. Online networks have also included policymakers to nurture research partnerships and build capacity. Smaller communities of practice have budded from the network.

Evidence for Action | Evidence of What Works

Robert Wood Johnson Foundation, USA

The Robert Wood Johnson Foundation (RWJF) is a philanthropic organization that works in partnership with researchers, policymakers, and communities through an array of funding programs to build a national initiative in America called a Culture of Health (Robert Wood Johnson Foundation 2021).

Coproduction is not an explicit focus across all areas of RWJF's work. Rather, they call for proposals for specific initiatives where there is a need for on-the-ground community work and fund coproduced research projects where there is a strong community voice in the project. RWJF staff remain engaged with the projects as collaborators and encourage the inclusion of community perspectives while independent third parties manage the coproduction process.

Evidence for Action (E4A) is a signature program of the RWJF that involves investigator-initiated research to assess the impact of programs, policies, and practices on health and well-being, with a particular focus on research that will help advance health equity (Evidence for Action (E4A) 2021). E4A funds and provides technical assistance to researchers and organizations working with communities to develop rigorous evaluations of innovative interventions to identify actionable strategies and priorities.

One call for proposals sought to gather empirical evidence from global initiatives whose approaches have been effective in improving health, or the determinants of health, by improving gender equity, and that have the potential to be adapted and implemented in the US. Applicants were invited from around the world – particularly those who have first-hand knowledge of evidence-based approaches to gender equity in their countries, and who would collaborate with US-based partners to study the adaptation of these approaches to a US setting. Project teams included researchers working alongside policymakers, practitioners, or members of impacted communities, from both the intervention's home country and the US.

INVOLVE | Public and Patient Involvement

National Institute for Health Research, United Kingdom

The National Institute for Health Research (NIHR) works in partnership with the National Health Service, universities, local government, other research funders, patients, and the public to deliver and enable world-class research to improve the health and wealth of the UK and low- and middle-income countries through responsive and commissioned research.

The NIHR has long engaged and involved patients, carers, and the public to improve the reach, quality, and impact of their research. They see a key role for these groups in all processes by which research is identified, prioritized, designed, conducted, evaluated, and disseminated. However, the NIHR sought new ways of evolving and improving patient and public involvement. They saw the application of coproduction in health and social care research as more than simply robust engagement, but rather as a deliberative process that requires public members and practitioners to be involved on an equal footing throughout every stage of the design and delivery of research.

INVOLVE is a national advisory group to support public involvement in the NHS, public health, and social care research (INVOLVE 2021). INVOLVE, in partnership with colleagues from across NIHR and beyond, led the development of five principles for coproducing research that were adopted and embedded across the processes, procedures, and culture of the NIHR and have guided NIHR's approach to coproduction: sharing of power; including all perspectives and skills; respecting and valuing the knowledge of all those working together on the research; reciprocity so everyone benefits; and, building and maintaining relationships.

Coproduction is practiced in different ways across the NIHR. In both research projects or research infrastructure, patients, carers, and the public participate in the application and decision-making process. Not only are proposals reviewed by patients, carers, and public members, these stakeholders also sit on funding panels. The path to impact statements on project applications require the inclusion of public and patients.

One example is a research design service, which provides advice and guidance on research proposals, and has a patient and public involvement team that works coproductively with public members on the team. Public members chair meetings, develop project plans, co-host podcasts, deliver presentations, and lead sessions designed to reflect the extent to which the team is adhering to the coproduction principles.

DISCUSSION

This brief review of the literature, and examples of coproduction by funders around the world, demonstrates the range of opportunities for funders to support coproduction. Most of the work – at least that is publicly visible – seems to focus internally on the programs that funders offer; there is little about externally facing work where funders actively influence the research system in which they operate to enable coproduction. We suggest this is a significant opportunity.

Before funders take on coproduction in earnest, we suggest they consider – conceptually and practically – the commitments they are willing to make, the role they are willing (or are able) to play, and what success will look like. We cover these considerations briefly below before discussing the internally focused program work and externally facing enabling and advocacy role.

Funders in Coproduction: General Considerations

Funders should consider the different ways in which coproduction may change their practice. It is easy to think that coproduction just makes sense, but generating knowledge coproductively can bring unanticipated challenges – ranging from different conceptualizations of what coproduction means in practice, to divergent ideas for realizing goals and evaluating outcomes that emerge through coproduction (Arnott et al. 2020a), to managing the tensions that naturally arise from the differing interests of participants involved in coproduction (Oliver et al. 2019).

The recognition of tensions inherent in coproduction leads to a discussion of power relations (Fransman et al. 2018; Hickey 2018) and issues of equity. Funders can encourage a diversity of knowledge, skills, and perspectives by requiring that knowledge users are involved at every stage in the coproduction of research. Funders must also act to support fair and equitable partnerships by setting expectations through their funding conditions followed by active monitoring, noting the positional authority different stakeholders have in decision-making, and moderating power dynamics to see that all views are invited and valued. This is difficult work, but it is important to be vigilant in monitoring power differentials that show up in coproduction, and redress these to build trust among all of the participants (Hickey 2018).

Another consideration for funders is the extent to which they are willing to get involved in facilitating coproduction. For example, while it may sound beneficial for a funder to broker partnerships, there is a risk of too much intervention (Arnott et al. 2020a; Cordero et al. 2008) that could introduce unintended outcomes. Moreover, enhanced program and relationship management capability will be needed, not only for administering coproduction grants but to facilitate coproduction throughout the project.

Conceptualizing coproduction also means re-thinking what success looks like. It may require redefining impact and how it is measured (Campbell and Vanderhoven 2016). By its nature, coproduction is a non-linear, fluid research process that evolves through interactions between researchers and knowledge users. It requires flexibility, allowing the research to evolve to increase the utility of the knowledge that is produced. It should be no surprise that coproduction will be different in each research project. As such, the solutions or outcomes may be unexpected. There is a range of writing specifically on coproduction and impact, not all of it about funders specifically but nevertheless useful (e.g., Pain et al. (2015)).

Internally Focused Funder Processes to Support Coproduction

A number of insights for funders that want to support or participate in coproduction emerged from the literature review and conversations with funders, which we briefly summarize here – from program design and the review processes, to training and capacity building, to implementation and monitoring and reporting.

Among the elements funders should consider in the design of grants that incorporate coproduction is the support of relationship-building, even to the extent of matching researchers and knowledge users. Important is clarifying expectations about what coproduction entails, and incentivizing true and equitable partnerships. Funders should dedicate resources to support the partnerships, allow adequate time and resourcing for partnership building, and consider funding an inception phase where researchers and knowledge users may be coming together for the first time to plan and develop research proposals.

It will take much more time to coproduce research, especially if it involves multiple stakeholders. Funders should build extra time in their timelines and consider lengthening the duration of grants to allow sufficient time for coproduction. Additional time and resources will also be needed to maintain effective engagement between the researchers and knowledge users throughout the duration of the projects.

There are also important considerations at the application stage (Matso and Becker 2014), where in traditional research the precise specification of research questions and the methods necessary to produce the required evidence are important (Campbell and Vanderhoven 2016). Traditional grant opportunities advantage researchers that have already defined a problem (Matso and Becker 2014). By contrast, coproduction necessitates engagement of knowledge users at the start of projects to define the problem and shape the research questions. As noted above, this could be achieved by awarding a separate planning grant, or staging the research coproduction process to include problem framing (Fransman et al. 2018). In regular grants – as opposed to planning phase grants – program managers should require documentation from applicants that shows problems have been robustly defined with knowledge users (Matso and Becker 2014).

Assessment of coproduction proposals is another important area of consideration for funders (Matso and Becker 2014). Coproduction represents a qualitatively different form of research, and therefore the frameworks and criteria required to assess effectively the merits of such proposals need to be qualitatively different too (Campbell and Vanderhoven 2016). Assessments should include ethical considerations and the nature and strength of the partnership (Fransman et al. 2018). In addition, leads of review processes should be carefully chosen and supported, and membership of review panels need to be thought through. Panels should include experts in participatory processes (Matso and Becker 2014), and all should be trained in knowledge translation approaches such as coproduction (Fransman et al. 2018; Holmes et al. 2012). There is also good reason to include potential knowledge users in the adjudication process (Arnott et al. 2020a; Frank et al. 2014; McLean and Tucker 2013; Scarrow et al. 2017).

We noted little in the literature about training in coproduction, and there are few resources for researchers to learn about knowledge translation generally (Cooper et al. 2017). It is worth considering investing resources to train both researchers and knowledge users in coproduction. Coproduction requires researchers to demonstrate reflective learning and to use skills such as facilitation and participatory engagement (Campbell and Vanderhoven 2016); knowledge users could make use of these skills as well. An opportunity for capacity building is the development of coproduction capabilities amongst established researchers, PhD supervisors and early career researchers (Campbell and Vanderhoven 2016). Funders who offer fellowship awards could provide such training; there is also an advocacy or influence role for funders with universities in this regard, which we discuss below. Beyond formal training, capacity building through sessions on partnership principles, and organizing mutual learning events with knowledge users on partnerships could be helpful (Fransman et al. 2018).

Funders should also consider implementation support (Arnott et al. 2020b). Implementation specialists and skilled project managers will be critically important in managing the coproduction process. Funders are also encouraged to become directly involved where appropriate to their mandate, e.g., proactively supporting quality interactions between researchers and knowledge users (Matso and Becker 2014), as well as fostering the development of new partnerships and acting as a broker within and across projects (Sibbald et al. 2014).

Lastly, processes for monitoring and evaluating progress on coproduction projects deserve a rethink. Funders could promote learning by encouraging research teams to reflect on lessons and failures in the narrative section in progress reports (Fransman et al. 2018), including adjustments to the research project made in partnership with knowledge users to increase the chances of a successful outcome. Equally important, funders should invite independent evaluation of their own research coproduction activities, including funding and capacity-building programs.

The above potential actions for funders could be significant in terms of benefit, but also in terms of changes to organizational strategy and funding practice. As noted, clarity is required in the conceptualization of coproduction and what it means for a funder, including its role in research, and the commitments it is prepared to make to ensure coproduction of research is successful.

Externally Facing Systems-Level Activities to Enable Coproduction

Our review of the literature and funder examples focused primarily on what research funders can do: in other words, what they have direct control over; for example, the creation of coproduction funding opportunities. But we suggest there is also a role for funders in areas they cannot necessarily control but that they can influence, in this case to catalyze the conditions for successful coproduction.

Research ecosystems are complex and funders are one among many players (Arnott et al. 2020b; Holmes et al. 2017). If coproduction is not embraced in the larger research system, funders' efforts in coproduction will not reach their potential, nor achieve maximum benefits. For example, researchers are not rewarded or promoted for spending time developing relationships, and universities do not necessarily train researchers in coproduction: funders could advocate here. All of the program work discussed above could be complemented by externally facing engagement by funders, including sparking debates on different ideas of impact or advocating on issues of equity and ethics in coproduction (Arnott et al. 2020a).

Research funders could also influence the system by studying their own practice and publishing: there are few, if any, examples of funders publishing detailed empirical evaluations of their attempts to link research to decisions (Matso and Becker 2014; McLean and Tucker 2013). Another important area for funders is advancing the scholarship of coproduction; they can do this through funding programs, but we suggest there is an important advocacy role here.

Finally, funders could have a great deal of influence by joining forces to collaborate and learn from each other (Campbell and Vanderhoven 2016) and from related work (e.g., examples of initiatives relating to patient engagement but not specially termed coproduction include Strategy for Patient Oriented Research (SPOR) SUPPORT Units (Canadian Institutes of Health Research 2021), a national initiative led by the Canadian Institutes of Health Research, and the US-based Patient-Centered Outcomes Research Institute (PCORI) (Patient-Centred Outcomes Research Institute (PCORI) 2021)). Funders could also learn from very relevant but largely separate well-established literature – including community-based research, patient engagement in healthcare, and action research – and act on what they learn to bring about much-needed change to traditional research systems.

FUTURE RESEARCH

There are a number of questions to be answered related to research coproduction (Arnott et al. 2020b):

- To what extent do different modes or intensities of coproduction yield different results?
- To what extent and how does coproduction improve decision quality and outcomes?

- How can research–practice partnerships, at different scales, link together to advance actionable knowledge?
- To what extent are funder programs effective for promoting research coproduction and how can they be improved?

The study of partnership formulation is another opportunity (Sibbald et al. 2014), as are further exploration of the assumption that closer interaction between research and practice is necessarily better, and how the outcomes of coproduction can be achieved at scale when it so reliant upon repeated in-person interaction and trusted relationships (Arnott et al. 2020a).

CONCLUSION

The involvement of knowledge users in science is important, but it is complex (Matso and Becker 2014). Funders are ideally placed to both understand the complexity, and develop the necessary expertise to facilitate successful coproduction.

Despite this ideal positioning, there is little in the literature about funders' approaches to, and experiences of, coproduction. Perhaps this is not surprising, given the few case studies available on how funders are implementing and evaluating strategies to increase the use of knowledge more generally (McLean et al. 2018; Riley et al. 2011).

However, the recent literature reviewed for this chapter, the five examples of funders' activities, and the developing funder coalitions referred to above indicate a growing interest and an increasing sense of the action by funders, individually and collectively, to support research that benefits citizens and society. We suggest that coproduction specifically offers an opportunity for funders to make bold changes to research funding and research practice – and the broader research system – to realize this benefit.

REFERENCES

1. African Institute for Policy Development (AFIDEP). (2021). *The Evidence Leaders in Africa*. [Online]. https://www.afidep.org/programme/evidence-leaders-in-africa-ela (accessed 31 August 2021).
2. Arnott, J., Kirchhoff, C., Meyer, R., Meadow, A., and Bednarek, A. (2020a). Sponsoring actionable science: what public science funders can do to advance sustainability and the social contract for science. *Current Opinion in Environmental Sustainability* 42: 38–44. doi: 10.1016/j.cosust.2020.01.006.
3. Arnott, J.C., Neuenfeldt, R.J., and Lemos, M.C. (2020b). Co-producing science for sustainability: Can funding change knowledge use? *Global Environmental Change* 60: 101979. doi: 10.1016/j.gloenvcha.2019.101979.

4. Campbell, H.J. and Vanderhoven, D. (2016). *Knowledge that Matters: Realising the Potential of Co-Production*. Manchester:N8 Research Partnership. https://eprints.whiterose.ac.uk/99657/1/FinalReport-Co-Production-2016-01-20.pdf.

5. Canadian Institutes of Health Research. (2021). *SPOR SUPPORT Units*. [Online]. https://cihr-irsc.gc.ca/e/45859.html (accessed 31 August 2021).

6. Cooper, A., Shewchuck, S., and MacGregor, S. (2017). *Social Science Funding Agencies' Promotion and Support of Knowledge Mobilization and Research Impact: An International Study. RIPPLE Research Report*. Kingston. http://www.ripplenetwork.ca/wp-content/uploads/2019/03/Projects/1_FA_Project/AERAPaperCooperetalFundingAgencies2017.pdf.

7. Cordero, C., Delino, R., Jeyaseelan, L., Lansang, M.A., Lozano, J.M., Kumar, S., Moreno, S., Pietersen, M., Quirino, J., Thamlikitkul, V., Welch, V.A., Tetroe, J., Ter Kuile, A., Graham, I.D., Grimshaw, J., Neufeld, V., Wells, G., and Tugwell, P. (2008). Funding agencies in low- and middle-income countries: support for knowledge translation. *Bulletin of the World Health Organization* 86: 524–534. doi: 10.2471/blt.07.040386.

8. Dodson, J. (2017). *Building Partnerships of Equals: The Role of Funders in Equitable and Effective International Development Collaborations*. London:UK Collaborative on Development Science. https://www.ukcdr.org.uk/wp-content/uploads/2017/11/Building-Partnerships-of-Equals_-REPORT-2.pdf.

9. Durose, C., Beebeejaun, Y., Rees, J., Richardson, J., and Richardson, L. (2012). *Towards Coproduction in Research with Communities. (Connected Communities)*. Arts and Humanities Research Council. https://www.research.manchester.ac.uk/portal/files/33424282/FULL_TEXT.PDF.

10. Evidence for Action (E4A). (2021). E4A website. [Online]. https://www.evidenceforaction.org.

11. Frank, L., Basch, E., Selby, J.V., and Patient-Centered Outcomes Research Institute. (2014). The PCORI perspective on patient-centered outcomes research. *JAMA* 312: 1513–1514. doi: 10.1001/jama.2014.11100. (accessed 11 January 2022).

12. Fransman, J., Hall, B., Hayman, R., Narayanan, P., Newman, K., and Tandon, R. (2018). *Promoting fair and equitable research partnerships to respond to global challenges*. Rethinking Research Collaborative. https://rethinkingresearch-partnerships.files.wordpress.com/2018/10/fair-and-equitable-partnerships_research-report-public.pdf.

13. Graham, I.D., McCutcheon, C., and Kothari, A. (2019). Exploring the frontiers of research co-production: the Integrated Knowledge Translation Research Network concept papers. *Health Research Policy and Systems / BioMed Central* 17: 88. doi: 10.1186/s12961-019-0501-7.

14. Hickey, D.G. (2018). The potential for coproduction to add value to research. *Health Expectations* 21: 693–694. doi: 10.1111/hex.12821.

15. Holmes, B., Scarrow, G., and Schellenberg, M. (2012). Translating evidence into practice: the role of health research funders. *Implementation Science: IS* 7: 39. doi: 10.1186/1748-5908-7-39.

16. Holmes, B.J., Best, A., Davies, H., Hunter, D., Kelly, M.P., Marshall, M., and Rycroft-Malone, J. (2017). Mobilising knowledge in complex health systems: a call to action. *Evidence & Policy: A Journal of Research, Debate and Practice* 13: 539–560. doi: 10.1332/174426416X14712553750311.

17. Holmes, B.J., Bryan, S., Ho, K., and McGavin, C. (2018). Engaging patients as partners in health research: lessons from BC, Canada. *Healthcare Management forum/ Canadian College of Health Service Executives = Forum gestion des soins de santé / Collège canadien des directeurs de services de santé* 31: 41–44. doi: 10.1177/0840470417741712.

18. Holmes, B.J., Schellenberg, M., Schell, K., and Scarrow, G. (2014). How funding agencies can support research use in healthcare: an online province-wide survey to determine knowledge translation training needs. *Implementation Science: IS* 9: 71. doi: 10.1186/1748-5908-9-71.

19. International Development Research Centre. (2021a). *Innovating for maternal and child health in Africa*. [Online]. https://www.idrc.ca/en/initiative/innovating-maternal-and-child-health-africa (accessed 31 August 2021).

20. International Development Research Centre. (2021b). International Development Research Centre website. [Online]. https://www.idrc.ca/en (accessed 31 August 2021).

21. INVOLVE. (2021). *Guidance on co-producing a research project.* [Online]. https://www.invo.org.uk/posttypepublication/guidance-on-co-producing-a-research-project (accessed 31 August 2021).

22. Matso, K.E. and Becker, M.L. (2014). What can funders do to better link science with decisions? Case studies of coastal communities and climate change. *Environmental Management* 54: 1356–1371. doi: 10.1007/s00267-014-0347-2.

23. McLean, R.K., Graham, I.D., Bosompra, K., Choudhry, Y., Coen, S.E., Macleod, M., Manuel, C., McCarthy, R., Mota, A., Peckham, D., Tetroe, J.M., and Tucker, J. (2012). Understanding the performance and impact of public knowledge translation funding interventions: protocol for an evaluation of Canadian Institutes of Health Research knowledge translation funding programs. *Implementation Science: IS* 7: 57. doi: 10.1186/1748-5908-7-57.

24. McLean, R.K.D., Graham, I.D., Tetroe, J.M., and Volmink, J.A. (2018). Translating research into action: an international study of the role of research funders. *Health Research Policy and Systems / BioMed Central* 16: 44. doi: 10.1186/s12961-018-0316-y.

25. McLean, R.K.D. and Tucker, J. (2013). *Evaluation of CIHR's Knowledge Translation Funding Program*. Canadian Institutes of Health Research. https://cihr-irsc.gc.ca/e/documents/kt_evaluation_report-en.pdf.

26. Moser, S.C. (2016). Can science on transformation transform science? lessons from co-design. *Current Opinion in Environmental Sustainability* 20: 106–115. doi: 10.1016/j.cosust.2016.10.007.

27. National Health and Medical Research Council (NHMRC). (2021). NHMRC website. [Online]. https://www.nhmrc.gov.au (accessed 31 August 2021).

28. Oliver, K., Kothari, A., and Mays, N. (2019). The dark side of coproduction: Do the costs outweigh the benefits for health research? *Health Research Policy and Systems / BioMed Central* 17: 33. doi: 10.1186/s12961-019-0432-3.

29. Pain, R., Askins, K., Banks, S., Cook, T., Crawford, G., Crookes, L., Darby, S., Heslop, J., Holden, A., Houston, M., Jeffes, J., Lambert, Z., McGlen, L., McGlynn, C., Ozga, J., Raynor, R., Robinson, Y., Shaw, S., Stewart, C., and Vanderhoven, D. (2015). *Mapping Alternative Impact: Alternative Approaches to Impact from Co-produced Research.* Durham University: Centre for Social Justice and Community Action. https://www.durham.ac.uk/media/durham-university/research-/research-centres/social-justice-amp-community-action-centre-for/documents/Mapping-Alternative-Impact-Summary-Report.pdf.

30. Patient-Centred Outcomes Research Institute (PCORI). (2021). *PCORI website.* [Online]. https://www.pcori.org (accessed 31 August 2021).

31. Research on Research Institute. (2021). *Research on Research Institute website.* [Online]. https://researchonresearch.org (accessed 31 August 2021).

32. Riley, C., Matso, K., Leonard, D., Stadler, K., Trueblood, D., and Langan, R. (2011). How research funding organizations can increase application of science to decision-making. *Coastal Management* 39: 336–350. doi: 10.1080/08920753.2011.566117.

33. Robert Wood Johnson Foundation. (2021). *Robert Wood Johnson Foundation USA website.* [Online]. https://www.rwjf.org (accessed 31 August 2021).

34. Scarrow, G., Angus, D., and Holmes, B.J. (2017). Reviewer training to assess knowledge translation in funding applications is long overdue. *Research Integrity and Peer Review* 2: 13. doi: 10.1186/s41073-017-0037-8.

35. Sibbald, S.L., Tetroe, J., and Graham, I.D. (2014). Research funder required research partnerships: a qualitative inquiry. *Implementation Science: IS* 9: 176. doi: 10.1186/s13012-014-0176-y.

36. Smits, P.A. and Denis, J.L. (2014). How research funding agencies support science integration into policy and practice: an international overview. *Implementation Science: IS* 9: 28. doi: 10.1186/1748-5908-9-28.

37. Tembo, D., Morrow, E., Worswick, L., and Lennard, D. (2019). Is co-production just a pipe dream for applied health research commissioning? An exploratory literature review. *Frontiers in Sociology* 4: 50. doi: 10.3389/fsoc.2019.00050.

38. Tetroe, J.M., Graham, I.D., Foy, R., Robinson, N., Eccles, M.P., Wensing, M., Durieux, P., Legare, F., Nielson, C.P., Adily, A., Ward, J.E., Porter, C., Shea, B., and Grimshaw, J.M. (2008). Health research funding agencies' support

and promotion of knowledge translation: an international study. *The Milbank Quarterly* 86: 125–155. doi: 10.1111/j.1468-0009.2007.00515.x.

39. The African Academy of Sciences. (2021). *The African Academy of Sciences website*. [Online]. http://www.aasciences.africa (accessed 31 August 2021).

40. The Australian Prevention Partnership Centre. (2021). *The Australian Prevention Partnership Centre website*. [Online]. https://preventioncentre.org.au (accessed 31 August 2021).

41. Transforming Evidence for Policy and Practice. (2021). *Transforming Evidence for Policy and Practice website*. [Online]. http://transforming-evidence.org (accessed 31 August 2021).

CHAPTER 6

Building Blocks for Research Coproduction

Reflections and Implications

Jo Rycroft-Malone, Ian D. Graham, Anita Kothari, and Chris McCutcheon

INTRODUCTION

Our starting point in the creation of this book was to provide a roadmap, evidence, and some practical advice about conducting research that explicitly responds to knowledge user needs in order to produce research findings that are useful, useable, and used. The long history and continued challenge of research not making a timely difference to practice, service delivery, or policy provides the motivation to think and act differently in the research endeavor. In conceptualizing practice and knowledge production as synergistic and inextricably linked, our proposition is that we have a greater chance of creating evidence-informed solutions to real world problems that will be implemented.

The turn to research coproduction is becoming increasingly popular, at least in name, if not always in deed. As the contents of this book demonstrate, taking an authentic research coproduction approach requires a particular mindset,

Research Coproduction in Healthcare, First Edition. Edited by
Ian D. Graham, Jo Rycroft-Malone, Anita Kothari, and Chris McCutcheon.
© 2022 John Wiley & Sons Ltd. Published 2022 by John Wiley & Sons Ltd.

significant consideration to, and enactment, of a collaborative research lifecycle, and sustained investment in building and maintaining meaningful relationships. In this final chapter, we reflect on some of the themes that thread throughout this book, including the building blocks and conditions necessary for research coproduction. In doing so we also highlight both the challenges and opportunities that research coproduction offers, including issues requiring further refinement and development.

RESEARCH COPRODUCTION: A PRINCIPLES-BASED APPROACH

Research coproduction is not a research method. As a number of authors have demonstrated (Langley et al. Chapter 3.3, Cooke et al. Chapter 3.1, Graham et al. Chapter 4.1) research coproduction is a framing – an approach to the research lifecycle that focusses as much on processes as outcomes. Langley et al. (Chapter 3.3) extend this idea further to suggest that research coproduction is "a way of being not a way of doing." As such, research coproduction can draw on multiple methods from different paradigms but these need to be framed around a flexible set of agreed principles. Some examples of these principles have been shared by authors drawing on their own and other's work (e.g., Hickey et al. (2021), Plamondon et al. Chapter 2.2, Sibley et al. Chapter 2.3, Cooke et al. Chapter 3.1, Langley et al. Chapter 3.3, Hutchinson et al. Chapter 3.5,) and include sharing power, valuing different sources of knowledge and viewpoints equally, reciprocity and mutuality, and inclusivity. It is these principles that establish a foundation. Therefore, the starting point for any research coproduction journey is an active dialogue amongst partners about vision, motivations, demands, priorities, and expectations. Reaching an agreement about a set of principles establishes a way of working that will provide the touchstones for the partnership and projects.

It is this principles-based approach that extends the concept of user engagement in research to one of research coproduction. As a values-driven approach to knowledge generation it is about *working with* rather than simply *engaging in*. This level of partnership extends throughout the whole research lifecycle rather than engagement in specific aspects of it (Hoekstra et al. 2020). Research coproduction reflects the shift away from a two-communities framing of knowledge production (Kothari et al. Chapter 1), to broader societal changes, including the democratization of science where citizens drive the agenda and knowledge users and researchers are equal partners. Greater user engagement and leadership in research also aligns with an increasing emphasis across research systems to reduce waste, as Chalmers and Glasziou (2009, p. 86) point out *"An efficient system of research should address health problems of importance to populations and the interventions and outcomes considered important by patients and clinicians."* As such, the arguments for partnering with knowledge users in the research process are practical and moral.

As the evidence for principles-based coproduction research grows and develops, so too will learning and practical wisdom about what a set of core principles might include and how best to operationalize those principles – in particular, how they work at different levels of a research coproduction partnership and how to evaluate the faithfulness to those principles throughout the research process.

STAKEHOLDERS: AN INCLUSIVE AND FLEXIBLE APPROACH

We advocate an inclusive view of who the stakeholders might be that become partners in research coproduction. Critically, stakeholders can be anyone who might use research findings to influence decisions (knowledge users), be impacted by the use of the findings, or simply be interested in the research process and/or its findings (see Kothari et al. Chapter 1). For example, through an inclusive lens, health system decision-makers are one type of stakeholder (Cooke et al. Chapter 3.1, Bowen et al. Chapter 3.4, Hutchinson et al. Chapter 3.5), whilst patients and the public (Ludwig and Banner Chapter 3.2) are another; but, within these broad categories there will be different perspectives and interests. Stakeholders may be individuals, teams, organizations, or communities. Additionally, stakeholders will be more or less obvious, visible or heard. As such, work is required to reach out to work with diverse stakeholders, and ensure clarity about role and contribution depending on the nature of the partnership and project. As Plamondon et al. (Chapter 2.2) point out, people, groups, and communities occupy complex social locations (positionality) which influence and shape what they bring to the research coproduction process. Therefore, who is involved and how they partner requires careful navigation as partnerships are being established, throughout the research lifecycle and, potentially, an enduring relationship.

Given the ebb and flow of the research process, the role and contribution of different partners will likely be dynamic and change through different phases based on interests and expertise. However, the literature treats knowledge users as a homogenous group. We are reminded by Bowen et al. (Chapter 3.4) that "one size will not fit all." Not only is it important to understand up front how different partners wish to provide input, it is also critical that flexibility is built into the research design, the allocation of resources, and the project management approach (Graham et al. Chapter 4.1) so that differing types of input, at different stages, can be accommodated (McCutcheon et al. Chapter 4.2). Future studies could examine the best type of engagement for different types of project.

Additionally, further investigations might dive deeper to uncover differences among, say, policymakers, practitioners, or patients, and what this might mean for expertise and shared decision-making throughout the research lifecycle.

MEANINGFUL PARTNERSHIP: ESSENTIAL INGREDIENTS

The golden thread throughout this book has been how research coproduction is dependent on, and a function of, developing, nurturing, and sustaining meaningful partnerships. Whilst partnerships are not new given the long tradition of participatory research, partnership working framed around a set of agreed principles is one of research coproduction's essential ingredients – it is intentionally and deliberately egalitarian. As Sibley et al's review (Chapter 2.3) showed, most facilitators and barriers to research coproduction were related to processes associated with managing research partnerships. As such, partnership is the context in which the research coproduction endeavor has the potential to flourish, or not.

As a values-driven approach for engaging in the research cycle, the quality of the partnership is critical. Several authors have pointed to the factors that influence both the establishment and maintenance of partnerships (e.g., Plamondon et al. Chapter 2.2, Sibley et al. Chapter 2.3, Cooke et al. Chapter 3.1, Ludwig and Banner Chapter 3.2, Hutchinson et al. Chapter 3.5). Given there are reactive and proactive routes into the research process, including being initiated by researchers, through a researcher and knowledge user collective, and/or via knowledge users, the conditions for start-up are variously established and will likely influence the research trajectory (Hutchinson et al. Chapter 3.5). As Plamondon et al. (Chapter 2.2) argue, early attention needs to be directed towards cultivating an understanding of the position and motivation of stakeholders. Fundamentally, this requires the exploration and sharing of power in philosophy and action; and ideally a shift towards equity. Traditionally (and typically), power has resided in researchers and funders, rather than with knowledge users. As such, within the context of research coproduction there is still much to learn about the practical strategies that should be adopted to stop replicating colonial ways of doing research. In this book authors provide some helpful ideas. For example, Langley et al. (Chapter 3.3) provide examples of tools, practical strategies, and approaches that include creative ways of facilitating more equitable engagement in the research process. Additionally, Cooke et al. (Chapter 3.1) and Graham et al. (Chapter 4.1) remind us to build in the practical features of project management to enable power-sharing, such as being attentive to investigator status, establishing a democratic governance framework, and building flexibility into timelines. Importantly, deliberate reflection on issues of power and balance are required throughout the research lifecycle.

A deliberative process, in which people come together to gain greater under-standing of each other, provides the platform upon which decisions about the mechanics of the research process, such as design and approach, can be negoti-ated. If a shared understanding is not reached early on, it is likely to lead to ten-sions throughout the research journey. Critically, relationship-building takes work and has to be the focus of significant effort and time, which can result in tension and possible trade-offs between productivity and inclusion (Boaz et al. 2018). Unfortunately, this critical platform-building work is not an activity that typically attracts funding, unless it is part of an existing infrastructure or part-nership arrangement (Bowen et al. Chapter 3.4, Hutchinson et al. Chapter 3.5, Holmes and Jones Chapter 5.3), which risks compromising the attention and time that is put into the foundations of meaningful research coproduction.

Maintaining meaningful partnerships will be a function of the early estab-lishment work, in which clarity and agreement has been reached about the goals, approach, and respective roles of each partner in the research process. Additionally, appropriate structures and processes are needed to sustain produc-tive research coproduction partnerships. Authors have highlighted a number of conditions that contribute to this, which include: ensuring partners have access to appropriate resources and have the capacity to partner; training and support is provided and accessible; there is genuine organizational (as well as individual) buy-in; communication style and approaches that support partnership working and governance arrangements that allow for agility. There are also soft factors which are important, including that the "chemistry is right" (Hutchinson et al. Chapter 3.5), and that mutuality allows for constructive dialogue and an inten-tional effort to maintain a trusting relationship. Finally, we also advocate that sustaining research coproduction partnership working requires a good dose of humility – particularly on the part of those who have a research persona, where both cultural and scientific humility are needed.

The chapters in this book present a wealth of experiential evidence about how research coproduction happens and what success might look like; however, there is still more to do to build the research evidence base about partnership work. Several authors have noted the challenges associated with both the quality and quantity of evaluation and the reporting of working in partnership (e.g., Sibley et al. Chapter 2.2 and McLean et al. Chapter 4.3). McLean et al. (Chapter 4.3) have outlined a number of questions of relevance to evaluating the partner-ing experience of knowledge users and researchers, and the impact of that expe-rience, including a new evaluation framework. There is also a potential to fill a gap in coproduction evaluation by building and evaluating a set of indicators for successful research coproduction partnerships from a multi-stakeholder, multi-context perspective.

We suggest that the consequences of developing meaningful partnerships can extend beyond a particular research lifecycle. The potential spin-offs from projects that are coproduced and meet knowledge users' needs might whet the appetite for wider collaboration in new initiatives or projects (McCutcheon et al. 4.2). Sustained engagement with genuine power-sharing and shared learning may create a resilience in the partnership that could ignite new and unexpected ideas and outcomes. This possibility provides both an incentive and reward for investing in the partnership as an essential ingredient.

SYSTEM ARCHITECTURE: THE CONTEXT OF RESEARCH COPRODUCTION

As all of the chapters in this book have highlighted, context matters. However, there is not just one context for research coproduction. They include: the operating context, research or science, politics, practice, the social, emotional, and ethical contexts, and so on. Aggregated, these contexts represent the research coproduction ecosystem. There has been an increasing turn to viewing the conduct of research and its impact as both complex and adaptive. The architectures or ways in which those systems are organized provide the conditions and spaces that more or less facilitate connectivity and offer the resources and assets that can result in collaborative action and research coproduction (Rycroft-Malone et al. 2016). Architecture, as chapter authors have demonstrated, is relevant at both the project (e.g., Cooke et al. Chapter 3.1) and organizational partnership levels (e.g., Bowen et al. Chapter 3.4, Hutchinson et al. Chapter 3.5).

Funders and funding are a critical feature of the research coproduction system's architecture. Funders are both enablers and influencers (Holmes and Jones Chapter 5.3). As such, it is not just the funding programs on offer that can provide support for research coproduction, but it is also the way in which funders act to drive behavior change in the research system. Furthermore, funders are in an ideal position to support capacity and capability building to undertake high quality research coproduction and build the evidence base. Providing opportunities for organizations, through infrastructure awards such as that described by Cooke et al. (Chapter 3.1) in the funding of Applied Research Collaborations (previously Collaborations for Leadership in Applied Research and Care [CLAHRC]), and for individuals through, for example, fellowships such as Knowledge Mobilisation Fellowships in England (NIHR) and the Evidence Leaders in Africa scheme (Holmes and Jones Chapter 5.3), are ways in which funders can drive developments in skill and competence and build the architecture. Fundamentally, funding for research coproduction needs to be programmatic: funders should make resources available for foundational activities, such as relationship-building, as well as supporting coproduction, such as training opportunities, right through the research lifecycle, including knowledge mobilization and dissemination.

Another key part of the system is the academy. The way in which the research and science system has traditionally operated can be counterproductive to meaningful research coproduction. Rewards, and therefore incentives, for researchers are often at odds with those for knowledge users. The most obvious is, as Burton and Elin (Chapter 5.1) pointed out, that universities have particular expectations for academic promotion that value particular types of activity and output, such as publishing papers in high-ranked journals. Some of these expectations are beginning to shift through external influences. For example, the San Francisco Declaration On Research Assessment (DORA) is encouraging signatories to move away from metrics such as impact factors: funders wishing to see the full breadth of a researcher's contributions in their curriculum vitae, including their contributions to broader society, can use their "Résumé for Researchers." There is also evidence to show that researchers themselves are adding collaborations with knowledge users to their curriculum vitae, thus demonstrating both the breadth of their partnership working and the impacts from those relationships (Boland et al. 2020). However, much of what is outlined in this book requires more radical system change if it is to become embedded. Fundamentally, this will require a shift in the academy's values to recognize the importance of researching through partnership arrangements. This shift should align well with fulfilling a higher education institution's role as a civic institution.

There are certain features of the system that provide the oil – in some cases, the glue – for research coproduction. Research ethics approval systems and processes is one such element. Given the often developmental and incremental approach to developing research coproduction proposals, details emerge through interaction and doing. Typically, ethical review boards/panels want detail upfront. Additionally, the people involved in research might be viewed as participants in traditionally framed research projects, whereas in coproduction projects they might have a dual role as partner and participant, which gives rise to questions about appropriate consent mechanisms. Whilst all research needs to uphold the highest standards of ethical propriety, we argue that the differences that coproduction research presents for ethical scrutiny require more accommodating perspectives and approaches, whilst maintaining rigor and robustness. Testing the system over time with different types of research coproduction projects should allow mutual learning in this respect.

Navigating and managing the many interfaces in the architecture of a research coproduction ecosystem is also seen as an important ingredient by a number of contributors, particularly those in Section 3. Having the capacity and ability to work across, including up and down, organizational boundaries is important to the research coproduction effort. Whilst members of the research coproduction team must work across different interfaces, investment in particular boundary-spanning roles might be worthwhile, particularly where research coproduction is a feature of an academic-service organizational partnership (Hutchinson et al. Chapter 3.5). Often there is little incentive within organizations for knowledge users to become research team members. Boundary-crossing roles could include knowledge users working in academia and/or researchers being embedded in services. There has been increasing interest in the potential of hybrid roles, variously labeled as researchers in residence, intermediaries, embedded researchers, relationship brokers (Bowen et al. 2017; Ward et al. 2021). People adopting these positions can assume the concomitant roles of facilitator, broker, translator, and researcher. However, putting these roles into action can be challenging, including managing fit, belonging, role strain, role conflict, and navigating different stakeholders' expectations. Additionally, those occupying these boundary-spanning roles need highly tuned skills and expertise. Fundamentally, there is still much to learn about their potential contribution to the research coproduction endeavor, which needs further rigorous evaluation, including the costs and benefits to organizations and to the individuals themselves.

Whilst conducting research is often viewed as an individual activity, the turn to more inclusive and interdisciplinary approaches to applied research, including those outlined in this book related to research coproduction, with emphasis on the multiple contexts of research practice is needed. As Sibley et al. (Chapter 2.3) summarize, typically it is system factors that are identified as barriers to research coproduction processes and readiness to apply findings. Conversely however, it is also the features of the systems, including the people who occupy them, that can be harnessed to improve the conditions for potentially successful research coproduction partnerships, projects, and programs. As both the practice and evidence base for health-related coproduction develops and matures, so too will our understanding of how to best develop facilitative ecosystems, including how we might usefully evaluate the influence of these systems on all aspects of the research coproduction lifecycle. It is therefore particularly important that research teams build in evaluation of research coproduction processes, specifically those that can explain what works, for whom, and in what circumstances, and to also provide rich descriptions of the conditions in which coproduction was operationalized.

SUPPORTING PEOPLE'S CAPABILITY FOR RESEARCH COPRODUCTION

As the contents of this book have demonstrated, meaningful research coproduction is an involved activity; moreover, there is still much to learn about how best to do it. An area where there is a particular knowledge gap is our understanding of the competencies, preparation, and support required for people as individuals and team members to be involved in, and conduct research coproduction. This gap is, in part, a function of a lack of systematic and accumulated learning to date: more effort on how to build competence and capability is needed. As the evidence base and our experience grows in quantity and quality so too will our ability to develop more specific competency frameworks and curricula. Currently, we have frameworks to draw on from health services research, knowledge translation, and allied fields – such as, improvement and implementation science (Burton and Elin Chapter 5.1) – as well as a growing wealth of experiential knowledge (Cassidy et al. Chapter 5.2). There is also a growing recognition that it may be necessary to enhance knowledge users' capability to partner with researchers (Ludwig and Banner Chapter 3.2, Bowen et al. Chapter 3.4).

Given the principles-based and solution-focussed approach we advocate in this book, research coproduction should not be associated with any particular research methodology (Burton and Elin Chapter 5.1). As such, coproduction requires a broad range of competencies that are research-related, personal, and relational; or, to put it another way, competencies that relate to doing, as well as being. Given the requirements of authentic and sustained partnership-working, communication skills, emotional intelligence, and the ability to negotiate and resolve conflict, as well as honed interpersonal skills, will be as critical to successful research coproduction as expertise in operationalizing particular research methods. These are the types of "soft skills" that are hard to put into action; for that reason it is possible that not everyone will be able to master and/or be comfortable with research coproduction.

The expectations about the mastery of skills related to core research coproduction competencies will likely differ, depending on the role being played in the team and the composition of individuals on the team. Whilst we suggest that training and support are needed just as much for researchers as for knowledge users, the skills needed may differ between individuals and groups, and throughout the research lifecycle. This requires a deliberate focus on ensuring clarity about the role and expectations of each team member, and an understanding of where there may be gaps in skills and knowledge so that an appropriate plan can be put into place to support development needs. This type of mapping is as relevant for knowledge users as it is for researchers.

Burton and Elin (Chapter 5.1) have identified an increased focus on meeting the competencies needed for research coproduction, which will require revisions to the way in which research training is organized, what is in the curricula, when during the training is it provided, and how it is accessed. Cassidy et al. (Chapter 5.2) described how they "stumbled on" opportunities of "learning as you go" through one-off projects; there is a need for a better framing of the learning experience, including attention to how it is funded. There is a strong experiential basis to build on, including some helpful learning points outlined by Cassidy et al. (Chapter 5.2). Work now needs to be done to systematize this knowledge and develop learning and development opportunities that are directly relevant to the distinctiveness of a research coproduction approach.

BUILDING SYSTEMS CAPABILITIES FOR RESEARCH COPRODUCTION

In order to develop the potential for more embedded research coproduction we also need to look towards how we build the capacity and capabilities of systems: how to scale up activity from individual project partnerships. As Bowen et al. (Chapter 3.4) observe, most research partnerships are not between, for example, a particular university and health service, but typically between one or more researchers and a manager within a specific service or program. As they articulate, this results in some vulnerabilities, not least the absence of full institutional buy-in; and, in practical terms, engagement and partnerships being more exposed to challenges such as staff turnover. There are some examples of inter-organizational partnerships in this book, such as that described by Hutchinson et al. (Chapter 3.5) within an Australian regional health system, and others outlining the regional Applied Research Collaborations (ARCs) in the United Kingdom (although the extent to which ARCs and their predecessor CLARHCs foster genuine research coproduction could be questioned) (Cooke et al. Chapter 3.1). However, these types of organizational arrangement are relatively rare. Whilst we do not underestimate the effort and investment that is required to position and develop organizational level partnerships, as Bowen et al. (Chapter 3.4) and Hutchinson et al. (Chapter 3.5) describe, the mutual benefits of conducting research coproduction within these types of system partnerships may well counterbalance the costs.

There is also work to do to develop the infrastructure within organizations to support research coproduction as an institutional and inter-organization approach to knowledge generation. This would require a philosophical commitment by institutions, as well as the appropriate resources. We outlined earlier that one of the catalysts to research coproduction would be access to appropriate funding mechanisms; however, perhaps there is also more to consider about how different types of partner need to develop their infrastructure to support and incentivize this way of working. This infrastructure may be different dependent on the type of knowledge user (patient, policy maker, provider, industry) and service, and the level of partnership (project, program, community, health system). Equally, the academy needs to revisit its value proposition and consider what mechanisms and structures might nurture, incentivize and reward engaged scholarship.

JUDICIOUS COPRODUCTION

As Ostrom herself cautions "co-production is not, of course, universally advantageous" (Ostrom 1996, p. 1082). This is a sentiment expressed by other commentators, including reference to the "dark side of coproduction" (Oliver et al. 2019) and, as a result, the potential risk of getting "lost in the shadows" (Williams et al. 2020). Whilst Oliver et al. (2019) point out some of the challenges of engaging in coproduction, Williams et al. (2020) remind us that the propensity to label any forms of collaboration as coproduction (what they term "cobiquity") is counterproductive and misaligned with the fundamental tenets of working coproductively. As we outlined earlier in this chapter, it is the principles-based approach, driven by a set of values, that extends the concept of engagement and collaboration to one of research coproduction. It is this values-driven, power-sharing approach to knowledge generation that results in working with, rather than simply engaging in.

Some may suggest we describe an idealized vision of research coproduction. However, the authors in this book have also highlighted the challenges and pitfalls of research coproduction; including, for example, conflict, dissatisfaction, not being listened to, resource intensiveness, and gaining buy-in from all partners (e.g., Sibley et al. Chapter 2.3). Oliver et al. (2019) also drew our attention to some of the challenges, risks, and costs. Future studies might focus on identifying the risks, and mitigating strategies, that different types of knowledge user and researcher experience when involved in coproduction. It is important that we continue to open up our research coproduction efforts to critique and challenge as we learn and develop capacity and expertise. We are certainly not suggesting that research coproduction is a panacea; conversely, we do suggest that framing research efforts through a coproduction lens also needs judicious application (McCutcheon et al. Chapter 4.2).

CLOSING THOUGHTS

Our intent with this book was to curate some useful advice, and the related literature, on how to navigate the research coproduction lifecycle, including an exposition of the conditions required to facilitate success. Despite a long history of community participation in research, research coproduction within a healthcare context is relatively young, and as such there is still much to learn. As we have outlined, we come from a position of research coproduction being more than collaboration in a research project. It is a principles-based approach which requires exploration and sharing of power so that an equitable partnership provides the conditions for the research process. The implications of this equitable approach to research challenges our current systems of research production. Our research systems, and the institutions within them, will require structural change to accommodate and embed authentic research coproduction.

We are not blind to the fact that many of the authors in this book come from privileged positions and have researcher personae. However, our examples have been taken from lived experience and our writing teams have partnered with knowledge users as authors. We should also acknowledge that we present a Global North view of research coproduction; the voices of those from the Global South have not been included in this edition.

There are still many questions about how to evaluate research coproduction, including those related to processes, outcomes, and the impact of a co-produced research lifecycle: intended or unintended, achieved, proximal, or distal. An area of particular inquiry is how to best assess the enactment of research coproduction against its underpinning principles. This will be important learning and will be foundational to improving future research practice.

Whilst McFarlane and Salsberg have reviewed some of the conceptual underpinnings of research coproduction (Chapter 2.1), we note there is no overarching theory of research coproduction. In that respect, our view of research coproduction is theoretically pluralist. As we reflect on the content of the book, including this final chapter, we see the beginnings of a conceptual platform. Research coproduction has emerged from a more socially constructed view of knowledge generation and use, and we also acknowledge that systems made up of structures, as well as people, play an important facilitative role. In this respect, we are reminded of Best and Holmes (2010)'s three generations of thinking about how to convert knowledge into action: linear, relational, and systems. These generations represent an increasing shift from knowledge transfer to a more distributed and deliberative process and perspective. But does this conceptualization now go far enough? We argue that it might be time to extend these generations to a fourth, which we frame as "democratization."

This fourth generation of thinking acknowledges the fundamental principles of research coproduction: all have an equal voice and role to play throughout the research lifecycle. This requires an inclusive approach in which power is equally shared. Given much research is currently initiated and led by researchers, it is researchers who have the greatest capacity and responsibility for change. This book provides the building blocks and tools for a more democratized approach to the research process and, as a consequence, the potential for generating evidence-informed solutions to real-world problems that will more rapidly translate into better care and health.

REFERENCES

1. Best, A. and Holmes, B. (2010). Systems thinking, knowledge and action: towards better models and methods. *Evidence & Policy: A Journal of Research, Debate and Practice* 6: 145–159. doi: 10.1332/174426410X502284.

2. Boaz, A., Hanney, S., Borst, R., O'Shea, A., and Kok, M. (2018). How to engage stakeholders in research: design principles to support improvement. *Health Research Policy and Systems / BioMed Central* 16: 60. doi: 10.1186/s12961-018-0337-6.

3. Boland, L., Brosseau, L., Caspar, S., Graham, I.D., Hutchinson, A.M., Kothari, A., McNamara, K., McInnes, E., Angel, M., and Stacey, D. (2020). Reporting health research translation and impact in the curriculum vitae: a survey. *Implementation Science Communications* 1: 20. doi: 10.1186/s43058-020-00021-9.

4. Bowen, S., Botting, I., Graham, I.D., and Huebner, L.A. (2017). Beyond "two cultures": guidance for establishing effective researcher/health system partnerships. *International Journal of Health Policy and Management* 6: 27–42. doi: 10.15171/ijhpm.2016.71.

5. Chalmers, I. and Glasziou, P. (2009). Avoidable waste in the production and reporting of research evidence. *Lancet* 374: 86–89. doi: 10.1016/s0140-6736(09)60329-9.

6. Hickey, G., Brearly, S., Coldham, T., Denegri, S., Green, G., Staniszewska, S., Tembo, D., Torok, K., and Turner, K. (2021). *Guidance on co-producing a research project*. Southampton: INVOLVE. https://www.learningforinvolvement.org.uk/wp-content/uploads/2021/04/NIHR-Guidance-on-co-producing-a-research-project-April-2021.pdf. (accessed 11 January 2022).

7. Hoekstra, F., Mrklas, K.J., Khan, M., McKay, R.C., Vis-Dunbar, M., Sibley, K.M., Nguyen, T., Graham, I.D., SCI Guiding Principles Consensus Panel, and Gainforth, H.L. (2020). A review of reviews on principles, strategies, outcomes and impacts of research partnerships approaches: a first step in synthesising the research partnership literature. *Health Research Policy and Systems / BioMed Central* 18: 51. doi: 10.1186/s12961-020-0544-9.

8. Oliver, K., Kothari, A., and Mays, N. (2019). The dark side of coproduction: Do the costs outweigh the benefits for health research? *Health Research Policy and Systems / BioMed Central* 17: 33. doi: 10.1186/s12961-019-0432-3.

9. Ostrom, E. (1996). Crossing the great divide: coproduction, synergy, and development. *World Development* 24: 1073–1087. doi: 10.1016/0305-750X(96)00023-X.

10. Rycroft-Malone, J., Burton, C.R., Wilkinson, J., Harvey, G., McCormack, B., Baker, R., Dopson, S., Graham, I.D., Staniszewska, S., Thompson, C., Ariss, S., Melville-Richards, L., and Williams, L. (2016). Collective action for implementation: a realist evaluation of organisational collaboration in healthcare. *Implementation Science: IS* 11: 17. doi: 10.1186/s13012-016-0380-z.

11. Ward, V., Tooman, T., Reid, B., Davies, H., and Marshall, M. (2021). Embedding researchers into organisations: a study of the features of embedded research initiatives. *Evidence & Policy: A Journal of Research, Debate and Practice*. doi: 10.1332/174426421X16165177580453.

12. Williams, O., Sarre, S., Papoulias, S.C., Knowles, S., Robert, G., Beresford, P., Rose, D., Carr, S., Kaur, M., and Palmer, V.J. (2020). Lost in the shadows: reflections on the dark side of co-production. *Health Research Policy and Systems / BioMed Central* 18: 43. doi: 10.1186/s12961-020-00558-0.

Index

Note: Page numbers followed by "*f*" refers to figures and "*t*" refers to tables.

Research Coproduction in Healthcare, First Edition. Edited by
Ian D. Graham, Jo Rycroft-Malone, Anita Kothari, and Chris McCutcheon.
© 2022 John Wiley & Sons Ltd. Published 2022 by John Wiley & Sons Ltd.